Noninfectious Diseases of Wildlife

Noninfectious Diseases of Wildlife

EDITED BY **GERALD L. HOFF,** Ph.D.
JOHN W. DAVIS, D.V.M., Ph.D.

The Iowa State University Press / **AMES, IOWA, U.S.A.**

 Composed and printed by The Iowa State University Press

First edition, 1982

Library of Congress Cataloging in Publication Data
Main entry under title:

Noninfectious diseases of wildlife.

Includes bibliographies and index.
1. Wildlife diseases. I. Hoff, Gerald L. (Gerald Lawrence), 1945- . II. Davis, John William, 1917.
SF997.N66 639.9′6 81-11789
ISBN 0-8138-0990-8 AACR2

Contributors

MORLEY W. BARRETT, B.S.A., M.Sc.
Biologist, Fish and Wildlife Division, Alberta Department of Recreation, Parks and Wildlife, Lethbridge, Alberta, Canada

GORDON A. CHALMERS, D.V.M., D.P.V.R.
Pathologist, Veterinary Services Division, Alberta Department of Agriculture, Lethbridge, Alberta, Canada

JOHN E. COOPER, D.V.M.
Pathologist, Royal College of Surgeons of England, Lincoln's Inn Fields, London, England

GERALD E. COSGROVE, M.D.
Pathologist, Department of Pathology, Zoological Society of San Diego, San Diego, California 92112

JOHN W. DAVIS, D.V.M., Ph.D.
Professor, Department of Veterinary Science, Virginia Polytechnic Institute and State University, Blacksburg, Virginia 24061

R. N. T. W. FIENNES, M.A., M.R.C.V.S.
Head, Pathology Department, Zoological Society of London, Nuffield Institute of Comparative Medicine, Regent's Park, London NW1 4RY, London, England

ROLF HARTUNG, Ph.D.
Professor, Department of Environmental and Industrial Health, University of Michigan, School of Public Health, Ann Arbor, Michigan 48104

DIANE M. HOFF, B.S.
Kansas City, Missouri

GERALD L. HOFF, Ph.D.
Chief, Office of Epidemiological Services, Kansas City Health Department, Kansas City, Missouri 64109

ROBERT L. JARVIS, Ph.D.
Assistant Professor, Department of Fisheries and Wildlife, Oregon State University, Corvallis, Oregon 97331

FREDERICK W. OEHME, D.V.M., Ph.D.
Professor of Toxicology, Medicine, and Physiology and Director, Comparative Toxicology Laboratory, Kansas State University, Manhattan, Kansas 66506

S. J. PROCTOR, D.V.M., Ph.D.
Research Scientist, Pathology, Wellcome Research Laboratory, Burroughs Wellcome Company, Research Triangle Park, North Carolina 27709

L. C. SATTERFIELD, B.S.
Research Associate, Biology Division, Oak Ridge National Laboratory, Oak Ridge, Tennessee 37830

DANIEL O. TRAINER, Ph.D.
Acting Vice Provost, College of Natural Resources, University of Wisconsin, Stevens Point, Wisconsin 54481

JOEL D. WALLACH, D.V.M.
Associate Professor, Department of Nutrition, National College of Naturopathic Medicine, Portland, Oregon 97204

JOSEPH G. ZINKL, D.V.M., Ph.D.
Assistant Professor, Department of Clinical Pathology, School of Veterinary Medicine, University of California, Davis, California 95616

Contents

Preface

As an environmental and ecological factor, disease exerts direct and indirect influences upon the survival of individual wild animals and on population dynamics. During the past 20 years emphasis has been given to the infectious and parasitic diseases of free-ranging and captive wildlife. This can be partially attributed to the concern with diseases transmissible to man or domestic livestock and partially to the training of the investigators. As a result there has been a tremendous expansion of knowledge, with several journals and a number of texts providing ready access to this expanding data base.

During this time, noninfectious diseases received less attention. Lead poisoning of waterfowl and pesticide poisoning of wild mammals and birds were probably the most prominent noninfectious diseases studied. With increased interest in capturing, transporting, accommodating, and breeding wild animals, postcapture complications and genetic disorders became evident. Various intervention programs had to be designed to cope with physiologic derangements, such as cardiac and respiratory failure, stress, shock, hyper- and hypothermia, capture myopathy, and nutritional deficiencies. Sound management practices became necessary not only for captive animals but for free-ranging wildlife as well.

Consequently, the diverse nature of noninfectious diseases in wildlife has produced a widely scattered literature. This is a result primarily of the more varied backgrounds of the investigators as compared to those of workers in the infectious and parasitic disease fields. Such diversity is reflected by the contributors to this book. This first edition represents an experimental effort to bring together some of the diffuse knowledge on noninfectious diseases of free-ranging and captive wildlife. Issue may be taken with the choice of topics; however, predominant diseases, as well as some diseases of lesser prominence, are presented. The resulting text we hope will be of value to wildlife disease investigators, wildlife managers, veterinarians, and university students.

Noninfectious Diseases of Wildlife

1 General Toxicology

ROLF HARTUNG

POISONINGS have probably contributed significantly to disease in wild animals throughout the course of their evolution. However, because of an increased level of industrialization, and intensified reliance on the use of chemical substances for environmental modification, man has greatly increased the occurrence of poisoning among wild animals. The overall impact is still somewhat difficult to assess, but there are several well-documented examples which indicate that specific environmental toxicants have caused or contributed to drastic declines in several species (Henry, 1975; King and Flickinger, 1977; Ratcliffe, 1970).

DOSE-RESPONSE RELATIONSHIP. The concept that dose and duration of exposure are related to the observed effect in animals is central to the discipline of toxicology. The most simplistic dose-response curves relate the proportion of a population that dies after exposure to single doses of a toxicant. The dose-response curve describes the variability of a population in its response to a specific material. Dose-response curves are analyzed statistically by relatively complex regression procedures, such as probit analysis (Finney, 1964). Simplified methods of analysis have been developed by Lichtfield and Wilcoxon (1949) and others.

The median lethal dose (LD_{50}), median lethal concentration (LC_{50}), and median tolerance (TL_m or TL_{50}) describe only the midpoint of a dose-response curve, but these measures have taken on a disproportionate importance in the evaluation of toxic effects. The slope of a dose-response curve is often ignored in discussions of toxicological evaluations. However, the slope of the curve is a measure of the variability in the response of a population to a toxic insult. Steep dose-response curves indicate a relatively uniform response, while shallow dose-response curves demonstrate the existence of a signficant gradient ranging from very sensitive to very resistant individuals.

The study of harmful effects of chemicals does not restrict itself to the evaluation of immediate lethality, but delves further into the responses of the organism to absorbed chemical substances. Toxic substances may produce dose-related changes in organ structure and function and in the activities of important enzymes; they may produce changes in growth rates, reproduction, or behavior. The studies of carcinogenicity, mutagenicity, and teratogenicity are special subdivisions of these types of analyses. For all of these phenomena the response is dose related for any one chemical substance. In these cases the midpoints of the dose-response curves are called median effective doses or concentrations (ED_{50} or EC_{50}).

It is meaningless to speak of a toxic substance unless one also specifies the dose at which toxicity is expected to occur. Even substances normally considered safe, such as water, triglycerides, carbohydrates, and sugar, may, under certain extreme conditions, produce disease or death and may, therefore, under those conditions be considered toxic substances. Other substances that produce significant toxicity at relatively low dose levels may be administered at exceedingly low doses at which no effect can be measured by any available experimental technique.

ABSORPTION, DISTRIBUTION, METABOLISM. The actual dose that is absorbed is of primary importance to an understanding of the effects in the exposed organism. The absorptive processes are significantly affected by the physical and chemical properties of the substance. Most toxic substances are absorbed by passive diffusion, and, therefore, their absorption depends on the rate by which they can move through the cell membrane, the concentration gradient across the cell membrane, and the duration of the exposure.

The absorption of various substances through biological membranes is influenced mainly by lipid solubility and molecular size. Within limits, as lipid solubility increases, the absorption rate increases (Overton, 1902; Scheuplein and Blank, 1971). However, as molecular weight increases, the absorption rate decreases. Materials of large molecular weight and low lipid solubility are probably absorbed mostly by other processes, such as phagocytosis or pinocytosis. These findings acquire importance under environmental conditions. When heavy metals are ingested in the form of inorganic salts, their rate of absorption tends to be low. For example, the absorption of mercury salts from the gastrointestinal tract is only a few percent in a mouse during the time those doses pass through the entire intestinal tract.

On the other hand, if the lipid solubility of mercury is increased by introducing it as methyl mercury chloride, the rate of absorption from the gastrointestinal tract increases significantly so that more than 95% of the administered dose is absorbed (Clarkson, 1972). Increased lipid solubility will allow for greater distribution to other body compartments so that methyl mercury is readily able to cross the blood-brain barrier and produce central nervous system effects (Takeuchi, 1972). This means that methyl mercury has a significantly higher bioavailability from environmental sources than does inorganic mercury. Within crude limits it is possible to predict the efficiency of absorption of various chemical substances by evaluating their lipid solubility in comparison to their water solubility in relation to their molecular size.

The higher the lipid solubility, the greater the potential for storage of the substance in lipid depots within the organism. The more water-soluble compounds tend to be characterized by functional groups that are readily ionizable, or that can at least convey considerable polarity to a molecule. Conversely, lipid-soluble compounds tend to lack or have only a few such functional groups. This also has the interesting consequence that compounds with high lipid solubility and extremely low water solubility tend to be resistant to metabolism within the host organism (Williams, 1959). As a result, such compounds tend to have simultaneously an efficient rate of absorption, a significant propensity to be stored in lipid depots, and a long biological half-life. Specific examples are DDT and PCB compounds.

Even at the most basic conceptual level, absorption, metabolism, and excretion of toxic compounds are influenced by a complex interplay of physical, chemical, and biological factors. When these factors are translated to a large organism, such as a bird or mammal, the factors involved in the *in vivo* dynamics of toxic substances become even more complex (Wagner, 1975).

By far the most significant route of absorption of toxic substances in wildlife is the oral route. When exposures involve particles or aerosols, these may be deposited on fur or feathers or inhaled. A large proportion of the substances that have been deposited on feathers or fur will be removed by preening and subsequently ingested. When aerosols consisting of droplets and particles above 10 microns in size are inhaled, these larger bodies tend to be lodged in the upper respiratory tract from where they may be removed by mucociliary action and, subsequently, swallowed (Casarett, 1975). Thus, the absorption of toxic substances by ingestion may take a number of direct and indirect routes in wild animals. Normally only extremely fine particles and gases are able to penetrate to the alveoli in mammals or to the parabronchi in birds.

The significance of the respiratory route of absorption in wildlife is not well established. However, there are some important toxicological differences between respiratory and oral absorption. While heavy metals are absorbed rather poorly from the intestinal tract, they are absorbed to a greater degree from the respiratory tract. Therefore, an equivalent inhaled dose will produce a much higher body burden than an ingested dose. It is also important to consider how materials are distributed after they have been absorbed by different routes. Materials that have been inhaled will be distributed via the general circulation. Materials that have been ingested will be transported by the hepatic portal system to the liver where significant metabolism may take place before the material is passed on to the general circulation.

In general, the metabolic pathways in the liver tend to make toxic substances more water-soluble. Oxidative and conjugating pathways tend to predominate (Williams, 1959). In many instances this metabolism may result in compounds that have a lower toxicity than the parent compound. However, there are numerous instances in which metabolites are much more toxic than the parent compound. Because of this fact, an absorbed toxic substance can affect the level of metabolic activity in the liver, which can have a significant effect on the outcome.

The nutritional status of an animal can have pronounced effects on this absorption. If a substance is ingested with food on a relatively full stomach, there is an increased chance of chemical reaction with stomach or gastrointestinal contents and an increased possibility of the metabolism of the ingested substance by gastrointestinal bacteria. Likewise, the food in the stomach acts as a dilutant so that absorption is slowed and peak blood levels are reduced. On the other hand, an empty stomach may greatly increase the speed of absorption so that much higher blood levels of the toxicant are reached.

Starvation can also produce indirect effects by reducing the amount of microsomal enzymes (mixed function oxidases) in the liver. This would greatly increase the toxicity of materials that are normally detoxified by the mixed function oxidases, while significantly decreasing the toxicity of materials that would have to be activated by the mixed function oxidases. These mixed function oxidases play a key role in the metabolism of many lipid-soluble organic compounds. Their activity may be greatly elevated when they are stimulated by many of the compounds that are normally metabolized by them. Therefore, exposures to halogenated aromatic hydrocarbons and similar compounds may be able to modify the toxicity of other compounds that are metabolized by the same pathway (Fouts, 1972).

FACTORS INFLUENCING TOXIC RESPONSES. A great number of factors affect the toxicity of most compounds. These may be divided into intrinsic factors, for example, species, sex, age, extent of individual variability, and extrinsic factors, such as nutrition, health history, temperature, stress, and many others. The most pronounced differences in the reaction to toxic substances are usually related to species differences. In general, closely related species tend to react similarly, while the further organisms are phylogenetically separated, the greater the likelihood that a substance may produce different effects on a quantitative as well as a qualitative basis (Albert, 1960). At the extreme, these differences have been utilized to a large extent in the selective use of toxic substances for environmental control. All pesticides and a large number of drugs have utilized these species differences to achieve selective toxicity. However, in a few cases even closely related species may have significantly different sensitivities to a specific toxicant. A highly substituted norbormide seems to have the greatest differential toxicity. For this compound, the LD_{50} for Norway rats, *Rattus norvegicus,* is 4.3 mg/kg. However, the LD_{50} for most other mammals, including some very closely related rodents, is about 1,000 mg/kg or greater (Roszkowski, 1965). Differences such as these are unusual.

Qualitative differences, especially in substances that affect the nervous system, are common. Morphine derivatives, which have a sedative effect in primates and many other species, produce a decidedly stimulatory effect in cats. Amphetamines and caffeine, which may produce stimulatory effects in adult humans, may produce a slight calming effect in children. Aside from these qualitative differences between the young and adult, there are often quantitative differences related to age. Young animals tend to absorb many substances more readily than adults, possibly because of a less well-defined intestinal barrier. In the subsequent distribution of the toxic substance, the blood-brain barrier is likewise not as well established in the young as it is in the adult. Consequently, the young may be more readily affected by lead and mercury.

Sex may affect the toxicity of some substances. For example, the female rat is more sensitive to selenium, while the male rat is more sensitive to lead (Hurst, 1958). Sex differences in the reaction to toxic substances have often been shown to be related to hormonal differences and have been reversed by the proper endocrinological alteration.

The dose-response curve clearly demonstrates the extent of individual differences. Closely inbred populations tend to have dose-response curves with rather steep slopes, indicating a relatively limited range of individual variabilities. Wild or outbred populations tend to have dose-response curves with shallower slopes, indicating a greater variability of response within the population.

Unusual dose-response curves may result if a portion of the population exhibits genetic differences with respect to enzymes, which may be important in the metabolism of specific toxic substances. These differences have been demonstrated in man for deficiencies of pseudocholinesterase, glucose-6-phosphate dehydrogenase, and methemoglobin reductase. Therefore, it is likely that other species might show deficiencies or singularities with respect to certain metabolizing enzymes, which might then render specific segments of those populations exquisitely sensitive to specific toxicants. Since the recognition of such genetically determined enzyme deficiencies often depends on the study of the rare individuals that react unusually, this type of study has so far only been done on humans and some species of laboratory animals. In more routine toxicity studies, unusually sensitive animals are eliminated from subsequent statistical analyses as "outlyers."

HAZARD IN RELATION TO TOXICITY. While toxicity is a property of the interaction of chemical substances with living organisms, hazard is related to the actual occurrence of a toxicologically significant event under natural conditions. While the toxicity of a compound can be readily elucidated by laboratory studies, and many techniques have been developed to uncover even very subtle events, the analysis of hazard is still largely intuitive and at best in its infancy. In evaluating the potential hazard of a toxic substance, one needs to consider the toxicity of the material in relation to the dynamic status of the individual organism in its environment. This means that the toxic substance must gain direct access to the individual at risk at sufficient concentrations and for a sufficient duration to cause toxicity. Whenever a toxic substance is not uniformly distributed in the environment, these concepts apply. A substance deposited on the forest floor will have a greater potential impact on terrestrial animals than arboreal animals.

In addition, toxic substances that occur in

discrete packets may be considerably more hazardous if they are able to attract an animal, while the hazard may be significantly reduced if the animal shows avoidance. Thus, an important factor in the effectiveness of commercial rodenticides lies in bait formulation and placement of bait stations. Subsequently, the effectiveness of a rodenticide depends heavily on whether the animal is able to learn to avoid the bait station and become bait-shy, or whether it never makes the connection between the toxic symptoms experienced and the consumption of the bait. Behavioral and ecological factors must be taken into account when one is trying to evaluate the impact of a toxic substance under environmental conditions. Therefore, most toxic substances destined for release into the environment should probably be tested in the laboratory as well as the field before they are released on a wider scale.

DYNAMICS OF TOXIC SUBSTANCES IN THE ENVIRONMENT. When a substance is released into the environment a number of forces start to act on it immediately. The most important of these are the dispersive forces that dilute the substance, largely by diffusion and turbulent mixing. Organic compounds are commonly changed by photooxidation and chemical or metabolic breakdown. Some materials, for example, DDT, PCB compounds, mirex, and dieldrin, are very resistant to these processes so that they have long persistence in the environment. At the other extreme, such materials as short-chain alcohols, organic acids, amino acids, and simple aldehydes may be rapidly broken down in the environment.

The potentially toxic trace elements, such as mercury, lead, cadmium, arsenic, and others, represent special cases. In the first place, their environmental persistence is infinite because, for practical purposes, they can neither be created nor destroyed. Problems do not appear to arise from normal global background levels with which all ecosystems have evolved, but are caused by the occurrence of localized, elevated concentrations resulting from man's activity or specific geological formations. Initially, when heavy metals are released from industrial processes into the environment, there tend to be a number of rapid changes in their chemistry as environmental buffering agents and chelators make their effects felt (Huckabee and Blaylock, 1973). In general, this tends to concentrate these heavy metals in soil or in aquatic sediments. However, both mercury and arsenic can be methylated by microorganisms in sediments. Even though the proportions of the total amount of mercury in the environment that may be in a methylated state at any time is small, this form is taken up much more rapidly by fish and other aquatic organisms so that it can subsequently enter the food web for other aquatic wildlife. Even though these elements can undergo chemical transformation, any elevated concentrations of them have to be dispersed by mixing, diffusion, or deep sedimentation to reduce their bioavailability.

DETERMINATION OF ENVIRONMENTAL EFFECTS. Most reports of poisonings of birds or mammals in the environment describe mortalities caused by excessive release of industrial pollutants, pesticides, or oils. Even under these circumstances, it is often difficult to establish the magnitude of the mortalities, and frequently it may not be possible to establish the nature of the causative agent. Sometimes, there is a tendency to categorize mortalities that cannot be ascribed to known parasitic, bacterial, or viral diseases as "poisonings" by a process of elimination. This procedure is to be discouraged. Since cause-effect relationships need to be established for other disease categories for proper diagnosis, a similar scientific attitude should prevail toward the diagnosis of cases of poisoning.

When mortalities due to toxic substances occur sporadically, the determination of environmental effects becomes more difficult. It is unlikely that such deaths would come to the attention of field personnel, because of the difficulty in finding the dead animals involved and the great probability that it would not be possible to mount the analytical effort to establish whether these individual deaths were due to toxic agents.

Animal populations may also be affected without any evidence of direct mortality. A depression in reproductive performance may readily produce declines in animal populations. In the case of the eggshell thinning problem caused by chlorinated hydrocarbon pesticides, the effect was fairly obvious in retrospect (Ratcliffe, 1970). Nevertheless, it required several years for these findings to become accepted. A field census is too imprecise to detect small changes in population density and can usually be applied only to limited areas. In addition, the population densities of most noneconomic wildlife species are virtually unknown.

Effects of toxic agents on animal behavior may indirectly produce increased predatory pressure, resulting in population declines. Bellrose (1959) presented data which suggested that low-grade lead poisoning in waterfowl reduced their mobility, which could result in increased losses due to predation. Again, the impact on total populations is difficult to ascertain because of lack of precision in determining the effects on population numbers. Effects of economic poisons or pollutants on food or other requisites can also influence populations with similar measurement problems.

For each of these problems the dilemma facing the investigator is that the present methods of environmental evaluation have to contend with large-scale variations, so that large sample sizes are required to detect early changes. By the time these changes become obvious, the severity of the observed effect is often unacceptable. The effort required to remedy such a situation is usually enormous. A significant level of improvement in environmental surveillance, combined with more sophisticated testing requirements, including limited field tests for chemicals that are to be released into the environment on a large scale, should greatly reduce the environmental impact of toxic substances.

REFERENCES

Albert, A. 1960. Selective toxicity. Wiley, New York.

Bellrose, F. C. 1959. Lead poisoning as a mortality factor in waterfowl populations. Illinois Natur. Hist. Surv. Bull. 27:235–288.

Casarett, L. J. 1975. Toxicology of the respiratory system. In L. J. Casarett and J. Doull. Toxicology. Macmillan, New York.

Clarkson, T. W. 1972. Biotransformation of organomercurials in mammals. In R. Hartung and B. D. Dinman. Environmental mercury contamination. Ann Arbor Sci. Publ., Ann Arbor.

Finney, D. J. 1964. Statistical method in biological assay. 2nd ed. Hafner, New York.

Fouts, J. R. 1972. Some studies and comments on hepatic and extrahepatic microsomal toxication-detoxication systems. Environ. Health Perspect. 2:55–66.

Henry, C. J. 1975. Research, management, and status of the osprey in North America. World Conf. on Birds of Prey, Vienna, 1975:199–222.

Huckabee, J. W., and B. G. Blaylock. 1973. Transfer of mercury and cadmium from terrestrial to aquatic ecosystems. Adv. Exp. Med. Biol. 40:125–160.

Hurst, W. E. 1958. Sexual differences in the toxicity and therapeutic action of chemical substances. In A. L. Walpole and A. Spinks. The evaluation of drug toxicity. Little, Brown, Boston.

King, K. A., and E. H. Flickinger. 1977. The decline of brown pelicans on the Louisiana and Texas Gulf Coast. Southwest Natur. 21:417–431.

Lichtfield, J. T., Jr., and F. Wilcoxon. 1949. A simplified method of evaluating dose-effect experiments. J. Pharm. Exp. Therap. 96:99–113.

Overton, E. 1902. Beitrage zur allgemeinen Muskel- und Nervenphysiologie. Arch. ges. Physiol. 92: 115–280.

Ratcliffe, D. A. 1970. Changes attributable to pesticides in egg breakage frequency and eggshell thickness in some British birds. J. Appl. Ecol. 7:67–115.

Roszkowski, A. P. 1965. The pharmacological properties of norbormide, a selective rat toxicant. J. Pharm. Exp. Therap. 149:288–299.

Scheuplein, R. J., and I. H. Blank. 1971. Permeability of the skin. Physiol. Rev. 51:702–747.

Takeuchi, T. 1972. Biological reactions and pathological changes in human beings and animals caused by organic mercury contamination. In R. Hartung and B. D. Dinman. Environmental mercury contamination. Ann Arbor Sci. Publ., Ann Arbor.

Wagner, J. G. 1975. Fundamentals of clinical pharmacokinetics. Drug Intelligence Publ., Hamilton, Ill.

Williams, R. T. 1959. Detoxication mechanisms. 2nd ed. Wiley, New York.

2 *Plants Poisonous to Free-living or Caged Mammals and Birds*

FREDERICK W. OEHME
JOHN W. DAVIS

POISONOUS PLANTS are found throughout the world, and have been associated with man since before the time of Christ. The Bible indirectly refers to the poisonous properties of some plants, and during medieval times plants were used for ulterior motives. However, as man became more civilized, his knowledge of poisonous plants centered on their importance to livestock production. In the United States, little information was available regarding the toxic properties of poisonous plants before 1894; since then numerous field and experimental investigations have documented the variety and complexity of the toxic chemicals found in plants (Arnold, 1968; Chopra et al., 1965; Everist, 1974; Forsyth, 1968; Gardner and Bennetts, 1956; Hurst, 1942; Kingsbury, 1964; Muenscher, 1951; Shone and Drummond, 1965).

Because of the economic input of livestock production, the hazard of poisonous plants to meat-producing animals and related farm livestock has been an important part of agriculture and veterinary medicine. The literature abounds with regional and general reviews of the potential toxicity of specific plants to livestock and other farm animals (Beath et al., 1953; Buck et al., 1976; Clare, 1952, 1955; Clarke and Clarke, 1967; Core et al. 1961; Duncan and Jones, 1949; Duncan et al., 1957; Durrell et al., 1952; Evers and Link, 1972; Featherly, 1945; Gilkey, 1968; Harden, 1961; Huffman et al., 1956; Hulbert and Oehme, 1968; Hyatt et al., 1953; Kingsbury, 1958; Lee and Doyle, not dated; Liener, 1969; Massey, 1954; McLeun and Nicholson, 1958; Oehme, 1973; Radeleff, 1970; Sampson and Malmsten, 1942; Watt and Bryer-Brandwijk, 1962; Welch and Morris, 1952; West and Emmel, 1952). Plants potentially toxic to dogs, cats, and other small domestic animals have also been reviewed (Oehme, 1977).

CONDITIONS OF POISONING. Plant toxicities occur through the ingestion of forages in sufficient quantity or during stages of growth when significant amounts of the toxic principle are present. In domestic livestock, most cases of plant poisoning occur in the early spring before the usual forage becomes plentiful, or during periods in summer or fall when pasture grasses become dry and brown because of drought or other climatic conditions. Under these circumstances, poisonous plants may be found in moist meadows or along the banks of streams running through pastures. Normal pasture land may not harbor toxic plants, but such forage may grow along fence rows or in the margins of grazing areas.

Some plants may contain unusual irritating chemicals that are liberated in the plant juices or sap when animals browse or brush against them during normal transit through fields. A review of the toxic components of plants used for food has been produced (Liener, 1969).

Climate and Soil. Because of climatic conditions and soil types, plants are usually confined to definite geographic areas. If the ecology of an area is altered by mechanical, climatic, or other means, plants normally found in limited amounts may become abundant and, therefore, troublesome (Hulbert and Oehme, 1968). Overgrazed pastures and disturbed fields favor the invasion of previously scarce plants that often are poisonous. Coupled with the scarcity of normal forage due to climatic or other conditions, the invading plants may become attractive to grazing animals and their consumption is favored.

In such instances, parts of the plant not previously consumed and parts of the plant high in toxin content may be consumed (Table 2.1). The toxin of water hemlock is most abundant in the root stock or in the roots; these parts are likely to cause poisoning when the soil is sufficiently wet that they are readily pulled out of the ground or are easily trampled, liberating the toxin into surrounding waters. Poisoning from lupine usually occurs through eating the seed. Plants that retain their succulent nature and mature late in the season may be particularly dangerous for animals that are seeking forage during times of drought.

Contrary to popular belief, wild animals are not always capable of differentiating between toxic and nontoxic plants (Fowler, 1975). While some plant species may taste bitter or emit odors that would normally repel most animals, these inhibitions may be overridden when forage becomes scarce and hunger is common. However, that losses in wildlife due to plant poisonings are unusual is attested to by the scarcity of documented information about such poisonings.

Adaptation, Learned Behavior, Species Resistance. Wild animals appear to demonstrate some ability to differentiate between toxic and nontoxic plants or to limit consumption of the toxic variety to nonharmful amounts. This characteristic is generally thought to occur through a learning process in animals living in a geographic area where certain toxic plants are present. Poisoning, however, may occur if conditions force the animals to move to strange environments with subsequent exposure to unfamiliar toxic plants. Similar observations have occurred in livestock. Cattle or horses raised in a specific locale may safely pasture fields containing a variety of toxic plants, but if new animals are placed in the field, toxicity may promptly occur. If local cattle or sheep are driven or moved to strange pastures, the incidence of toxicity from plants found in those fields increases dramatically. Since wild animals have learned to live with toxic plants by adaptation or learning, poisoning usually does not occur unless abnormal conditions reduce their forage below maintenance levels or artificial conditions are present in confined wild animals to force them to eat the toxic material.

In certain animal species, wild animals are not affected by plants that routinely produce toxicity in domestic species. Elk, *Cervus canadensis;* ruffed grouse, *Bonasa umbellus;* white-tailed deer, *Odocoileus virginianus;* and other species have fed freely on mountain laurel, *Kalmia latifolia, Rhododendron* sp., and other related plants known to contain toxic constituents (Table 2.1). These wild species will often consume the buds, leaves, and limited amounts of twigs from these plants, especially during winter.

Despite the adaptation, learned behavior, and species resistance observed in some wild animals, a variety of toxic plants have been shown to contain poisonous principles in one or more parts of the plant (Table 2.1). Hence, the potential for wild and caged animals to become poisoned from exposure to such forages is present. Yew, *Taxus baccata,* toxicity has been recorded in pheasants, *Phasianus colchicus* (Jordan, 1964), and a yew toxicity described in a kangaroo (Kohler and Grunberg, 1960). Poisoning due to *Pieris japonica* was observed in zoo animals (Gillis et al., 1961). Locoism in elk has been observed (Adcock and Kness, 1969). Such reports confirm that wild animals can be poisoned by plants and suggest that depending upon the plant species, climatic and growth conditions, and the animal species involved, the amount of poisonous plant necessary to produce toxicity or death varies greatly.

Anatomical and Physiological Differences. When considering the hazard of poisoning in wild mammals and birds, differences in anatomy and physiology among various species become important. The obvious differences between wild mammals with rumens and those without provide some variation in the rate of ingestion of plants, degree and rapidity of absorption of toxic components, and the general degree of the toxicity pattern. More marked differences occur when variations between mammals and birds are considered. The general digestive tract anatomy and its functioning offer variations. The general metabolic rate and temperature are usually greater in birds, and enzymatic processes in the liver and other body tissues provide additional variations.

The avian kidney also differs from its mammalian counterpart in anatomy and physiology, hence its capability to excrete ingested plant toxins. The liver and the kidney are constructed of lobules with a central vein and are supported by the usual arterial and portal blood. The glomeruli are small in birds and their filtration capability is remarkably lower than that of mammals. Therefore, excretion of toxins is reduced in birds. The enzymatic activity of the tubules, however, is much higher than that in mammals; this offers the opportunity for increased excretion in birds. The end product of protein metabolism in birds is uric acid, which is precipitated as crystals in the tubules because of the resorption of water and bases. This process enables the bird to excrete waste products and at the same time save water; filtration and resorption are not necessary to the same extent as in mammals. The filtration-resorption system of mammals does not exist in birds, as the tubular apparatus in birds is functionally superior to the glomerular apparatus of mammals (Feldman and Kruckenberg, 1975).

The blood from the posterior intestinal tract of birds passes directly to the kidneys without being previously filtered by a lymph organ or the liver, as it is in mammals. This blood contains many of the absorbed substances from the intestinal tract, and plant toxins and other nephrotoxic substances can act directly on avian kidneys. Although pathology may reveal damage to the avian tubular system, the glomeruli are not usually involved in nephrotoxic kidney changes. There is probably a much higher spontaneous recovery rate in the tubular system of birds than in mammals, since following toxic insult to the tubular system of birds no obvious clinical signs may be present (Feldman and Kruckenberg, 1975).

Table 2.1. Some Plants, Shrubs, and Trees That Can Cause or Have the Potential for Causing Poisoning in Wildlife (Modified from Fowler, 1975)

Plant	Toxic Plant Part	Poisonous Principle and Signs of Poisoning
Lobelia sp., lobelia	leaves, stems, fruit	Alkaloid; gastroenteritis, nervous system depression or stimulation, sudden death
Narcissus sp., daffodil	bulbs	
Laburnum vulgare, golden chain	leaves, seeds	
**Taxus* sp., yew	needles	
Delphinium sp., larkspur	leaves, seeds	
Solanum sp., European bittersweet, nightshade	unripe berries, leaves	
Colchicum autumnuale, autumn crocus	leaves	
Euphorbia sp., poinsettia, euphorbia, spurge, snow-on-the-mountain	leaves, milky sap	Resinoid; dermatitis, gastroenteritis, nervous system stimulation
Kalmia latifolia, mountain laurel	leaves	
Rhododendron sp., azalea, rhododendron	leaves	
Melia azedarach, China berry	fruits	
Ricinus communis, castor bean	beans and leaves	Phytotoxin; diarrhea, shock syndrome
Abrus sp., precatory bean, rosary bean	bean	
Robinia pseudoacacia, black locust	leaves	
Thevetia peruviana, yellow oleander	leaves	Cardioactive glycoside; cardiac irregularities, diarrhea, vomiting
**Nerium oleander,* oleander	all parts	
**Digitalis purpurea,* foxglove	leaves	
Convollaria majalis, lily of the valley	leaves and flowers	
Dieffenbachia seguine, dumbcane	stems	Oxalate crystals, water-soluble toxin; salivation, stomatitis
Colocasia sp., elephant ear	stems, leaves	
Philodendron sp., philodendron	stems, leaves	
Aesculum sp., buckeye, horse chestnut	leaves and fruit	Glycoside; nervous system stimulation, gastroenteritis
Daphne sp., daphne	bark, leaves, fruit	
**Prunus* sp., chokecherry, wild cherry	leaves, pits	Hydrocyanic acid (HCN); dyspnea, convulsions, bright red venous blood
Heteromeles sp., toyon, Chistmas berry	leaves	
Senecio sp., tansy ragwort, groundsel	leaves	Pyrrolizidine alkaloid; hepatopathy
Lantana camara, lantana	foliage	Hepatotoxin; hepatopathy
Datura sp., angel's trumpet, jimsonweed	leaves, seed	Atropinelike alkaloids; mania, dilated pupils
Hedera helix, English ivy	leaves, berries	Saponin; gastroenteritis
Nicotiana sp., tobacco	leaves	Nicotine; nervous stimulation, then depression
Ligustrum vulgare, privet	leaves, berries	Unknown; gastroenteritis
Hydrangea macrophylla, hydrangea	leaves	
**Astragalus* sp., locoweed	think all parts of plant above ground	Not specifically known; jerky uncoordinated movements, weight loss, final stages acutely nervous, weak, unable to eat and drink
**Oxytropis* sp., locoweed	think all parts of plant above ground	Not specifically known; jerky uncoordinated movements, weight loss, final stages acutely nervous, weak, unable to eat and drink
**Crotalaria* sp., crotalaria	tops of plant, seeds	Alkaloid; slow weight loss, weakness, stupor
**Asclepias eriocarpa,* woolly-pod, broad-leafed milkweed	whole plant above ground	Resinoid; dullness, weakness of hindquarters, staggering, convulsions until death, initial rapid heartbeat

* Have caused poisoning in wildlife.

These interacting but distinct factors affect the widely diverse and controversial nature of plant poisonings in wild mammals and birds. They complicate an already unclear situation that is further confused by the widely differing toxicity that might be expected with the same poisonous plant exposure in different species of mammals and birds. The variety of plants capable of producing toxicity and the diversity of clinical syndromes that might be expected are a direct consequence of the species variability and wide diversity in the conditions under which plant toxicity may occur.

A sampling of the plants reported toxic for mammals and birds is given in Table 2.1. All these plants are potentially hazardous to wildlife, and the large number of other uncultivated plants found in forests and uninhabited areas offers the potential for an additional listing of currently unrecognized species capable of producing poisonings.

Toxic Principles. It may be seen that a number of toxic principles are recognized, and the clinical effects observed may vary from mild digestive tract signs to acutely severe and fatal nervous disorders. Deer may be poisoned by eating chokecherry, *Prunus melanocarpa,* although small amounts may be consumed without apparent harm. The diversity of the herbivore diet may be a saving influence. Deer browse on many different shrubs and herbs, thus diluting the cyanide in the chokecherry to levels compatible with life. The cyanogenetic glycosides present in the cherry seeds release cyanide upon digestion. These seeds are only dangerous if the seed capsule is broken by seed-eating birds, or by animals that customarily chew their food prior to swallowing. The principal manifestations of cherry seed poisoning are acute signs, with rapid respiration, convulsions, and coma leading to death.

A number of plants contain hepatotoxic substances, among them the pyrrolizidine alkaloids. These alkaloids taste bitter, a fact that normally inhibits grazing by wildlife. However, drought conditions may force animals to eat the poisonous plant species, resulting in toxicity.

Fungi are associated with a variety of forage and livestock poisonings. One species of fungus, *Aspergillus flavus,* grows on grains and other seed-bearing plants, and produces a toxin known as aflatoxin. Birds are very susceptible to this toxin and may be affected in a variety of ways. Signs include anorexia, ataxia, and depression. Death may occur. The liver is primarily affected, with necrosis and bile duct proliferation. The chemical is also considered a very potent hepatocarcinogen. No treatment is available for aflatoxicosis, but the reduction of stress, adequate dietary protein, and lipotropic agents may be helpful if illness is detected in animals in confined areas.

Cultivated plants may produce problems in caged mammals or birds that are offered parts of these plants by nondiscriminating zoo visitors. Wildcats are suggested as being especially sensitive to the ivies, *Hedera* sp., *Philodendron* sp., and *Dieffenbachia* sp., which may cause irritation to the mucous membranes, salivation, difficult and labored respiration, debilitation, and listlessness. No specific treatment is available, but general supportive measures should be used on these and other toxicities that are due to dangerous ornamental plants.

Blue-green algae toxin may occur in drinking water, in ponds, and in fish tanks. Vomiting, muscular tremors, convulsions, prostration, paralysis, and death occur. The onset is rapid and there is no known treatment. A variety of other toxic sources from plants must be considered as hazards for wild mammals and birds, and it is likely that with increasingly sensitive observations and opportunities, these will be recognized and recorded.

PATHOGENESIS AND SIGNS. Since plants contain many different chemicals, they are capable of producing a variety of clinical syndromes (Table 2.1). It is therefore important to understand that there is no unique group of signs by which plant poisonings in wild mammals and birds may be recognized. However, the sudden onset of illness without a visible cause should provide sufficient reason for including possible toxicity in the list of investigated etiologic agents. In the absence of fever, and with acute disorders of the digestive tract or central nervous system leading to loss of weight or prostration, plant poisoning may be suspected. Other clinical signs often produced by plant poisonings include general distress, repeated attempts to defecate, stomach or intestinal irritation, and an increase or variability in the heart rate. These general signs are often followed by weakness, labored breathing, collapse, and coma with death following within hours.

Just as the type of signs produced by poisonous plants may differ, so the severity and degree of clinical signs will fluctuate considerably and depend upon the kind of plant eaten, the amount consumed, the stage of plant growth and the type of soil and other climatic-environmental factors, the amount and kind of other feed consumed at the same time, and the individual tolerance of the animal species to the specific poison. The greatest variable appears to be the chemical composition of the plant during the growing season and the specific localization of toxic compounds in various portions of the plant during stages of growth.

Toxicities in wild and caged birds due to naturally occurring materials have been briefly described in other reviews (Feldman and Kruckenberg, 1975; Hartung, 1971; Petrak, 1969; Seneviratna, 1969). Since the diets of even closely related species of birds can be quite diverse, signs of intoxication resulting from feeds, plants, or fungi-contaminated waters may also be variable. Generally, signs of intoxication in birds are those of digestive disturbance. Vomiting, anorexia, emaciation, salivation, diarrhea, pasting of the vent, straining, impacted crop, and a progressively enlarging abdomen are among the signs most often seen.

PATHOLOGY. There is considerably more information available about the gross and microscopic lesions observed with plant poisonings in wild or caged mammals and birds. The nature of the poisoning frequently results in the animals being found in the terminal stages of poisoning or often when death has already ensued. Hence, the documentation of clinical signs is scarce, while the pathology observed is usually based on careful and detailed reports of the subsequent laboratory studies on the various plant intoxication syndromes.

DIAGNOSIS. As in the diagnosis of illness from any etiologic agent, successful diagnosis employs a number of procedures, observations, and techniques that are aimed at eliminating some potential causes and confirming certain observations, lesions, or laboratory findings that suggest the involvement of general or specific poisonous plants. Infectious, parasitic, and other nontoxic causes may be eliminated by clinical laboratory examinations, direct smears of droppings or feces, microbiological cultures, and thorough evaluation of the clinical history and physical examination findings.

Documentation. A successful diagnosis related to poisonous plants requires the careful documentation of management practices, the age and species of animal affected, a competent description by appropriately trained persons of the clinical signs and pathologic lesions, proper botanical identification of the suspected plant or plants, and possible laboratory confirmation of the presence in tissues of the poisonous principle from the suspected plant. Theoretical extrapolation of the possibility of the affected animal's ingesting sufficient quantities of the available plant to be toxic may be correlated with literature documentation of toxic doses or the experimental reproduction of toxicity and clinical signs and lesions produced by feeding trials. Study of the environmental factors surrounding the suspected toxicity, including geographic location, stage of growth, soil conditions, and climatic variations, all serve to reinforce the possibility of the plant in question being the toxic entity. Subsequent calculation of the required lethal dose based on the animal's weight and growth conditions of the plant and the final extraction and identification of the plant's poisonous principle in the animal's tissues serve as final diagnostic confirmation. Although all these requirements are difficult to meet in any one instance, the multidisciplinary input from various specialists is important too. This assures that the final diagnosis is "real" and scientifically confirmed.

Clinical Syndromes. Since plants may contain many different poisonous principles, there are no specific clinical signs or series of clinical syndromes that may be used to recognize plant poisonings. However, poisonings should be suspected if there is a sudden onset of illness with no visible cause and many animals in a herd show a similar disorder simultaneously. The involvement of the central nervous sytem, digestive tract, or other body systems may suggest a particular poisonous principle and indicate the necessity to review the available forage for its presence. Rapid and severe loss of weight in a group of animals, leading to weakness and eventual prostration, is also suggestive of plant poisoning, especially when coupled with poor feeding conditions or climatic circumstances favoring the ingestion of otherwise ignored poisonous plants. These clinical syndromes, including variation in heart rate, digestive tract dysfunctions, diarrhea, repeated attempts to pass feces, labored breathing, and general distress, may be present in various combinations that lead to weakness, collapse, coma, and eventual death.

Poisoning from glycosides may produce increased weakness, with staggering and collapse in affected animals. Respirations may increase and progress to gasping and eventual respiratory distress. Other signs may include incoordination, muscular tremors, bloat, convulsions, and death from respiratory and/or cardiac failure. The variety of clinical signs produced by various plants containing specific toxic principles are given in Table 2.1.

Occasionally, bright red venous blood may be observed on necropsy. This is a valuable diagnostic sign, although this color may remain only for several hours following death. Such bright red blood is suggestive of cyanide toxicity. Cyanide may be released from within the plant by freezing, wilting, or crushing, but rumen and digestive tract microflora also may cause enzymatic release of the cyanide from cyanide-glycoside–containing plant species. Young plants and sprouts tend to contain more glycosides than older plants, and plants grown in the shade contain more of the cyanide principle than those exposed to the sun. Because of its volatility, cyanide is usually not retained in plant or animal tissues for any considerable length of time after cutting of the plant or death of the animal. This reduces the possibility of securing chemical analysis of plant or animal tissues to assist in diagnosis.

The final confirmation of plant toxicity should be by laboratory identification of the incriminated poisonous principle in the affected animal's tissues. Unfortunately, laboratory techniques for the identification of the varied and complex plant materials are not readily available, nor are the specific toxic principles in the variety of plants available for animal and bird consumption chemically characterized in significant quantity. Cyanide, nitrate-nitrite, mycotoxins, and isolated alkaloids and glycosides may be identified if sufficient analytical capability is available. Liver, digestive tract content, and occasionally blood may be utilized for such laboratory procedures. When coupled with pathologic lesions, grossly or microscopically, that further suggest or support specific chemical etiologies, the diagnosis of specific plant poisonings may be made with relative confidence and accuracy.

TREATMENT. From a practical standpoint, the treatment of free-living wild animals suffering from plant poisoning is extremely difficult. Even in instances of caged mammals and birds, treatment is at best supportive and frequently nonspecific. However, treatment in caged animals is more effective, since the opportunity for early treatment is greater and restraint and treatment facilities permit more definitive and thorough care than is possible in the wild state. Because of difficulty in diagnosis, however, a cautious optimism and guarded prognosis is only realistic in most cases of toxicity.

Whenever toxicity due to poisonous plants is a possibility, the affected animals should be removed from the browsing area as soon as possible. Such movement should be accomplished quietly and without undue excitement, although this is often difficult in the native state with animals not used to being handled. If a particular animal cannot be removed from the area containing the suspected poisonous plant, it should be made comfortable in that locale and protected from the environment; feed and water should be provided readily.

Once the animal is under relative control, the classic principles of toxicity treatment should be implemented: any unabsorbed plant material should be removed from the digestive tract, specific or general poison antidotes should be given, and elimination of the absorbed toxic principle should be hastened. General supportive measures to keep vital body functions active and to maintain general homeostasis are an important and necessary part of successful therapy.

Removal of Unabsorbed Poison. Prevention of further absorption of the toxic principle from the plant and elimination of the unabsorbed poison may be accomplished by the use of laxatives and by giving absorbants that will bind the unabsorbed toxin in the digestive tract. Mineral oil may be given through a stomach tube at the dose of ½ to 3 liters, depending on animal weight. Saline laxatives may also be given, with 25–1,000 gm of sodium sulfate or magnesium sulfate given orally as a 20% solution. Twenty to 30 ml of milk of magnesia may also be utilized. Such treatment will produce diarrhea and may be contraindicated if a severe purging action is already present due to the toxicity. Activated charcoal (250–5500 gm) is an effective binding agent for various toxic principles present in the digestive tract and prevents their absorption and promotes elimination in the feces.

Antidotes. Specific antidotes are generally not available for the wide variety of toxic principles found in poisonous plants. Some suggested individual treatments may be employed as given in Table 2.2, but the most specific therapy is employed with cyanide toxicity. Sodium nitrite and sodium thiosulfate have been effective in treating all species of animals suffering from cyanide toxicity.

Elimination of Absorbed Poison. The toxin already absorbed may be hastened in its normal elimination through the kidneys or other excretion routes. Providing ample water for affected animals, even in the presence of diarrhea, helps urinary flow and increases the excretion of water-soluble toxins. Such fluids are best administered orally with a stomach tube or, if the animal is drinking water, by making ample quantities available. Fluid therapy and administration of diuretics also may increase urine flow.

Supportive Therapy. Since most toxic animals will be seen in the later stages of poisoning and specific antidotes are not available for most plant toxins, the use of intelligent and aggressive supportive therapy will be most effective in the

Table 2.2. General Clinical Signs and Recommended Treatments for Wild or Caged Mammals and Birds That Have Been Poisoned by Plants

Plant	General Clinical Signs	Recommended Treatment
Produce Primarily Gastrointestinal Effects		
Kalmia latifolia, mountain laurel	Salivation; vomiting; weakness; inability to stand; coma.	Mineral oil, laxatives; stimulants.
Solanum nigrum, black nightshade	Marked thirst; diarrhea; anorexia; weakness; irregular gait; inability to stand; coma.	Laxatives; physostigmine; philocarpine; stimulants.
Quercus sp., oak	Anorexia; weight loss; dry scaly muzzle; hard, mucoid feces; weakness.	Symptomatic treatment; stimulants; blood transfusions and fluid therapy.
Senecio sp., ragwort	Dropsy; anorexia; rough haircoat; diarrhea; marked straining; rapid weight loss; coma.	Symptomatic treatment.
Veratrum sp., western false hellebore	Excessive salivation; polyuria; irregular gait; vomition; cardiac arrythmias; shallow respirations, congenital anomalies.	Rest and oxygen administration. Symptomatic treatment.
Produce Primarily Central Nervous System Stimulation		
Dicentra cucullaria, Dutchman's breeches	Excessive salivation; weakness; trembling; convulsions.	Parenteral calcium-magnesium-phosphorus IV; mild cathartic.
Delphinium sp., larkspur	Hypersensitivity; muscular trembling; collapse; prostration; convulsions; constipation; bloat; excessive salivation sometimes noted.	Physostigmine (2.2 grains) + strychnine (1.1 grain) in 20 ml water given SC per 500 kg.
Astragalus sp., *Oxytropis* sp.,-locoweed	Very excitable and irritable; abnormal gait; separate from herd; head held peculiarly; disturbed vision; chronic loss of flesh; weakness; prostration; convulsions.	Laxatives; sedatives; quiet.
Lupinus sp., lupine	Nervousness; loss of muscular control; frothing of the mouth; convulsions; difficulty breeding; congenital anomalies.	Sedatives; laxatives. Potassium permanganate: 2–4 ml/kg (1: 10,000) solution, gastric lavage. Physostigmine salycyclate: horse and cow—30–120 mg SC, IM; sheep—5–20 mg SC, IM.
Nerium oleander, oleander	Overstimulation of the vagus; abdominal pain; vomiting; diarrhea; tremors; progressive paralysis; coma.	Atropine sulfate; emetic; gastric lavage. Symptomatic treatment.
Conium maculatum, poison hemlock	Muscle twitch; weakness; rapid, shallow respiration; coma; congenital anomalies.	Laxatives; tannic acid; stimulants. Supportive treatment.
Cicuta sp., water hemlock	Violent spasms resulting in rapid respiration and heart rate; coma.	Artificial respiration; sedatives.
Eupatorium rugosum, white snakeroot	Marked trembling; incoordination; weakness; inability to stand.	Laxatives; stimulants.
Centaurea solstitialis, yellow star thistle	Lip twitching; involuntary chewing; mouth open; inability to swallow or hold food in mouth; mechanical damage to lips.	Symptomatic treatment.

Table 2.2. *(cont.)*

Plant	General Clinical Signs	Recommended Treatment
Produce Primarily Central Nervous System Depression		
Robinia pseudoacacia, black locust	Anorexia; depression; weakness; posterior paresis; irregular pulse; labored breathing.	Digitalis; symptomatic treatment. Supportive therapy.
Xanthium strumarium, cocklebur	Red mucous membranes; labored rapid breathing; inability to stand; depression; coma.	Oil and lard PO; stimulants; adsorbants. Physostigmine 5–30 mg IM repeated in ½–1 hour.
Crotalaria sp., crotalaria	Slow weight loss; weakness; stupor.	Supportive therapy.
Zigadenus sp., death camas	Rapid depression; increased pulse and respiration; coma.	Atropine sulfate (4.4 mg) + picrotoxin (17.6 mg) in 5 ml water given IV per 100 kg. Repeated every 2 hours for 2–3 injections.
Thermopsis rhombifolia, false lupine	Depression; anorexia; marked stiffness; tucked up appearance of abdomen; congenital anomalies.	Sedatives; laxatives. Potassium permanganate: 2–4 ml/kg (1: 10,000) solution, gastric lavage. Physostigmine salicylate: horse and cow—30–120 mg SC, IM; sheep—5–20 mg SC, IM.
Equisetum sp., horsetail	Weakness; diarrhea; rapid weight loss; incoordination; coma.	Thiamine hydrochloride 100–200 mg SC for several days. Symptomatic treatment; supportive therapy.
Asclepias subverticillata, whorled milkweed	Incoordination; depression; shallow respiration; inability to stand; coma.	Symptomatic treatment.
Produce Primarily Blood Alterations		
Cyanide (*Triglochin* sp., arrowgrass; *Prunus* sp., chokecherry)	Initial excitement and muscle tremors, followed by pronounced polypnea and dyspnea; salivation; lacrimation; voiding of feces and urine; gasping for breath; clonic convulsions. Blood is bright cherry red.	Sodium nitrite (1%) 16 mg/kg IV, followed with 20% sodium thiosulfate 30–40 mg/kg IV. Repeat treatment with sodium thiosulfate only. Or 20% sodium nitrite (10 ml) + 20% sodium thiosulfate (30 ml), 0.09 mg/kg IV.
Dicoumarol (*Melilotus* sp., sweetclover)	Stiffness and lameness; subcutaneous hemorrhages all over body, especially over bony prominences; gastrointestinal bleeding and anemia.	Vitamin K_1 5 mg/kg IM for 5 days.
Nitrate-nitrite (*Amaranthus* sp., pigweed; *Avena sativa,* oat hay; *Brassica napus,* rape; *Sorghum vulgare,* sudan grass; *Zea mays,* corn)	Salivation; diarrhea; anoxia (dyspnea, cyanotic mucous membranes; rapid, weak pulse); blood typical dark brown (methemoglobinemia).	4% methylene blue 10 mg/kg IV.
Produce Primarily Epithelial Damage		
Tetradymia sp., horsebrush	Photosensitization.	Topical ointments; keep out of sun; graze at night.
Hypericum perforatum, saint-john's-wort	Photosensitization.	See horsebrush.
Setaria lutescens, foxtail, *Stipa* sp., needlegrass; *Aristida* sp., poverty grass; *Trifolium incarnatum,* crimson clover	Mechanical injury.	Symptomatic treatment.

recovery process of affected animals. Animals should be kept warm by means of shelter and dry environments. Respiratory support should be maintained to keep normal oxygenation of body tissues ample and to support normal organ function. Cardiac activity must be maintained at a normal rate and body fluids and vascular parameters must be within physiological ranges. Electrolyte balance is especially important, since acidosis is a common effect of intoxications. Appropriate relief for pain due to abdominal irritation or other injuries should be provided. Increased or decreased central nervous system activity should be stabilized to appropriate levels. Convulsions may be treated with sedatives, and central nervous system depression may be reversed by utilizing stimulants. However, since sedatives and anesthetics affect vital functions, drugs having this effect must be used with caution to avoid further depressing already sick animals. Especially in the wild state, sick mammals may be more susceptible to anesthetic effects than healthy domestic species. Nervous system, muscular, or generalized weakness may be treated with appropriate stimulating drugs, but caution must also be used to avoid undesirable side effects that may be more pronounced in wild mammals and birds.

The variety of clinical signs produced by toxic plants may serve to weaken or aggravate the primary toxic effect of the poisonous principle. Such clinical alterations should be treated appropriately, but with reason and understanding of the basis for their occurrence and potential harm. For example, persistent diarrhea may be treated with appropriate drugs to reduce fluid loss, but the effect on retarding elimination of unabsorbed toxin from the digestive tract also must be considered. Further, the increased susceptibility of the diarrhea-affected digestive tract to secondary infections may suggest the application of antimicrobial agents to reduce the incidence of bacterial complications. Suggested treatment for some plants that may cause toxicity in wild and caged mammals and birds are listed in Table 2.2.

PREVENTION OF PLANT POISONINGS. Prevention of plant poisoning in caged animals is largely a function of management. Elimination of poisonous plants from environments within or around the cage will prevent the animal from accidentally ingesting toxic forage or prevent visitors from using the opportunity to "feed" toxic plants to caged animals through fences. Appropriate structure of cages and the providing of "buffer zones" between observers and animal may prove valuable. In zoos utilizing the free-roaming concept that permits birds and nonaggressive mammals to move at will throughout the zoo environment, providing abundant nontoxic feeds usually prevents the animals from seeking other possibly toxic forage. Absolute safety should be assured by eliminating all toxic plants from the zoo grounds.

If exposure is unavoidable, certain toxic plant principles may be reduced in toxicity by the proper management of feeding procedures. High levels of concentrates in the feed tend to prevent the liberation in the digestive tract of cyanide from cyanide-containing plants. The high level of concentrate must be consumed within several hours of exposure to the toxic cyanide. Large quantities of dextrose also tend to reduce the harmful effects of cyanide. Forage intended for animal feeding and known to contain hazardous levels of cyanide may be utilized with safety if placed in a silo with sufficient water to ensure a degree of fermentation. Other plants known to contain oxalic acid (halogeton and greasewood) may be reduced in toxicity by simultaneously feeding calcium at two to three times normal dietary levels.

Prevention of plant toxicities in free-living mammals and birds is considerably more difficult, since ample opportunity exists for indiscriminate and diverse browsing of forage throughout the environment. A shortage of desirable browse is perhaps the most frequent condition that results in free-roaming animal losses from ingestion of toxic plants. Most poisonous plants are sufficiently low in palatability so that poisonings usually occur only if animals are forced to graze on the less desirable plants. Occasionally, management practices or activities of neighboring livestockmen result in trimmings or other portions of toxic plants being placed in forage areas and made available to wild mammals and birds.

If sufficient quantity and variety of browse is permitted to grow on natural range areas, the presence of these desirable forages will reduce the invasion and growth of poisonous plants, making fewer toxic species available to wild animals. However, whether proper browse can be maintained for wildlife depends on the management of available areas for feeding. Control treatments with chemicals, burning, or mechanical and biological control measures should be applied before feed production occurs in order to reduce the spread of toxic plants already present in the area.

CONCLUSION. Poisonous plants available to wild or caged mammals and birds are extremely diverse. This results in variable syndromes being produced in affected animals, with clinical signs and necropsy findings reflecting the biological effect of the poisonous principle or principles consumed. Because of the relative isolation of wild mammals and birds, specific and abundant documentation of toxic effects from poisonous plants in these species is not well recorded. Most information is obtained by extrapolation from experimental findings in laboratory animals or from reported cases occurring in large domestic animals.

It is likely that future social development will see more interest taken in the health of free-roaming animals, and with it interest in hazards to which wild mammals and birds are exposed. Increased observations of the "life style" of wild animals will probably result in increasing awareness and documentation of toxicities due to environmental compounds such as those found in poisonous plants. Increased environmental interest in wild species and knowledge of chemical-biological interactions will likely result in a greater understanding of the variety of effects that poisonous plants may produce. As more extensive zoo facilities are developed and as increasing study of wild animals in their native habitat occurs, curiosity will lead to increased speculation as to what various animals will eat. With curiosity a tendency for mischievousness will occur, and it is likely that zoo and caged animals will face a greater hazard from toxicity as a result of human ignorance.

These trends suggest a need for greater emphasis on the study and classification of toxic effects from poisonous plants in wild and caged mammals and birds. Just as the livestockman requires a rational knowledge of animal husbandry to develop his specialty, there is an obvious need to develop adequate information on the effects of poisonous plants to allow responsible personnel to successfully deal with plant intoxications in wild mammals and birds.

SOME SPECIFIC PLANT POISONINGS OF WILDLIFE

Pieris japonica Poisoning

ETIOLOGY. *Pieris japonica*

SIGNS. Diarrhea, colic, vomiting, and paralysis of the hindquarters in Barbary sheep, *Ammatragus lervia,* camel, *Camelus dromedarius,* black bear, *Ursus americanus,* and guanacos, *Lama guanico,* resulted after they had been fed *Pieris japonica* leaves by visitors to a zoo (Gillis et al., 1961).

Yew Poisoning

ETIOLOGY. *Taxus baccata*

SIGNS. Bennett's wallaby, *Protemnodon bennetti,* showed central nervous system signs. Early in the syndrome there was severe excitation with attempts to escape. A strong salivary flow occurred and mydriasis was followed by somnolence that was periodically interrupted by epileptic-like attacks. On closer examination a strong tachycardia with weak respirations and digestive tract bloat were noted (Kohler and Grunberg, 1960). Two of the kangaroos died within six hours after ingestion of the yew needles and two others died within 48 hours. The yew leaves were fed by a well-meaning warden at the zoo.

Yew produced extensive losses in pheasant chicks three to four weeks of age (Jordan, 1964). Clinical signs were few and far between prior to death. The chicks were initially in good condition with no sign of toxicity; however, one day 7 were found dead, followed by 10 dead the next day, 20 the third day, and 30 the fourth day.

PATHOLOGY. Gross pathological findings associated with *Taxus baccata* poisoning in pheasants consisted of a gastritis with some inflammation in the upper part of the duodenum (Jordan, 1964). The liver was engorged with blood, and the lungs were engorged to a lesser extent.

Gross pathological findings in kangaroos poisoned by *T. baccata* leaves consisted of a highly acute hyperemia in all parenchymatous organs, stomach dilatation, and tympany of the intestinal tract (Kohler and Grunberg, 1960). There was a light to medium acute intestinal inflammation of mucous membrane. In spots there was a hemorrhagic gastritis. Emphysema was also noted. The pancreas and thymus remnants had hemorrhages. A right side dilatation of the heart was present. A few small subepicardial hemorrhages were present over the right ventricle. The large veins of the body contained uncoagulated blood. In the head above the parietal bones, a subcutaneous bloody gelatinous edema was found, which may have been due to the trauma of the excitation period. The lactating mammary gland was very hyperemic and congested. Hyperemia occurred in the meninges. Edema occurred in the lung of one kangaroo.

Histological findings consisted of congestive hyperemia of the brain along with swelling of endothelial cells of the capillaries in the areas of hyperemia, especially in the cerebrum. The Virchow-Robin space contained little albumin. There was marked edema in the cerebellum; perivascular hemorrhages were seen in the area of the nucleus caudatus. Hemorrhages occurred, localized in the meninges, and manifested themselves mainly as discrete permeability interruptions that resulted in connective tissue being loosened and containing erythrocytes. Severe regressive changes occurred in the ganglion cells. The most affected cells were the small ganglion cells of the outer layer of the cerebrum and those of the ammonite. Pyknosis occurred in the ganglion cells in the cerebrum along with clumping of substance and, at times, an obvious enlargement of the nucleoli. Vacuolation was found in the ganglion cells. Occasionally cells were found in the Purkinje cell layer of the cerebellum ganglion cells. The molecular layer of the cerebellum often had dilated capillaries with swollen endothelial cells. Where Purkinje cells were damaged, there was an increase in the number of glial cells. Pericellular microglia proliferation was found in the ganglion cells of the medulla oblongata where edema also occurred.

The stomach and intestinal tract had inflammation of the mucosa with desquamation of the epithelium and inflammation with leukocytic infiltration. The mucous membrane was hyperemic. The small intestine contained an acute and partial necrotic enteritis. The lamina propria of the large intestine showed leukocytic and plasmatic infiltration and desquamation of the surface epithelium. The kidneys had a strong peristaltic hyperemia in all the parenchymatous tissues and in the marrow and crust layer. A significant dissociation of the kidney epithelium was present, especially in the tubuli recti, which contained albumin cylinders. The glomeruli appeared swollen. There was swelling of the epithelial cells which led to a restriction of the lumina. One kangaroo had epithelial necrosis with pyknosis of the nuclei in the marrow area and near the papillae, but there were some cells intact and in relatively good condition. The myocardium had hyperemia with a nearly complete infarction of the capillaries that contained red blood corpuscles. The liver appeared acutely congested with hydrops and dilatation. Focal degeneration of liver cells occurred. The lungs were completely hyperemic; there were focal hemorrhages in the alveoli. The lungs contained edema and there were focal hemorrhages inside the pancreas.

Gross pathology associated with deer poisoned by *T. baccata* consisted of inflammation of the mucosa and hemorrhages of the forestomachs (Kohler and Grunberg, 1960). The intestinal tract had inflammation of the mucosa of the duodenum and jejunum. The liver was severely congested. Both the auricles and ventricles of the heart showed dilatation and were tightly filled with blood. Hemorrhages occurred in the spleen. Edema was found in the lung.

Woolly-pod or Broad-leafed Milkweed Toxicity

ETIOLOGY. *Asclepias eriocarpa*

SIGNS. Wild cottontail rabbits, *Sylvilagus* sp., and domestic rabbits, *Oryctolagus caniculus,* after being fed broad-leafed milkweed, *Asclepias eriocarpa,* as either fresh or dried material developed progressive anterior paralysis (Vail, 1942). At first the rabbits assumed a humped position but later became prostrate and comatose and died in a matter of hours.

PATHOLOGY. Congested blood vessels with hemorrhage in the heart, liver, spleen, small intestine, stomach, and kidneys (Vail, 1942).

Locoism Toxicity

ETIOLOGY. *Astragalus* sp. and *Oxytropis* sp.

SIGNS. Locoism has been described in elk (Adcock and Keiss, 1969). The general clinical signs include emaciation, extreme weakness and depression, fine and coarse generalized muscular tremors, stumbling, and incoordination. One elk had posterior ataxia, hopped uphill with difficulty, and was unable to keep its hindlimbs together, with the result that they were splayed. The neck and head may repeatedly be flexed to one side. When elk were experimentally fed pelleted locoweed of *Astragalus* and *Oxytropis,* the only signs produced were a progressive weight loss and generalized depression in the later stages of the study. This illustrates the variability found among plants and the apparent fluctuation in toxicity due to stage of growth and environmental factors.

Pronghorn antelope have shown signs similar to those reported in cattle with locoism (Buechner, 1950). Hyperexcitability, rough hair coat, ataxia, and loss of weight were reported; occasionally blindness is noted and abortions may occur with death common.

PATHOLOGY. Adcock and Keiss (1969) consistently found emaciation and serous atrophy of adipose tissue on gross examination of elk with locoism. The liver was pale tan and had prominent individual lobules. The gray matter of the brain was pale. Renal cortices were pale and congestive mottling was noted. The lymph nodes throughout the body were swollen and pale. Occasionally pulmonary congestion and edema, excessive amounts of fluid in serous cavities, pale blood, and serous atrophy of bone marrow were observed.

Histological changes in affected elk consisted of swelling and fine vacuolation of the cytoplasm of neurons accompanied by axonal dystrophy (Adcock and Keiss, 1969). Neurons were affected throughout the cerebral cortex, basal nuclei, hippocampus, diencephalon, midbrain, pons, medulla oblongata, and cerebellum. Also affected were neurons of the spinal cord, gasserian ganglion, spinal ganglion, mesenteric plexus, and the ganglion cell layer and inner nuclear layer of the retina. The optic nerve head and optic nerve fiber layer of the retina contained dystrophic axons. Marked cytoplasmic swelling and vacuolation were seen in the epithelial cells of the choroid plexus, hepatocytes, acinar cells of the pancreas and salivary glands, follicular cells of the thyroid, and proximal tubular epithelium of the kidney. The lymph nodes contained collections of macrophages with vacuolated cytoplasm.

After elk were fed pelleted locoweed, *Astragalus* and *Oxytropis,* moderate progressive weight loss and depression occurred in the latter stages, but on gross examination there was pallor of the gray matter in the brain, a grayish-tan pallor of the hepatic parenchyma with accentuation of the lobular architecture, and a paleness of the renal cortex. Histopathological lesions in the brain, kidney, and liver were identical to those found in naturally occurring cases.

Pyrrolizidine Alkaloid Intoxication

ETIOLOGY. Rattle box, *Crotalaria* sp., and heliotrope, *Heliotropium* sp. (Fowler, 1975)

SIGNS. Seger et al. (1969) studied deer from an Audubon refuge in Louisiana which were suspected of being intoxicated with pyrrolizidine alkaloids from plants of the genera *Crotalaria, Heliotropium,* and *Senecio.* The deer were left from a white-tailed deer die-off in the coastal marshes of Louisiana following an extended period of below normal rainfall. After a few months, the deer showed typical signs of hepatoencephalopathy, including incoordination, blindness, convulsions, icterus, hemoglobinuria, and lack of fear of man. They become emaciated, anemic, and moribund.

PATHOLOGY. These animals were heavily parasitized with lice; the blood was thin and watery. The more distal marrow of the tibia and femur was yellow and gelatinous. There was little body fat left. There was serous atrophy of the cardiac and mesenteric adipose tissue. The liver was small and pale, and its surface appeared dull and somewhat granular. The kidneys were pale.

On microscopic examination a megalocytosis of the liver was found; there was hypertrophy of the hepatocytes. The nuclei of the affected cells were as much as 25 microns in diameter as opposed to normal-sized nuclei of 5 to 9 microns. The largest cells were found at the periphery of the lobes, but all cells in some lobes appeared affected. The nuclei membranes stained heavily in most cells because of the concentration of chromatin near the membrane. Single nuclei were enlarged near the nuclei membrane. Discrete acidophilic cytoplasmic globules up to 5 microns were found in some hepatocytes. Each globule was encased in a clear halo. Bile duct proliferation was minimal. There was some fibroplasia of Glisson's capsule and the portal triads. Necrosis was found in only individual hepatocytes.

This type of pathology parallels that found associated with pyrrolizidine alkaloid poisoning in sheep. *Crotalaria, Heliotropium,* and *Senecio* were found on the deer range and evidence of grazing the plants was noted. Little other forage was available for browsing.

Tutu Poisoning

ETIOLOGY. *Coriaria arborea*

SIGNS. Circus elephants, *Elephas maximus,* have been poisoned by tutu (Anderson, 1968). The first signs noted were excitement, ataxia, salivation, and a profuse watery diarrhea. Later central nervous system signs developed, with convulsions that began as trembling during which profuse salivation and diarrhea occurred. This progressed to a generalized shaking and loss of balance that caused the elephants to crash to the ground. While the animals were prostrate, they showed involuntary paddling of the limbs and appeared unconscious and in respiratory distress. The convulsions occurred every three to four minutes and lasted one to three minutes each. These were interspersed with periods of apparent normality during which the elephants could stand.

PATHOLOGY. Unavailable.

Tarbush Poisoning

ETIOLOGY. *Flourensia cernua*

SIGNS. Signs found associated with a pronghorn antelope, *Antilocapra americana,* die-off caused by tarbush poisoning were a slow unsteady gait, arched backs, a ruffled appearance to the hair, and general lethargy (Hailey et al., 1966). Affected antelope were able to run but could not attain their normal speeds. Grayish-black material adhered to the hair around the base of the tail and to the rear feet; it had the characteristic odor of tarbush.

PATHOLOGY. According to Hailey et al. (1966) gross lesions in pronghorn antelope as a result of tarbush, *Flourensia cernua,* were predominantly vascular and interstitial. Blood in the lungs tended to localize into a lobular pattern. Hemorrhagic effusions were found in the serosal surface of the omasum, rumen, and abomasum and along the mesenteric attachment of the small intestine. Serous fluid was found in the pleural cavity. In the 10 to 12 animals necropsied, there was congestive inflammation and necrosis of the gastrointestinal wall. Petechial hemorrhages in the abomasum of all animals were speculated to be a result of *Haemonchus contortus* infestation. Three of four pregnant females had resorbing fetuses in their uteri.

Rumen samples taken from nine animals necropsied revealed tarbush present in high percentages (six contained 94–99% tarbush, one 85%, one 10%, and one 1%). The tarbush portion of the samples was composed of leaves, stems, and buds. This area had three years of below-average rain fall and had been grazed severely by domestic stock as well as wildlife. Only tarbush, *F. cernua;* creosotebush, *Larrea divaricata,* and snakeweed, *Amphiachyrus dracunculoidis,* were readily available as forage.

Histopathology was confined to the vascular system and the gastrointestinal tract. Degeneration of the vascular endothelium of the pulmonary vessels and hemorrhage into the vessel walls and surrounding tissues were sometimes severe. One animal with pulmonary lesions had proliferated the visceral pleura adjacent to the areas of hemorrhage. The intestinal mucosa was necrotic in three of five animals that had been killed. Three of the five animals had dead embryos undergoing resorption.

Chokecherry Poisoning

ETIOLOGY. *Prunus melanocarpa*

SIGNS. Cyanide poisoning has been reported in an antelope from the ingestion of chokecherry, *Prunus melanocarpa* (Ogilvie, 1955). The affected antelope was stiff and slow in physical movements; weakness was obvious.

PATHOLOGY. Digestive tract contained grain and dry material mostly composed of new growth of chokecherry.

Algae Poisoning

ETIOLOGY. *Microcystis aeruginosa, Gloctrichus pisum, Anabaena flossaquae*

SIGNS. Brandenberg and Shigley (1947) found a number of dead deer near the shore of a lake in North Dakota where cattle had drunk water containing blue-green algae. Cattle had developed central nervous signs within 15 to 20 minutes after consuming the toxic water and died in one to four hours. When Smit (1950) experimentally poisoned small animals with the alkaloid of algae, sudden death ensued after oral administration of the algae. Acute signs noted were restlessness, anemia, dyspnea, a progressive paralysis, coma, and death. Chronic signs included listlessness, ascites, and loss of condition.

PATHOLOGY. Bishop et al. (1959) extracted a cyclic polypeptide from *Microcystis aeruginosa* that was capable of killing mice within two to three hours and was called the "fast death factor." A second toxic factor called the "slow death factor" was also isolated. It killed mice less rapidly.

Gillam (1925) found dead wild birds, horses, cattle, hogs, and poultry that had drunk from lakes that had green scum containing *Gloctrichus pisum.* Gross pathology found was a patchy congestion of the lungs and a small quantity of tarry-looking blood vessels in the heart.

In 1934 Fitch stated that a farmer found tame and wild ducks dead near a small lake containing algae. At one end of the lake the algae *Anabaena flossaquae,* had been piled up by the wind. Freshly collected algae, when given orally, killed one experimental rabbit; but after storage at refrigeration or room temperature, it was nontoxic. When given intraperitoneally, the material was uniformly fatal to rabbits, guinea pigs, and chickens, even after being kept for three weeks at refrigeration temperature. No macroscopic lesions, except congestion of the blood vessels of the peritoneum were seen at necropsy of the experimental animals. The toxin was not neutralized by *Clostridium botulinum* antitoxin A, B, or C.

O'Donoghae and Wilton (1951) presented two gulls, three ducks, and one blue finch that had died on a lake containing blue-green algae to a diagnostic laboratory. Poisoning occurred after the algae became concentrated along the shore as a result of gentle winds blowing toward the shore. All the specimens appeared dehydrated and were difficult to skin. Dilatation of the heart, which was full of blood, was a constant finding. The hearts were dilated in the two gulls and the duck and were infected and full of blood, the livers were slightly mottled, the crops and gizzards were empty, and very little material was found in the intestinal tract. In the finch the liver was mottled with a few necrotic foci, the spleen was darkened and mottled; the crop and gizzard were empty; there was some erosion of the gizzard and a slight to marked hemorrhagic inflammation of the mucous membrane of the intestine.

A two-month-old pig was inoculated with one quart of the algae water and died within 24 minutes. Necropsy revealed a moderate inflammation of the mucous membrane of the stomach and intestine. Histopathology revealed the liver as having early degeneration, and the cytoplasm was very granular in appearance. The spleen had slight hemorrhage and hemosiderin deposits. The kidneys showed marked cloudy swelling with slight hemorrhage. A rabbit given 5 ml of sterile filtrate of this toxic water intraperitoneally had a dark and mottled liver with a distended gallbladder. On histopathological examination there were degenerative changes in the liver and kidneys with hemosiderin deposits in them.

Necropsy findings in the small animals as recorded by Smit (1950) in acute deaths were blood-stained ascites, swelling of spleen, hyperemia of the kidneys; the liver was dark red and soft and had severe necrosis with associated blood stasis, and surface hemorrhages. Lesions in chronic cases were confined to the liver and varied with severity of the condition. Necrosis, fatty degeneration, hemorrhages, blood stasis, various stages of hepatic cellular regeneration, and marked ascites were found in animals with extensive cirrhosis. Cirrhosis of the liver was the principal lesion found.

Daubentonia Toxicity

ETIOLOGY. *Daubentonia punicea*

SIGNS. Emmel (1943) found that 6 to 18 *Daubentonia punicea* seeds killed homing pigeons. The pigeons died 8 to 12 days after consuming the seeds.

PATHOLOGY. Gross pathology showed a loss of tone in the musculature of the heart and gizzard and a brilliant green staining of the lining of the gizzard and duodenum. In chronic cases the spleen was enlarged approximately three times normal and was dark in color. The kidneys were enlarged and the liver was pale or greenish in color.

In acute cases the histopathology showed a necrotic enteritis involving tips of the intestinal villi, particularly the anterior portion, and degeneration of the remaining tissues of the intestine, liver, and kidneys. There were necrotic foci in the liver; necrosis of individual tubular cells and the tubules occurred in the kidneys. A necrotic inflammation was present in the mucosa of the proventriculus. There was degeneration in the proventriculus and pancreas and scattered areas of congestion in the spleen, liver, kidneys, and lungs. The spleen and liver contained numerous deposits of blood pigment.

Oleander Poisoning

ETIOLOGY. Common *Oleander, Nerium oleander*

SIGNS. Signs were noted in a pet two-toed sloth that had escaped from its cage and spent overnight in an oleander bush. Signs noted in the morning were cramping, profuse salivation, central nervous signs, and weakness (Miller, 1976). A black bear, *Ursus luteolus,* suspected of oleander poisoning had a severe gastroenteritis; the animal had vomited quite often and showed considerable distress. The bear had access to oleander leaves that had been put in the cage by an unsuspecting person (Ratigan, 1921).

Signs noted in experimentally poisoned monkeys were vomiting, polyuria, salivation, bradycardia, vaginal hemorrhage, abortion, anorexia, constipation, loss of body weight, narcosis, restlessness, weakness, and shallow and rapid respirations (Schwartz et al., 1974).

PATHOLOGY. In the bear there was thickening of the stomach wall and the mucous membrane was slate or purple colored. Blood clots were found in the duodenum, suggesting previous hemorrhagic inflammation in the stomach (Ratigan, 1921).

Pathology recorded by Schwartz et al. (1974) included leukocytosis; neutrophilia with increased potassium, glutamic-oxaloacetic transaminase, glutamic-pyruvic transaminase, blood urea nitrogen, and α globulins; and reticulocytopenia. Decreased calcium glucose, total serum protein, albumin, α gamma globulin levels and albumin-globulin ratios, hemorrhages, degeneration, necrosis, or all of these were observed in the heart, gastrointestinal tract, skeletal muscles, ovaries, adrenal glands, liver, kidneys, and pancreas. Pancreatic weights were significantly reduced and adrenal weights were significantly increased in the monkey receiving the highest amount of the toxic plant leaves.

Foxglove Poisoning

ETIOLOGY. *Digitalis purpurea* in farmed red deer, *Cervus elaphus*

SIGNS. May see dullness, weakness, bloody diarrhea or pungent fetid diarrhea, irregular heartbeat with an occasional extra systole; may find deer dead; may be loss in weight, and deer docile (Corrigall et al., 1978).

PATHOLOGY. Gross lesions noted were congestion and hemorrhagic consolidated patches in the lungs; excess pericardial fluid, auricles distended, ecchymoses around the coronary groove of the heart; meningeal vessels of the brain were observed; digestive tract had very fluid or bloody contents in the small and large intestines. Abomasitis and typhlitis were seen (Corrigall et al., 1978).

REFERENCES

Adcock, I. L., and R. E. Keiss. 1969. Locoism in elk. A disease resembling cerebral pseudolipiosis. Bull. Wildl. Dis. Assoc. 5:121–124.

Anderson, I. L. 1968. Tutu poisoning in two circus elephants. NZ Vet. J. 145–147.

Arnold, H. L. 1968. Poisonous plants of Hawaii. Tongg Pub. Co., Ltd., Box 2113 Honolulu.

Beath, O. A., C. S. Gilbert, H. F. Eppson, and I. Rosenfeld. 1953. Poisonous plants and livestock poisoning. Univ. of Wyoming, Wyoming Agric. Exp. Sta., Laramie. Bull. 324.

Bishop, C. T., E. F. L. J. Anet, and P. R. Gorham. 1959. Isolation and identification of the fast-death factor in *Microcystis aeruginosa.* Can. J. Biochem. Physiol. 37:453–471.

Brandenberg, T. O., and F. M. Shigley. 1947. Water blood as a cause of poisoning in livestock in North Dakota. J. Am. Vet. Med. Assoc. 110:384–385.

Buck, W. B., G. D. Osweiler, and G. A. Van Gelder. 1976. Clinical and diagnostic veterinary toxicology. 2nd ed. Kendall-Hunt, Dubuque.

Buechner, H. K. 1950. Life history, ecology and range use of the pronghorn antelope in Trans-Pecos, Texas. Am. Med. Nat. 43:257–354.

Chopra, R. N., R. L. Badwar, and S. Ghosh. 1965. Poisonous plants of India. Indian Council of Agric. Res., New Delhi.

Clare, N. T. 1955. Photosensitization in animals. Adv. Vet. Sci. 2:182–211.

______. 1952. Photosensitization in diseases of domestic animals. Rev. Ser. No. 3. Commonwealth Bureau Animal Health. Commonwealth Agric. Bureaux, Farnham Royal, Bucks, England.

Clarke, E. G. C., and M. L. Clarke. 1967. Garner's veterinary toxicology. 3rd ed. Williams & Wilkins. Baltimore.

Core, E. L., J. H. Reitz, and W. H. Gillespie. 1961. The poisonous plants of West Virginia. A preliminary report. Proc. W.Va. Acad. Sci. 33:29.

Corrigall, W., R. R. Moody, and J. C. Forbes. 1978. Foxglove, *Digitalis purpurea,* poisoning in farmed red deer, *Cervus elaphus.* Vet. Rec. 102:119–122.

Duncan, W. H., and T. J. Jones. 1949. Poisonous plants of Georgia. Univ. of Georgia, School of Vet. Med. Bull. 49(13).

______, P. L. Piercy, S. D. Feurt, and R. Starling. 1955/1957. Toxicological studies of southeastern plants. I. Leguminosae. II. Compositae. Econ. Bot. 9:243–255; 11:75–85.

Durrell, L. W., R. Jensen, and B. Klinger. 1952. Poisonous and injurious plants in Colorado. Colorado Agric. and Mechn. College, Fort Collins. Colorado Agric. Exp. Sta. Ext. Serv. Bull. 412–A.

Emmel, M. W. 1943. *Daubentonia punicea* (Cav.) DC. Poisoning in pigeons. J. Am. Vet. Med. Assoc. 102:294–295.

Everist, S. L. 1974. Poisonous plants of Australia. Azus and Robertson, Sydney.

Evers, R. A., and R. P. Link. 1972. Poisonous plants of the Midwest and their effects on livestock. U. of Illinois Press, Urbana.

Featherly, H. I. 1945. Some plants poisonous to livestock in Oklahoma. Oklahoma Agric. Exp. Sta., Cir. C–118.

Feldman, B. F., and S. M. Kruckenberg. 1975. Clinical toxicology of domestic and wildlife caged birds. Vet. Clin. N. Am. 5:653–673.

Fitch, C. P. 1934. Waterbloom as a cause of poisoning in domestic animals. Cornell Vet. 24:30–39.

Forsyth, A. A. 1968. British poisonous plants. H. M. Stationery Office, London.

Fowler, M. E. 1975. Toxicities in exotic and zoo animals. Vet. Clin. N. Am. 5:685–698.

Gardner, C. A., and H. W. Bennetts. 1956. The toxic plants of western Australia. West Australian Newspapers, Ltd., Perth.

Gilkey, H. M. 1958. Livestock-poisoning plants. Oregon Agric. Exp. Sta. Bull. 564.

Gillam, W. G. 1925. The effect on livestock of water contaminated with fresh water algae. J. Am. Vet. Med. Assoc. 67:780–784.

Gillis, W. T., W. Ball, and W. Ball, Jr. 1961. Pieris poisoning in zoo animals. Michigan State Univ. Vet 22:24–26.

Hailey, T. L., J. W. Thomas, and R. M. Robinson. 1966. Pronghorn die-off in Trans-Pecos, Texas, due to tarbush, *Flourensia cernua,* poisoning. J. Wildl. Manag. 30:488–496.

Harden, J. W. 1961. Poisonous plants of North Carolina. North Carolina Agric. Exp. Sta. Bull. 414.

Hartung, R. 1971. Effects of toxic substances. In J. W. Davis, R. C. Anderson, L. Karstad, and D. O. Trainer. Infectious and parasitic diseases of wild birds. Iowa State Univ. Press, Ames.

Huffman, W. T., E. A. Moran, and W. Binns. 1956. Poisonous plants. USDA Yearbook of Agric.

Hulbert, L. E., and F. W. Oehme. 1968. Plants poisonous to livestock. 3rd ed. Kansas State Univ. Print. Serv., Manhattan.

Hurst, W. E. 1942. The poison plants of New South Wales. 1942. NSW Poisonous Plant Committee, Sydney.

Hyatt, M. T., R. G. Brown, and J. W. Herron. April 1953. Some plants of Kentucky poisonous to livestock. Circ. 502, College of Agric. and Home Econ., Univ. of Kentucky and USDA, Lexington.

Jordan, W. J. 1964. Yew, *Taxus baccata,* poisoning in pheasants, *Phasianus colchicus.* Tijdschr. Diergeneeskd. 1:187–188.

Kingsbury, J. M. 1958. Plants poisonous to livestock. A Review. J. Dairy Sci. 41:875–907.

______. 1964. Poisonous plants of the United States and Canada. Prentice-Hall, Englewood Cliffs.

Kohler, H., and W. Grunberg. 1960. Yew poisoning in a kangaroo. Arch. Exp. Vet. Med. 14:1149–1162.

Lee, O. C., and L. P. Doyle. ND. Indiana plants poisonous and injurious to livestock. Purdue Univ. Agric. Ext. Serv., Lafayette, Ext. Bull. 240.

Liener, I. E. 1969. Toxic constituents of plant foodstuff. Academic Press, New York.

Massey, A. B. 1954. Poisonous plants in Virginia. V.P.I. &. S.U. Agric. Ext. Serv. Blacksburg, Bull. 222.

McLeun, A., and H. W. Nicholson. 1958. Stock poisoning plants of the British Columbia ranges. Can. Dept. Agric. Publ. 1037.

Miller, R. M. 1976. Oleander poisoning in a sloth. 1976. J. Zoo Anim. Med. 7:11.

Muenscher, W. C. 1951. Poisonous plants of the United States. 2nd ed., Macmillan, New York.

O'Donoghae, J. G., and G. S. Wilton. 1951. Algae poisoning in Alberta. Can. J. Comp. Med. 15:193–198.

Oehme, F. W. 1973. Chemical toxicities in farm animals. Proc. 77th Annu. Meet., U.S. Anim. Health Assoc. 216–230.

______. 1977. Chemical and physical disorders. In R. W. Kirk. Current veterinary therapy VI. W. B. Saunders, Philadelphia.

Ogilvie, S. 1955. Chokecherry toxic to an antelope. 1955. J. Mammal. 36(1):146.

Petrak, M. L. 1969. Diseases of cage and aviary birds. Lea & Febiger, Philadelphia.

Radeleff, R. D. 1970. Veterinary toxicology. Lea & Febiger, Philadelphia.

Ratigan, W. J. 1921. Oleander poisoning in a bear. J. Am. Vet. Med. Assoc. 60:96–97.

Sampson, A. W., and H. E. Malmsten. 1942. Stock-poisoning plants of California. Univ. of California College Agric. Exp. Sta., Berkeley, Bull. 593.

Schwartz, W. L., W. W. Bay, J. W. Dollahite, R. W. Storts, and G. Russell. 1974. Toxicity of *Nerium oleander* in the monkey, *Cebus apella*. Vet. Pathol. 11:259–277.

Seger, C. L., J. D. Newson, E. E. Roth, and W. R. Hutchinson, Jr. 1969. Chronic toxic hepatitis in deer from a Louisiana coastal marsh. Bull. Wildl. Dis. Assoc. 5:295–296.

Seneviratna, P. 1969. Diseases of poultry including cage birds. John Wright and Sons, Ltd., Bristol.

Shone, D. K., and R. B. Drummond. 1965. Poisonous plants of Rhodesia. Rhod. Agric. J. 62:1–64.

Sixteen plants poisonous to livestock in the western states. 1958. USDA, Farmers Bull. No. 2106.

Smit, J. D. 1950. S. Afr. Indust. Chem. 4:66. As cited by J. M. Watt and M. G. Breyer-Brandwijk. The medicinal and poisonous plants of Southern and Eastern Africa. E. S. Livingstone, Ltd., Edinburgh.

Vail, E. L. 1942. Woolly-pod or broad-leafed milkweed, *Asclepias eriocarpa*, poisoning of rabbits. N. Am. Vet. 23:539–542.

Watt, J. M., and M. G. Breyer-Brandwijk. 1962. The medicinal and poisonous plants of Southern and Eastern Africa. E. S. Livingstone, Ltd., Edinburg.

Welch, H., and H. E. Morris. 1952. Range plants poisonous to livestock in Montana. Montana State College Agric. Exp. Sta., Bozeman, Circ. 197.

West, E., and M. W. Emmel. 1952. Poisonous plants in Florida. Univ. of Florida Agric. Exp. Sta., Gainesville, Bull. 510.

3 *Lead Poisoning of Waterfowl*

DANIEL O. TRAINER

LEAD POISONING, or plumbism, has been recognized as a morbidity and mortality factor of man and domestic animals for centuries. It has been theorized that the Roman civilization deteriorated largely as a result of lead poisoning in the ruling class; lead was used for manufacturing cooking utensils of the wealthy and in lead pipes for their plumbing systems.

Lead poisoning is a major ecologic factor affecting wild waterfowl populations of North America, and it is a significant mortality factor of waterfowl in all of the major flyways. The disease is caused by the ingestion of spent lead pellets that localize in the gizzard, where they are abraded and the lead is absorbed by the bird.

For more than a century, lead poisoning has been documented as a cause of death among wild avian populations in North America. In 1874, a die-off of waterfowl due to lead poisoning occurred in Texas (Phillips and Lincoln, 1930). Since that epornitic, there have been reports of this malady in waterfowl from all of the major continental flyways: the Pacific Flyway (Bowles, 1908), the Central Flyway (Mohler, 1945), the Atlantic Flyway (Grinnell, 1901), and the Mississippi Flyway (Shillinger and Cottam, 1937). An excellent comprehensive review of lead poisoning as a cause of mortality in waterfowl populations of North America was published by Bellrose in 1959.

Not only has lead poisoning been reported for many years from various parts of North America, it has also affected every major species of waterfowl in North America at one time or another (Bellrose, 1959). Dabbling ducks, especially the mallard, *Anas platyrhynchos,* and pintail, *A. acuta,* have been the major victims although populations of diving ducks, geese, and swans have also suffered significant mortality. The magnitude of losses during lead poisoning die-offs varies greatly, with some epornitics involving hundreds and even thousands of birds. A summary of the numbers and kinds of waterfowl that have succumbed to lead poisoning prior to 1959 is presented by Bellrose (1959).

More than 50 years ago, Dr. E. L. O'Roke of the University of Michigan described the significance of lead poisoning to waterfowl (Pirnie, 1935). He stated, "Considering the enormous quantity of lead that there must be in the vicinity of blinds that have been shot over for decades, it is reasonable to conclude that the potential danger of lead poisoning is great and should be considered in any waterfowl [management] program. In this writer's opinion, lead poisoning is a disease which takes the greatest toll of adult ducks in this section of the country."

Lead poisoning of waterfowl is most common in North America, but it also occurs in other parts of the world, such as New Zealand (Wisely and Miers, 1956) and Great Britain (Beer and Stanley, 1965). It has also been reported as a serious problem in captive animals (Bazell, 1971; Zook et al., 1972). In captive populations both birds and mammals can be involved, and the cause is not usually lead pellets but a variety of other sources, including putty, paint, and atmospheric lead pollution.

Using mortality surveys as well as fluoroscopy and gizzard studies, Bellrose (1959) estimated that one-quarter of the mallard population in North America carried lead pellets in their gizzards and were potential lead poisoning victims. It was also estimated that 4% of the mallard population of North America, 700,000 birds, were lost annually. This number exceeds the total hunting season harvest for many states. Bellrose (1959), Peterburs (1974), and others further extrapolated that lead poisoning annually claimed 2 to 3% of the total fall waterfowl population, or 2 to 3 million birds. Precise data on the annual mortality due to lead poisoning are lacking, but available information is sufficient to conclude that losses are significant and serious. Sublethal levels of lead have altered behavior, reproduction success, and disease susceptibility in mammals, but limited experimental studies in waterfowl have produced inconclusive results. Therefore, the sublethal effects of lead in waterfowl remain speculative at this time.

Lead poisoning in wildlife is not limited to waterfowl; there have been reports of lead poisoning in a variety of wild birds, including the pheasant, *Phasianus colchicus;* mourning dove, *Zenaidura macroura;* bobwhite quail, *Colinis virginianus;* and birds of prey. Small numbers of birds were involved, and lead poisoning was not considered a major cause of death in these species (Benson et al. 1974; Hunter and Rosen, 1965; Locke and Bagley, 1967; Westemier, 1965).

Consumption of flesh from waterfowl with lead poisoning does not constitute a hazard to human health. Many epornitics occur during the hunting season, yet there are no documented cases of lead poisoning in hunters. Transmission studies in experimental animals and the chemical analysis of tissues from intoxicated birds indicate that the flesh of lead-poisoned ducks does not constitute a hazard to humans (Jordan and Bellrose, 1951).

ETIOLOGY. The causative agents of lead poisoning are spent lead pellets, and the severity of the toxicity is related to the number of pellets ingested. Ingested pellets pass to the gizzard where they are retained and abraded by gizzard action. The adaptation of the avian digestive tract to use small stones or other small solid objects for grinding food makes the gizzard an unfortunate repository for lead pellets.

The toxicity of ingested pellets is due to the lead fraction in the pellet alloy. Gizzard action and abrasion of pellets result in absorption and circulation of complex lead compounds in the blood (Chisolm, 1971). During a "normal" daily intake of lead, approximately 90% passes through the intestinal tract and is not absorbed. The small amounts of absorbed lead are excreted via the urogenital tract and there is no net retention of lead in the body. When abnormal levels of lead are absorbed, the rate of absorption may exceed the rate at which lead can be excreted and the lead is concentrated and stored in bones. As the level of lead intake increases, the amount storable in bones is exceeded and levels of lead in the soft tissues increase. Chemical analysis of soft tissues can be used for diagnosis, and the greatest concentrations of lead occur in the liver where values in toxic birds can be 40 times those of normal birds (Coburn et al., 1951).

EPIZOOTIOLOGY. Lead is a ubiquitous element and a natural constituent of soil, water, vegetation, animal life, and air. Common sources of lead poisoning in domestic and human populations include lead pigments in paints, putty, earthenware pottery, industrial pollution, and gasoline exhaust.

As noted previously, the source of lead for intoxication of wild avian species, especially waterfowl, is the ingestion of spent lead pellets that have missed their target and settled on the bottom of ponds, rivers, and lakes. Because of the concentrated nature of waterfowl hunting, as well as some of the feeding characteristics of waterfowl, birds ingest these pellets while feeding or obtaining grit. The pellets localize in the gizzard where they are abraded by gizzard action and the lead is absorbed via the intestinal tract. Lead absorption from pellets embedded in muscle of wounded birds is minimal and does not result in intoxication (Machle, 1940).

Factors Affecting Accessibility of Lead Pellets. Lead poisoning of waterfowl is usually a seasonal malady, and mortality is prominent during migration in spring and fall when large numbers of birds are concentrated in heavily hunted waterfowl areas. Peak mortality occurs in late fall. In the Midwest, where lead toxity is most common, a number of ecologic factors are involved. Accumulations of lead pellets occur in heavily hunted areas. For concentrations of lead pellets to be accessible to birds, a firm bottom is necessary. In many well-known waterfowl areas, the bottom is soft and muddy; lead pellets deposited in these areas sink into the mud and are not accessible to birds. A solid-surfaced bottom of sand, gravel, or other solid substance is essential for the retention of pellets. These "solid bottoms" are often found where springs or flowing streams exist. In late fall, with the advent of freezing temperatures, ice forms and covers much waterfowl habitat, making it unavailable to birds. Areas that do not freeze or freeze last are usually those with flowing water or springs. This situation, combined with a solid bottom, makes these sites prime areas for waterfowl concentrations, available lead pellet concentrations, and lead poisoning. During spring, a similar situation develops, since the first sites that are free of ice are those with moving water. The first migratory birds to arrive utilize these areas and the opportunity for exposure to lead pellets exists.

Another factor that affects waterfowl accessibility to lead pellets is the depth of the water. Water levels affect waterfowl distribution and concentrations. Low water levels tend to concentrate birds into limited areas as well as expose lead pellets and make those that normally would be covered by deep water accessible to the birds. Water depth is especially important to dabbling species because of their feeding behavior and the limitations of feeding in water less than 15 inches deep. When water depths are two feet or more, most birds cannot reach the bottom to feed; therefore, pellets are inaccessible to them. Lead poisoning die-offs can be and have been predicted by utilizing data on water levels and depths, temperatures, migration, and waterfowl concentrations.

It was first documented by Jordan and Bellrose (1951) that diet played an important role in gizzard action, lead abrasion, and absorption. The physical rather than the nutritional form of the diet influences the severity of the intoxication. A solid food, such as whole corn, results in extensive gizzard action, which in turn results in maximum lead pellet abrasion and toxicity. At the other extreme, a soft food, such as leafy aquatic plants, for example, duck weed, coontail, pondweed, or commercial duck pellets, results in limited gizzard activity, lead pellet abrasion, and toxicity.

The number of pellets required to produce morbidity and mortality in waterfowl varies among individual birds, as well as with the size, species, sex, and age of the bird and its diet. Olney (1960) concluded that 60 to 80% of adult wild mallards with one pellet were likely to succumb if they were on a diet of wild seeds. Jordan and Bellrose (1951) reported that one or two lead pellets (No. 6 shot) were sufficient to cause lead poisoning in more than half of the mallards fed a whole corn or seed diet. If, however, the diet was composed of soft leafy plants, five or six pellets were needed to produce morbidity. Similar results were recorded for Canada geese, *Branta canadensis.* Four or five pellets of No. 4 lead shot were sufficient to kill a Canada goose on a whole corn diet; however, if the bird was on a commercial soft mash diet, more than 20 lead pellets were needed to produce intoxication (Cook and Trainer, 1966).

The number of pellets detected in gizzards of birds that died of lead poisoning varies considerably. During a Canada goose die-off involving more than 400 birds, the number of lead pellets detected in gizzards ranged from 9 to 110 per goose, with an average of 13 pellets per bird (Trainer and Hunt, 1965). More than 50 lead pellets per gizzard, range 0 to 201, were detected in 200 whistling swans, *Olor columbianus,* during an epornitic (Trainer and Hunt, 1965). Similar variation has been reported for ducks dying of lead poisoning, and as many as 200 lead pellets have been detected in a single bird.

Factors Affecting Ingestion of Lead Pellets. Why birds ingest lead pellets is not understood. Some theorize that the ingestion of lead pellets by waterfowl is accidental and that birds accidentally ingest pellets with food material. Others feel that lead pellets resemble certain aquatic seeds and that they are ingested deliberately by birds. Both explanations are valid; birds pick up pellets both accidentally and intentionally. Isolated cases of lead poisoning involving small numbers of pellets are probably the result of accidental ingestion, but during epornitics when large numbers of pellets (sometimes in the hundreds) are detected in the gizzards of birds, the pellets are ingested as seeds. Thus, the type of aquatic vegetation in the area becomes another important factor in the epizootiology of this malady.

To illustrate the potential for lead pellet accumulation, one only needs to consider the art of waterfowl hunting. It takes an average of five shots per hunter to kill a duck. The average duck hunter uses No. 6 shot in a 12-gauge gun, and each shell contains approximately 280 pellets; if six ducks are harvested per acre, there are 8,400 pellets deposited per acre per year. This is an average, and pellets actually accumulate more in areas of intensive hunting; therefore, the potential concentration of pellets deposited annually in popular hunting areas is obvious. In 1949, a survey to determine lead pellet concentration in prime waterfowl hunting areas of North America was conducted. Lake Puckaway in Central Wisconsin was the most heavily lead-laden site, and more than 25 years ago 118,048 pellets per acre were detected in this popular hunting area (Bellrose, 1959). The National Wildlife Federation estimates that 30 billion lead pellets, or more than 3,000 tons of spent pellets, are deposited annually by waterfowl hunters. Fortunately, much of this lead falls in sites where it is unavailable to waterfowl.

In addition to lead pellet detection in the gizzards of dead birds, live "normal" birds carry lead pellets. In Illinois, 5,000 ducks were examined by fluoroscopy and 10% of these birds had lead pellets in their gizzards (Bellrose, 1959). Two-thirds of the lead-carrying birds had only one pellet. As part of a food habits study, more than 36,000 waterfowl gizzards were examined and 5.3% contained lead pellets. Again, two-thirds of the gizzards contained a single pellet. Gizzards sampled during the fall had the highest percentage of pellets present. This correlated with the seasonal prevalence of lead poisoning and suggests that most pellets deposited during the fall hunting season are not available to birds the following spring.

SIGNS. Clinical signs of lead poisoning in waterfowl vary with the species involved and the amount of lead absorbed (Cook and Trainer, 1966; Jordan and Bellrose, 1951). The rapid erosion and absorption of large amounts of lead result in acute intoxication, and birds often succumb displaying few or no signs of disease. The number and severity of signs increase as the duration of the disease increases. Classical signs of lead poisoning are depicted in chronic intoxication.

Classical signs of lead poisoning usually occur in the following sequence: anorexia and lethargy, diarrhea with greenish staining of feathers in the vent region, muscular weakness characterized by

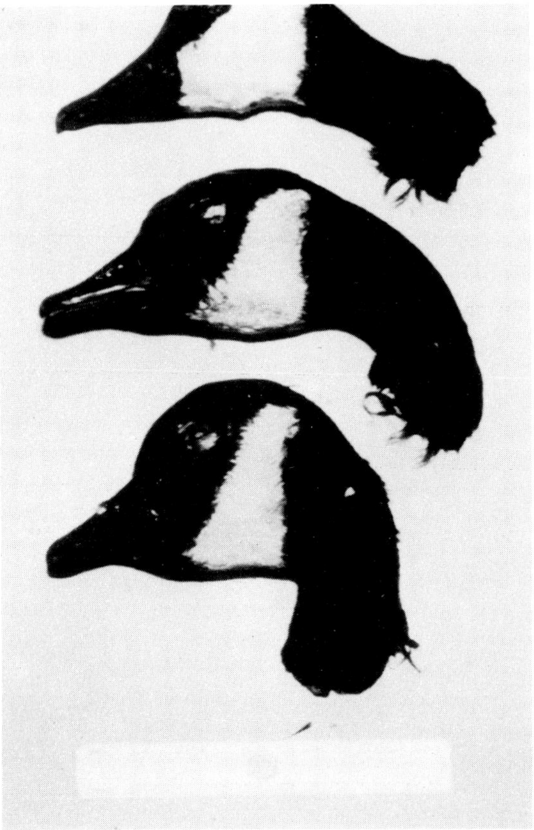

Fig. 3.1. Cephalic edema in Canada geese, *Branta canadensis:* the top specimen is normal, the middle specimen is moderate, and the bottom specimen is a severe case.

a "roof-shaped" position of the wings as they are held over the back and later a "wing drop" with wings extended downward, a marked cephalic edema with submandibular swellings (Fig. 3.1), emaciation, and flaccid paralysis. Experimentally, the first signs of disease occur two days after ingesting lead pellets. Depending on dosage, death can occur from 10 to as long as 72 days after exposure. There is a progressive loss of weight in birds with lead intoxication which resembles malnutrition. Birds absorbing a large amount of lead die rapidly with few signs and do not lose weight. Birds absorbing small amounts of lead have more extensive signs and lose 30 to 40% of their normal weight.

PATHOLOGY. The pathology of lead poisoning varies with the species involved, the level of lead consumed, the duration and extent of intoxication, and environmental factors such as diet.

Gross lesions of lead poisoning are similar to those produced by malnutrition (Jordan and Bellrose, 1951). Paralytic effects on gizzard muscles result in low food intake that contributes to this syndrome and the resulting pathology. Lesions are usually more prevalent and severe in chronic cases than they are in acute cases. Clemens et al. (1975) report a highly significant correlation between anorexia and loss of weight in experimental mallards with lead intoxication, but they also found that loss in body weight was due to the direct toxic effect of destruction on pectoral muscle.

Lesions of lead poisoning are similar in wild and experimental birds. These include emaciation; lack of fat deposits; muscular atrophy or razor keel; reduction of major flight muscles and flaccid muscle tissue; gallbladder distended to five times normal; impacted proventriculus (Fig. 3.2); greenish-brown, brittle horny pads of an atrophied gizzard; abraded lead pellets of various sizes and shapes in the gizzard (Fig. 3.3); enteritis; atrophied liver; flaccid heart; cephalic edema; edematous and enlarged salt glands; anemia and paleness of the entire body.

Histopathological findings in waterfowl vary with the degree of toxicity but often include the following:

Liver: Necrosis; congestion; large quantities of brownish, iron-containing pigment in the hepatic and Kupffer cells; varying degrees of edema and hepatic degeneration.
Kidney: Nephritis consisting of necrosis, and sloughing of tubular epithelium and brownish pigment in tubular epithelium cells; acid-fast intranuclear inclusion bodies in cells of the proximal convoluted tubules.
Heart: Patchy necrosis associated with hyaline or fibrinoid necrosis of blood vessel walls.
Lungs: Congestion and hemorrhage.
Brain: Edema in the Virchow-Robin spaces; edema of the meninges.
Gizzard: Patchy necrosis of muscle.
Pancreas: Irregular necrosis of acinar and islet tissues.
Blood: Anemia; erythrocyte changes, including anisocytosis, poikilocytosis, and a reduction in the number of erythrocytes.

All of these lesions are not detected in every case of lead poisoning, but they are often present in varying degrees in many cases; for more detailed descriptions of the pathology of lead poisoning consult Clemens et al. (1975), Coburn et al. (1951), Cook and Trainer (1966), Irwin and Karstad (1972), and March et al. (1976).

Microscopic lesions vary with the species; for example, in some ducks anemia and basophilic

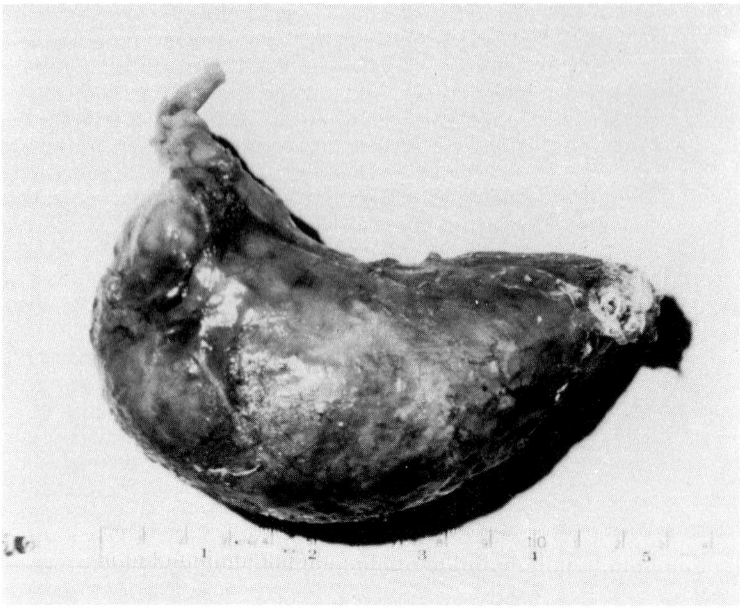

Fig. 3.2. A Canada goose, *B. canadensis*, proventriculus (esophagus) impacted with food.

stippling occur (Johns, 1934); these do not occur in the Canada goose (Cook and Trainer, 1966). Acid-fast inclusion bodies are common in kidney tubules of mallards but not in Canada geese (Locke et al., 1967).

DIAGNOSIS. A number of factors must be considered in order to make a diagnosis of lead poisoning in waterfowl. If a number of emaciated waterfowl with green diarrhea and edematous heads die during the fall or early winter in a heavily hunted area, lead poisoning should be suspected. The presence of eroded lead pellets in the gizzard, plus characteristic pathologic findings such as the presence of acid-fast intranuclear in-

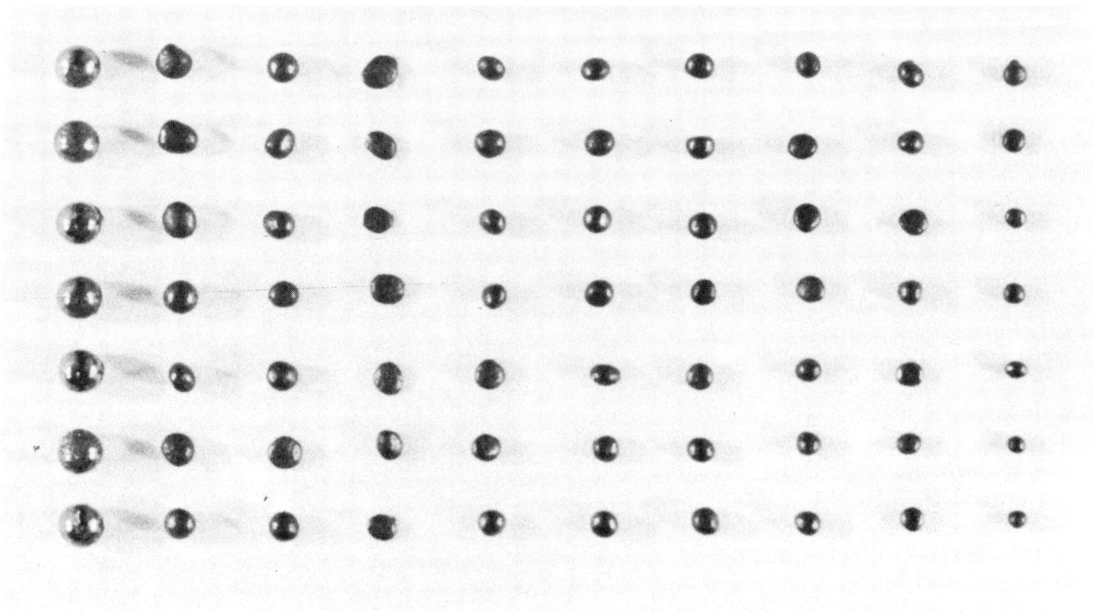

Fig. 3.3. Abraded lead pellets of various sizes and shapes from the gizzard of a lead-poisoned Canada goose, *B. canadensis*.

clusion bodies, would result in a tentative diagnosis of lead poisoning. A definite diagnosis depends on chemical analysis and confirmation of toxic lead levels.

Diagnostic lead levels vary between species and with the chemical test used. Liver or blood are the best tissues to use for chemical determinations. Lead levels in the liver, which are diagnostic in the Canada goose, range from 5 to 32 ppm (Cook and Trainer, 1966); in whistling swans, 18 to 37 ppm (Chupp and Dalke, 1964); and in mallards, 12 to 36 ppm (Coburn et al., 1951). Normal and toxic lead levels in blood have been determined for a variety of waterfowl (Clemens et al., 1975; Cook and Trainer, 1966; Irwin and Karstad, 1972; Trainer and Hunt, 1965).

Since lead is stored in the bones of birds, bones have been used as indicators of lead exposure. Interpreting the significance of lead levels in bone is difficult since the lead is "stored" in bone. Also, because of the time involved, it is impossible to determine the source of lead exposure. Bagley and Locke (1967) reported tremendous variation in "normal" baseline lead levels for a variety of avian species, further illustrating the difficulty of basing a diagnosis on any single factor, even lead levels.

If live birds are available for examination, the fluorescent erythrocyte test for lead poisoning can be used (Barrett and Karstad, 1971). This rapid simple test provides a reliable diagnostic method for lead intoxication.

Because of the ecological and chemical complexities associated with lead poisonings, it is important when making a diagnosis to consider environmental conditions, case history, signs, lesions, and chemical analysis.

TREATMENT AND CONTROL. The treatment of small numbers of birds with lead poisoning is possible and often practical. Chelating agents, such as calcium versenate and calcium disodium ethylenediaminetetraacetate (EDTA) have proven to be effective therapeutic antidotes for lead poisoning in man and wildlife. Calcium versenate is a chemical compound that forms a complex with lead replacing the calcium to form lead versenate, a soluble compound that is excreted in the urine. Calcium versenate has been used successfully to treat lead poisoning in swans (Rosen and Bonkowski, 1960) and other waterfowl (Wobeser, 1969). Calcium EDTA significantly reduces the lead level in blood and soft tissues, but has little effect on lead in bones or pellets in the gizzard. If pellets are in the gizzard, lead is constantly absorbed into the blood system; therefore, for treatment to be effective, it is necessary to treat intoxicated birds daily with chelating agents. Treatment is more effective in acute than in chronic lead poisoning. Also, if a bird develops an impaction, treatment is not effective. Treatment is practical for birds in captivity or for small numbers of wild birds.

It is sometimes possible to flush and siphon lead pellets from the gizzard. This is a laborious and time-consuming task; it can work but is only practical for small numbers of birds. The feeding of large amounts of grit can also be helpful, since it will sometimes cause birds to expel lead pellets. Impaction of the proventriculus renders these treatments ineffective and useless.

The most practical approach to controlling lead poisoning in wild waterfowl is to prevent birds from using feeding and loafing sites with large accumulations of lead pellets. This can be done by utilizing conventional bird dispersement methods such as bomb-scare devices, harassment with aircraft, elimination of artificial feeding especially with whole corn, and the manipulation of water levels to make it difficult for birds to acquire lead pellets.

Other possible solutions to the lead poisoning problem include the harvesting and recycling of lead from areas that are heavily hunted. This has been undertaken on several occasions by hunting clubs where concentrations of lead were dense enough to make it economically feasible.

The most practical approach to this problem is the substitution of nontoxic shot (steel pellets) for lead pellets in shotgun shells used for waterfowl hunting. Beginning in 1976, the use of steel pellets for hunting ducks, geese, swans, and coots is being phased in by the various flyways according to a plan devised by the U.S. Department of Interior (USDI, 1976). These regulations are not universal in application, applying only to designated areas or states.

A serious debate concerning the merits of nontoxic shot has developed regarding nontoxic ballistics, effects on gun barrels, and killing ability. Recent studies indicate that nontoxic shot offers a reasonable solution to the problem of lead poisoning; requiring its use in known epornitic areas is recommended.

REFERENCES

Bagley, G. E., and L. N. Locke. 1967. The occurrence of lead in tissues of wild birds. Bull. Environ. Contam. Toxicol. 2:297–305.

Barrett, M. W., and L. H. Karstad. 1971. A fluorescent erythrocyte test for lead poisoning in waterfowl. J. Wildl. Manage. 35:109–119.

Bazell, R. J. 1971. Lead poisoning: Zoo animals may be the first victims. Science 173:130–131.

Beer, J. V., and P. Stanley. 1965. Lead poisoning in the Slimbridge wildfowl collection. Wildl. Trust Annu. Rep. 16:30–34.

Bellrose, F. C. 1959. Lead poisoning as a mortality factor in waterfowl populations. Illinois Natur. Hist. Surv. Bull. 27:235–288.

Benson, W. W., B. Pharaoh, and P. Miller. 1974. Lead poisoning in a bird of prey. Bull. Environ. Contam. Toxicol. 11:105–108.

Bowles, J. H. 1908. Lead poisoning in ducks. Auk 25:312–313.

Chisolm, J. J. 1971. Lead poisoning. Sci. Am. 224: 15–23.

Chupp, N. R., and P. D. Dalke. 1964. Waterfowl mortality in the Coeur d'Alene River Valley, Idaho. J. Wildl. Manage. 28:692–702.

Clemens, E. T., L. Krook, A. L. Aronson, and C. E. Stevens. 1975. Pathogenesis of lead shot in the mallard duck. Cornell Vet. 65:248–285.

Coburn, D. R., D. W. Metzler, and R. Treichler. 1951. A study of absorption and retention of lead in wild waterfowl in relation to clinical evidence of lead poisoning. J. Wildl. Manage. 15:186–192.

Cook, R. S., and D. O. Trainer. 1966. Experimental lead poisoning of Canada geese. J. Wildl. Manage. 30:1–8.

Grinnell, G. B. 1901. American duck shooting. Forest and Stream Publishing Co., New York.

Hunter, B. F., and M. N. Rosen. 1965. Occurrence of lead in a wild pheasant, *Phasianus colchicus*. Calif. Fish Game 51:207.

Irwin, J. C., and L. H. Karstad. 1972. The toxicity for ducks of disintegrated lead shot in a simulated marsh environment. J. Wildl. Dis. 8:149–154.

Johns, F. M. 1934. A study of punctate stippling as found in the lead poisoning of wild ducks. J. Lab. Clin. Med. 19:514–517.

Jordan, J. S., and F. C. Bellrose. 1951. Lead poisoning in wild waterfowl. Illinois Natur. Hist. Surv. Biol. Notes 26:1–27.

Locke, L. N., and G. E. Bagley. 1967. Lead poisoning in a sample of Maryland mourning doves. J. Wildl. Mange. 31:515–518.

______., G. E. Bagley, and L. T. Young. 1967. The ineffectiveness of acid-fast inclusions in diagnosis of lead poisoning in Canada geese. Bull. Wildl. Dis. Assoc. 3:176.

Machle, W. 1940. Lead absorption from bullets lodged in the tissues: Report of two cases. J. Am. Med. Assoc. 115:1536–1541.

March, G. L., T. M. John, B. A. McKeown, L. Sileo, and J. C. George. 1976. The effects of lead poisoning on various plasma constituents in the Canada goose. J. Wildl. Dis. 12:14–19.

Mohler, J. 1945. Lead poisoning of geese near Lincoln. Neb. Bird Rev. 13:49–50.

Olney, P. J. S. 1960. Lead poisoning in wildfowl. Wildl. Trust Annu. Rep. 11:123–134.

Peterburs, W. B. 1974. A duck hunter speaks out on lead poisoning. Natl. Parks Conserv. Mag. 48: 22–25.

Phillips, J. C., and F. C. Lincoln. 1930. American waterfowl: Their present situation and the outlook for their future. Houghton Mifflin, Boston and New York.

Pirnie, M. D. 1935. Michigan waterfowl management. Michigan Dept. Conserv.

Rosen, M. N., and R. A. Bonkowski. 1960. A diagnostic technic and treatment for lead poisoning in swans. Calif. Fish Game 46:81–90.

Shillinger, J. E., and C. C. Cottam. 1937. The importance of lead poisoning in waterfowl. Trans. N. Am. Wildl. Natur. Res. Conf. 2:398–403.

Trainer, D. O., and R. A. Hunt. 1965. Lead poisoning of waterfowl in Wisconsin. J. Wildl. Manage. 29: 95–103.

United States Department of Interior. 1976. Final environmental statement—Proposed use of steel shot for hunting waterfowl in the United States. U.S. Dept. of Interior, Fish and Wildlife Serv., Washington D.C.

Westemeier, R. L. 1965. Apparent lead poisoning in a wild bobwhite. Wilson Bull. 78:471–472.

Wisely, B., and K. H. Miers. 1956. Lead poisoning in New Zealand waterfowl. NZ Wildl. Publ. 41:1–11.

Wobeser, G. 1969. Apparent favorable response of lead poisoning in a duck to treatment with a chelating agent. Bull. Wildl. Dis. Assoc. 5:120.

Zook, B. C., R. M. Sauer, and F. M. Garner. 1972. Lead poisoning in captive wild animals. J. Wildl. Dis. 8:264–272.

4 Polychlorinated Biphenyl (PCB) Compounds

JOSEPH G. ZINKL

POLYCHLORINATED BIPHENYL (PCB) compounds have many industrial uses. In addition, they have become widespread environmental contaminants as a result of leaks in containers, disposal of materials containing them, and accidental spillages. They are extremely fat-soluble but poorly water-soluble; thus, they concentrate in the fats of animals that ingest them and are concentrated in the animals at the top of the food chains.

ETIOLOGY. PCB compounds consist of a biphenyl nucleus to which varying numbers (1–10) of chlorine atoms are attached (Fig. 4.1). Commercial PCB compounds are mixtures of chlorinated biphenyl isomers and are marketed according to their chlorine content. The Aroclor compounds (Monsanto Corp.) are designated with the prefix 10 or 12 and a two-number suffix indicating their chlorine content. For example, Aroclor 1254 is a PCB mixture containing 54% chlorine. Other compounds have similar number designations to indicate their chlorine content. The most commonly used PCB compounds contain 42 to 54% chlorine (Nisbet and Sarofim, 1972).

Polychlorinated biphenyl compounds are chemically inert; resistant to chemical and heat degradation; and have low volatility, high dielectric constant, and high boiling point. Consequently, they are or have been used as insulators in capacitors and transformers; as fluids for heat transfer systems, hydraulic systems, gas turbines, and vacuum pumps; as fire retardants; as plasticizers; and in other products whose quality they have improved (Lloyd et al., 1976).

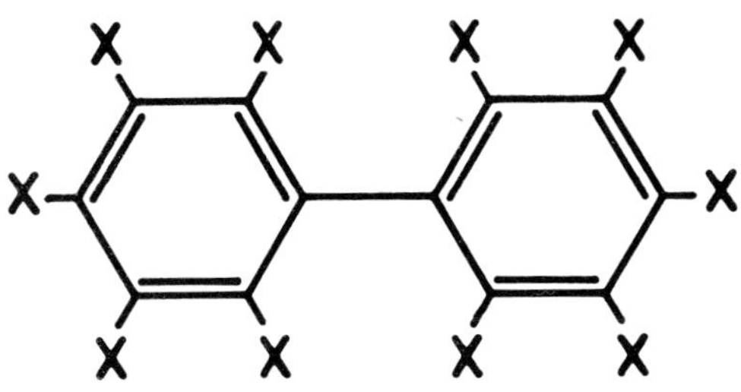

Fig. 4.1. A chlorinated biphenyl molecule is formed when each of the ten Xs represents either a hydrogen or chlorine atom. Commercial PCB compounds are mixtures of the 209 different isomers that can be formed.

EPIZOOTIOLOGY. PCB compounds contaminate the environment when they leak from sealed containers, are accidentally spilled, and are lost during the manufacture and disposal of products containing them or by vaporization and leaching from these products. They are spread through the environment by air, river, and ocean currents. In aquatic systems, PCB compounds can be widely dispersed from the source of pollution and are found in the water, sediments, fauna, and flora.

Like chlorinated hydrocarbon insecticides, PCB concentration in animals undergoes magnification through food chains. This causes the summit predators and scavengers, especially those associated with aquatic food chains, to have the highest PCB concentrations. Very high concentrations, up to 40 ppm, have been detected in the large predatory fish of the Great Lakes (Veith, 1975), the Hudson River (Nadeau and Davis, 1976), the Gulf of St. Lawrence (Pearce et al., 1973), and the Baltic Sea (Koeman et al., 1969). Herring gulls, *Larus argentatus;* herons, *Ardea cinerea;* and various species of cormorants have high PCB concentrations (Fox et al., 1975; Gress et al., 1973; Koeman et al., 1973; Prestt et al., 1970). Pelagic birds often have high PCB residue levels (Bourne and Bogan, 1972), as do raptors that feed on fish or other birds (Cromartie et al., 1975; Wiemeyer et al., 1975). Marine mammals, such as harbor seals, *Phoca vitulina;* ringed seals, *Pusa hispida;* sea lions, *Zalophus californianus;* and bottlenose dolphins, *Tursiopa truncatus,* have been found to contain moderate to high PCB concentrations (Addison and Smith, 1974; Anas, 1974; DeLong et al., 1973; Koeman et al., 1973). Polar bears, *Thalarctos maritimus,* have high PCB levels (Clausen et al., 1974).

In general, PCB concentrations in invertebrates are low and often not detectable. Several species of shrimp, however, have been found to contain up to 14 ppm of PCB compounds (Nimmo et al., 1971; Reimold, 1975). Also, in 1977, the Massachusetts Public Health Commission banned lobster fishing in the vicinity of New Bedford harbor because of high PCB contamination in the shellfish.

PATHOGENESIS. Environmental concentrations of PCB compounds are so low that acute poisoning is unlikely except in locations where an accidental spill occurs. Similarly, chronic exposure to these compounds is unlikely to cause extensive mortalities except in extremely susceptible species such as mink. Summit predators and scavengers, especially those associated with aquatic food chains, are most likely to be exposed to PCB concentrations of such magnitude that they may become chronically affected.

Toxicity of PCB compounds depends on the species, the percentage of chlorination of the PCB, and the route of exposure. Within 20 days after exposure to 5 ppb Aroclor 1254 in flowing sea water, 72% of juvenile pink shrimp, *Pinacus durorarum,* had died (Duke et al., 1970). Complete inhibition of oyster, *Crassostrea virginica,* shell growth occurred at exposure to 100 ppb Aroclor 1254, while lower concentrations of 10 ppb and 1 ppb caused 41% and 18% inhibition, respectively (Duke et al., 1970). For the scud, *Gammarus oceanicus,* mortality occurred at exposure levels of 1 to 10 ppb Aroclor 1254 (Wildish, 1970). Five ppb Aroclor 1254 caused mortality to pinfish, *Lagedon rhomboides,* and spot, *Lurostomus xantharus,* in 12 and 18 days, respectively (Hansen et al., 1971). Cutthroat trout, *Salmo clarki,* had a 96-hour LC_{50} with Aroclor 1221 of 1.17 ppm, while with Aroclor 1254 an exposure to 42.5 ppm was required to achieve a 96-hour LC_{50} (Stallings and Mayer, 1972).

Birds are most susceptible to PCB compounds of the mid-chlorination range (42 to 54%). The 5-day LC_{50} of Aroclor 1254 to bobwhite quail, *Colinis virginianus,* was 604 ppm. However, at the same exposure level pheasants, *Phasianus colchicus;* mallard ducks, *Anas platyrhynchos;* and Japanese quail, *Coturnix coturnix japonica,* were only one-third to one-half as sensitive (Heath et al., 1972; Hill et al., 1975). Acute oral LD_{50} of Aroclors 1242, 1254, 1260, and 1268 for 10-month-old male mallard ducks were greater than 2,000 mg/kg (Tucker and Crabtree, 1970). Tests with four species of blackbirds indicated that PCB compounds were about as toxic as DDE (toxicity of DDE was unspecified) (Dustman et al., 1971).

Among mammals, mink and monkeys are quite susceptible to PCB compounds. Mink, *Mustela vison,* died after being fed for 105 days with beef containing 3.54 ppm of PCB (Platonow and Karstad, 1973). Toxicity apears to be greater for mink when PCB-contaminated fish is fed than when an equal amount of PCB is added directly to the feed (Ringer et al., 1972). Rhesus monkeys, *Macaca mulatta,* after being fed 25 ppm Aroclor 1254 developed toxic signs (Allen, 1975). In contrast to mink and monkeys, only 50% of the rats, *Rattus norvegicus,* fed a ration containing 1,000 ppm of PCB compound for 8 months died (Kimbrough et al., 1972). Acute oral toxicities for most PCB mixtures administered to rats have been greater than 1 to 2 gm/kg (Grant and Phillips, 1974).

Reproduction. Polychlorinated biphenyl compounds are more likely to affect reproduction than cause direct mortality. Studies indicate that these compounds can adversely affect avian reproduction (Ax and Hansen, 1975; Call and Harrell, 1974; Dahlgren and Linder, 1971; Peakall and Peakall, 1973). The major effects are decreased production and hatchability of eggs and abnormal breeding behavior. The reduction in hatchability is not due to decreased fertility but rather to embryonic mortality during the last part of incubation (Briggs and Harris, 1973). Concentrations in the eggs in most of these experimental studies were 5 to 15 ppm. Concentrations of this magnitude have been found in eggs of wild birds (Blus et al., 1974; Risebrough et al., 1968; Ryder, 1974).

Embryonic mortality, cracked egg shells, and high mortality among newly hatched herring gulls of the Great Lakes may be due, in part, to PCB compounds (Gilman et al., 1977). Adult gulls of these areas are less tenacious in defending nest sites than gulls in less contaminated areas. In addition to PCB compounds there are many other chlorinated compounds in the waters of the Great Lakes, and perhaps interactions among contaminants are the cause of the poor reproductive success of the herring gulls.

Hays and Risebrough (1972) found roseate tern, *Sterna dougallii,* and common tern, *S. hirundo,* embryos and chicks from islands of Long Island Sound with feathering abnormalities, and bill and foot deformities. Concentrations in breast muscle ranged from 4.9 to 140 ppm, and fish taken from adults returning to the nesting areas had up to 3.2 ppm PCB concentrations. Experimentally, leg, toe, and bill deformities have been found in newly hatched domestic chickens, *Gallus gallus,* exposed to PCB compounds while in the egg (Tumasonis et al., 1973).

Peakall and Peakall (1973) considered the effects of environmental contaminants on avian reproduction to fall under three headings: 1) effects on the eggshell, 2) effects on the embryo, and 3) effects on parental behavior. To this list can be added the effects upon the newly hatched chick. Polychlorinated biphenyl compounds probably do not affect the quality of the eggshell (Peakall, 1975). The major influences of these compounds on wild birds are probably embryonic mortality and decreased hatchability. Possibly, PCB compounds also cause parents to be less tenacious at the nest by decreasing their nest attentiveness and by the destruction of eggs of normal shell thickness. Poisoning of young birds by PCB compounds in their food could occur. It is likely that very young chicks are more susceptible than adults, because their body fat is insufficient to store the lipid-soluble PCB compounds.

Among mammals, mink reproduction is suppressed when they are fed a diet containing only 0.64 ppm of PCB (Platonow and Karstad, 1973). Diets containing 30% Lake Michigan coho salmon, *Oncorhynchus kisutch,* which themselves contain PCB compounds caused reproductive failure in mink (Aulerich et al., 1973). Infant rhesus monkeys whose mothers had eaten a diet containing 0.5 and 5.0 ppm Aroclor 1248 throughout gestation and lactation experienced PCB poisoning (Carstens et al., 1977). White-footed mice, *Peromyscus leucopus,* after being fed 200 ppm of Aroclor 1254, experienced adult mortality, decreased numbers of litters, and decreased survival of newborn (Merson and Kirkpatrick, 1976). Litter size, however, was not affected. The PCB compounds could interfere with mammalian reproduction by affecting parental behavior both before breeding and during the neonatal period by reducing the function of the reproductive organs and by altering the responses of the neonates.

Interactions with Other Agents. Interactions between PCB compounds and other agents, chemical or infectious, may intensify the disease-producing capacity in wildlife species. The PCB concentrations in environmental samples often are positively correlated with concentrations of other chlorinated hydrocarbons. Stickel (1975) suggested that interactions among chlorinated hydrocarbons are additive rather than synergistic. It is possible that interactions between PCB compounds and other contaminants, such as DDE and dieldrin, could have effects on an animal that the individual compounds themselves would not.

Interaction of PCB compounds with a disease agent, duck hepatitis virus, was demonstrated by Friend and Trainer (1970). Mallard ducklings were fed Aroclor 1254 for ten days, followed by PCB-free feed for five days. These ducklings were more susceptible to the virus than control ducklings fed a PCB-free diet. A similar interaction may occur in abortions among California sea lions. San Miguel sea lion virus has been isolated from aborting females (Gilmartin et al., 1976). These animals and their aborted pups also have been found to contain higher concentrations of PCB compounds and DDT metabolites in their livers and blubber than normal animals (DeLong et al., 1973). It has been suggested that PCB compounds may increase susceptibility to infectious diseases by suppressing the immune system (Koller and Thigpen, 1973).

Stress and PCB Mobilization. Stress may cause PCB mobilization in contaminated animals and perhaps cause detrimental effects (Dahlgren et al., 1972; Stendell, 1975). Migration, molting, and a temporary decrease in food supply could cause PCB mobilization. The PCB compounds were mobilized to the livers of rats that were starved after having eaten a PCB diet for 20 weeks (Zinkl, unpublished). Cachectic cancer patients have been found to have higher serum PCB and DDE concentrations than nonpatients (Hesselberg and Scheer, 1974).

SIGNS. Animals acutely poisoned with PCB compounds have neurologic signs of tremors and convulsions preceding death (Stendell, 1975; Stickel, 1975). In subacute or chronic cases of PCB poisoning, weight loss, debilitation, edema, and signs of liver failure are seen. The signs associated with interactions of PCB compounds and other chemicals are likely diverse and depend on the nature and dosage of the chemicals. Interaction with infectious disease agents would likely manifest itself in signs of the disease rather than PCB toxicity. Certainly, interactions of these types should be considered in deaths among wild animals, although it would be extremely difficult to establish that an interaction has occurred.

PATHOLOGY. The most characteristic gross lesions in birds killed with PCB compounds are hydropericardium and edema. Ascites occurred in chickens fed 20 ppm Aroclor 1254 (Bayer and Bird, 1974), a level not much greater than that found in the diet of fish-eating birds from highly contaminated areas. Hydropericardium and edema have been found in herring gull chicks (Peakall, 1975). Since PCB compounds and other chlorinated hydrocarbons were present in the tissues, an interaction among contaminants might have occurred.

In both birds and mammals, PCB compounds cause atrophy of lymphatic tissue. The bursa of Fabricius and the spleen were atrophied in chicks fed PCB compounds (Flick et al., 1965; Vos and Koeman, 1970). Atrophy of the spleen, thymus, and lymph nodes occurs in mammals given these compounds (Allen, 1975; Kimbrough et al., 1972;

Vos, 1972). Lymphatic atrophy is probably the cause of the impaired ability of PCB-fed animals to produce antibodies.

Liver lesions are prominent in mammals and birds fed PCB compounds (Kimbrough et al., 1972; Koller and Zinkl, 1973; Vos, 1972). Grossly, the livers are enlarged, unusually firm, and light colored. The tissue may fluoresce under long-wave ultraviolet light as a result of increased porphyrin production (Goldstein et al., 1975; Vos and Koeman, 1970). Microscopically, necrosis, enlargement of cells, diffuse fibrosis, and bile duct proliferation are observed.

Skin lesions have been seen in monkeys, man, and rats that had eaten diets containing PCB compounds (Allen, 1975; Kikuchi and Masuda, 1976; Zinkl, 1977). Effects on the epidermal tissues in wild animals might also occur. Perhaps the feather abnormalities observed among terns of Long Island Sound (Hays and Risebrough, 1972) are due to dermal effects of PCB compounds.

DIAGNOSIS. The PCB compounds are detected by using a gas-liquid chromatograph (GLC) equipped with an electron capture detector. Lipid extracts that have been extracted into *n*-hexane and purified and concentrated by several additional procedures are injected into the GLC (White, 1976). Identification of environmental PCB compounds is accomplished by comparing retention times of major peaks with those of standards, usually commercial PCB compounds. Quantification of the PCB is accomplished by comparing the heights or areas of several major peaks with those of a standard PCB that has a similar chromatographic profile (Fishbein, 1972). Chromatographic profiles of environmental samples do not exactly resemble those of commercial PCB samples because the early, presumably less chlorinated peaks, are absent. Peak height ratios may also be altered. Most often, the profiles resemble those of the latter parts of Aroclor 1254, but samples with profiles similar to Aroclor 1242 and 1260 have been found (Fishbein, 1975; White, 1976).

Brain Tissue. In acutely poisoned animals, PCB concentration in brain tissue can be used for diagnosis. Residues of PCB compounds in the brains of blackbirds of several species given heavy doses of Aroclor 1254 were diagnostic (Stendell, 1975). Residues in the brains of birds that died varied from 349 to 763 ppm, while levels in the brains of birds that survived did not exceed 301 ppm. In studies with pheasants that had been administered 210 mg of Aroclor 1254 daily, residues of PCB in the brain tissue between 300 and 400 ppm generally indicated that death was due to PCB toxicosis (Dahlgren et al., 1972). Residue levels in very sensitive animals dying of PCB poisoning could be much lower than the above levels. For example, mink dying of PCB poisoning had residue levels in their brains of 11 ppm and 5 ppm (Aulerich et al., 1973; Platonow and Karstad, 1973). Some bald eagles, *Haliaeetus leucocephalus,* which had been found dead and had PCB residues in the brain of between 0.10 and 230 ppm, may have died from PCB toxicosis (Belisle et al., 1972; Cromartie et al., 1975).

Liver Tissue. Residue levels in liver tissue and in the entire body greater than 400 ppm are indicative of acute PCB poisoning (Koeman et al., 1973). Vos and Koeman (1970) found PCB concentrations as low as 120 ppm in the brains of chickens dying from PCB poisoning. The PCB concentrations were usually higher in the liver than in the brain. PCB may have been important in a die-off of common guillemots, *Uria aalge,* that occurred in the Irish Sea in 1969. The body burden of PCB in birds that died was about twice that in healthy birds that had been collected in the same area. Livers of birds that were shot and, presumably, were healthy contained only 0.9% the total body burden of PCB as compared to 22.5% for birds found dead. Residue levels in the brains were not determined (Parslow and Jefferies, 1973).

Age. In general, older animals have higher levels of PCB than younger animals (Bache et al., 1972; Bourne and Bogan, 1972; Veith, 1975). Adult females that have previously nursed young or laid eggs may have lower levels of PCB than males of the same age or females that have not lactated or laid eggs. This results from the excretion of part of the body burden through the lipids of milk or eggs (Clark et al., 1975; Dahlgren et al., 1971; Lincer and Peakall, 1973).

Many studies in birds have shown that reproduction is poor when PCB residues in eggs are between 5 and 15 ppm. Effects such as abnormal breeding behavior, decreased egg production, embryonic mortality, and reduced hatching success may occur when egg residues are at these levels (Peakall, 1975; Stendell, 1975; Stickel, 1975). Thus, PCB compounds should be considered responsible for decreased reproductive success when residue levels in eggs are about 10 ppm.

Species Susceptibility. Knowledge of species susceptibility to PCB compounds is necessary before the significance of residue concentrations in wild animals can be assessed. The extreme sensitivity of captive mink to these compounds suggests that wild mink and perhaps other mustelids may be threatened by PCB compounds. In addition, it is difficult if not impossible to determine what effect combinations of contaminants, such as PCB, DDT, DDD, DDE, dieldrin, aldrin, toxaphene, chloradane, hexachlorobenzene, hexachlorophene, polychlorinated terphenyls, chlorinated naphthalenes, chlorinated dibenzofurans, chlorinated dibenzodioxins, chlorinated phenols, and other contaminants might have on wildlife populations. Certainly, much more information concerning the individual and combined effects of these compounds is needed before the potential impact of PCB compounds on wildlife can be assessed.

TREATMENT, CONTROL, AND PREVENTION. In 1971, Monsanto Corporation restricted the sales of Aroclor products to closed-system uses only in an attempt to prevent further environmental contamination. In addition, Monsanto has produced PCB compounds, such as Aroclor 1016, which contain few of the higher-chlorinated isomers that are thought to be more toxic than the less-chlorinated isomers (Burse et al., 1974). Finally, in 1977, Monsanto ceased all production of these compounds (Anon., 1977). However, this suspension may be detrimental, since the Aroclor products contain fewer highly toxic contaminants, such as dibenzofurans, than do the foreign made PCB compounds (Vos and Koeman, 1970). Therefore, if foreign compounds are used to replace Aroclor products, continued environmental contamination by these and other agents may occur.

The use of nontoxic or less toxic substances to replace PCB compounds could further reduce environmental contamination. Continued search for products such as these has proved fruitful for some PCB uses. Perhaps complete replacement can be accomplished through further research.

Even with suspension of PCB sales and replacement with other substances, a large environmental burden of PCB compounds remains. The resistance of these compounds to degradation will result in their remaining in the environment for many years. Therefore, a problem will likely remain even if no additional environmental contamination occurs. Certainly, accidental leakage and spillage of PCB compounds into waterways must be avoided.

Treatment of birds poisoned by PCB is likely to be futile. Animals with a large amount of fat are probably less susceptible than thin animals. It might be possible to alternately starve and feed individual captive animals in order to decrease a high PCB burden in fat. Similarly, inducement of lactation or egg laying in females might be used to decrease body residues of PCB compounds.

REFERENCES

Addison, R. F., and T. G. Smith. 1974. Organochlorine residue levels in Arctic ringed seals. Variation with age and sex. Oikos. 25:335–337.

Allen, J. R. 1975. Response of the nonhuman primates to polychlorinated biphenyl exposure. Fed. Proc. 34:1675–1679.

Anas, R. E. 1974. DDT plus PCB's in blubber of harbor seals. Pestic. Monit. J. 8:12–14.

Anon. 1977. Untitled. Audubon Nov/Dec: 163.

Aulerich, R. J., R. K. Ringer, and S. Iwamoto. 1973. Reproductive failure and mortality in mink fed on Great Lakes fish. J. Reprod. Fertil. (Suppl.) 19:365–376.

Ax, R. L., and L. G. Hansen. 1975. Effects of purified polychlorinated biphenyl analogs on chicken reproduction. Poult. Sci. 54:895–900.

Bache, C. A., J. W. Serum, W. D. Young, and D. J. Lisk. 1972. Polychlorinated biphenyl residues: Accumulation in Cayuga Lake trout with age. Science 177:1191–1192.

Bayer, R. C., and F. H. Bird. 1974. Surface changes in the epicardium of chickens fed polychlorinated biphenyls. Poult. Sci. 53:737–741.

Belisle, A. A., W. L. Riechel, L. N. Locke, T. G. Lamont, B. M. Mulhern, R. M. Prouty, R. B. DeWolf, and E. Cromartie. 1972. Residue of organochlorine pesticides, polychlorinated biphenyls and mercury and autopsy data for bald eagles, 1969 and 1970. Pestic. Monit. J. 6:133–138.

Blus, L. J., B. S. Neely, Jr., A. A. Belisle, and R. M. Prouty. 1974. Organochlorine residues in brown pelican eggs: Relationship to reproductive success. Environ. Pollut. 7:81–91.

Bourne, W. R. P., and J. A. Bogan. 1972. Polychlorinated biphenyls in North Atlantic seabirds. Marine Pollut. Bull. 3:171–175.

Briggs, D. M., and J. R. Harris. 1973. Polychlorinated biphenyls influence in hatchability. Poult. Sci. 52:1291–1294.

Burse, V. W., R. D. Kimbrough, E. C. Villanueva, R. W. Jennings, R. E. Linder, and W. Sovocool. 1974. Polychlorinated biphenyls. Storage, distribution, excretion and recovery: Liver morphology after prolonged dietary ingestion. Arch. Environ. Health. 29:301–307.

Call, D. J., and B. E. Harrell. 1974. Effects of dieldrin and PCBs upon the production and morphology of Japanese quail eggs. Bull. Environ. Contam. Toxicol. 11:70–77.

Carstens, L. A., D. A. Barsotti, and J. R. Allen. 1977. Implications of polychlorinated biphenyl exposure in the infant nonhuman primate. Int. Symp. on Pathobiol. Environ. Pollut.—Animal Models and Wildlife as Monitors. Storrs, June 1–3.

Clark, D. R., Jr., C. O. Martin, and D. M. Swineford. 1975. Organochlorine insecticide residues in the free-tailed bat, *Tadarida brasiliensis,* at Bracken Cave, Tex. J. Mammal. 56:429–443.

Clausen, J., L. Braestrup, and D. Berg. 1974. The content of polychlorinated hydrocarbons in Arctic mammals. Bull. Environ. Contam. Toxicol. 12:529–534.

Cromartie, E., W. L. Riechel, L. N. Locke, A. A. Belisle,

T. E. Kaiser, T. G. Lamont, B. M. Mulhern, R. M. Prouty, and D. W. Swineford. 1975. Residues of organochlorine pesticides and polychlorinated biphenyls and autopsy data for bald eagles, 1971-72. Pestic. Monit. J. 9:11-14.

Dahlgren, R. B., and R. L. Linder. 1971. Effects of polychlorinated biphenyls on pheasant reproduction, behavior and survival. J. Wildl. Manage. 35:524-533.

______, Y. A. Greichus, and R. L. Linder. 1971. Storage and excretion of polychlorinated biphenyls in the pheasant. J. Wildl. Manage. 35:823-828.

______, R. J. Bury, R. L. Linder, and R. F. Reidinger, Jr. 1972. Residue levels and histopathology in pheasants given polychlorinated biphenyls. J. Wildl. Manage. 36:524-533.

DeLong, R. L., W. G. Gilmartin, and J. G. Simpson. 1973. Premature births in California sea lions: Association with high organochlorine pollutant residue levels. Science 181:1168-1170.

Duke, T. W., J. I. Lowe, and A. J. Wilson, Jr. 1970. A polychlorinated biphenyl (Aroclor 1254) in the water, sediment, and biota of Escambia Bay, Florida. Bull. Environ. Contam. Toxicol. 5: 171-180.

Dustman, E. H., L. F. Stickel, L. J. Blus, W. L. Riechel, and S. N. Wiemeyer. 1971. The occurrence and significance of polychlorinated biphenyls in the environment. Trans. N. Am. Wildl. Natur. Res. Conf. 36:118-132.

Fishbein, L. 1972. Chromatographic and biological aspects of polychlorinated biphenyls. J. Chromatogr. 68:345-426.

______. 1975. Toxicity of chlorinated biphenyls. Annu. Rev. Pharmacol. 14:139-156.

Flick, D. F., R. G. O'Dell, and V. A. Childs. 1965. Studies on chick edema disease. 3. Similarity of symptoms produced by feeding chlorinated biphenyl. Poult. Sci. 44:1460-1465.

Fox, G. A., A. P. Gilman, D. J. Hallett, R. J. Norstrom, F. I. Onuska, and D. B. Peakall. 1975. Herring gull productivity and toxic chemicals in the Great Lakes in 1975. Can. Wildl. Serv., Ms. Rep., Toxic Chemical Div. No. 34.

Friend, M., and D. O. Trainer. 1970. Polychlorinated biphenyl: Interaction with duck hepatitis virus. Science 170:1314-1316.

Gilman, A. P., G. A. Fox, D. J. Hallett, D. B. Peakall, and R. J. Norstrom. 1977. The herring gull as a monitor of Great Lakes contamination. Int. Symp. Pathobiol. Environ. Pollut.—Animal Models and Wildlife as Monitors. Storrs, June 1-3.

Gilmartin, W. G., R. L. DeLong, A. W. Smith, J. C. Sweeney, E. W. DeLappe, R. W. Risebrough, L. A. Garner, M. D. Dailey, and D. B. Peakall. 1976. Premature parturition in the California sea lion. J. Wildl. Dis. 12:104-115.

Goldstein, J. A., P. Hickman, V. W. Burse, and H. Bergman. 1975. A comparative study of two polychlorinated biphenyl mixtures (Aroclor 1242 and 1016) containing 42% chlorine on induction of hepatic porphyria and drug metabolizing enzymes. Toxicol. Appl. Pharmacol. 32:461-473.

Grant, D. L., and W. E. Phillips. 1974. The effect of age and sex on the toxicity of Aroclor 1254, a polychlorinated biphenyl, in the rat. Bull. Environ. Contam. Toxicol. 12:145-152.

Gress, F., R. W. Risebrough, D. W. Anderson, L. F. Riff, and J. R. Jehl, Jr. 1973. Reproductive failures of double-crested cormorants in Southern California and Baja California. Wilson Bull. 85:197-208.

Hansen, D. J., P. R. Parrish, J. I. Lowe, A. J. Wilson, Jr., and P. D. Wilson. 1971. Chronic toxicity, uptake, and retention of Aroclor 1254 in two estuarine fishes. Bull. Environ. Contam. Toxicol. 6:113-119.

Hays, H., and R. W. Risebrough. 1972. Pollutant concentrations in abnormal young terns from Long Island Sound. Auk 89:19-35.

Heath, R. G., J. W. Spann, E. F. Hill, and J. F. Kreitzer. 1972. Comparative dietary toxicities of pesticides to birds. U.S. Dept. of Interior, Bureau of Sport Fisheries and Wildlife Service, Special Sci. Rep. No. 152, Wildlife.

Hesselberg, R. J., and D. D. Scherr. 1974. PCB's and p,p′DDE in the blood of cachectic patients. Bull. Environ. Contam. Toxicol. 11:202-205.

Hill, E. F., R. G. Heath, J. W. Spann, and J. D. Williams. 1975. Lethal dietary toxicities of environmental pollutants to birds. U.S. Dept. of Interior, Bureau of Sport Fisheries and Wildlife Service, Special Sci. Rep. No. 191, Wildlife.

Kikucki, M., and Y. Masuda. 1976. The pathology of Yusho. In K. Higuchi. PCB poisoning and pollution. Academic Press, New York.

Kimbrough, R. D., R. E. Linder, and T. B. Gaines. 1972. Morphological changes in livers of rats fed polychlorinated biphenyl. Arch. Environ. Health 25:354-364.

Koeman, J. H., M. C. ten Noever de Braun, and R. H. de Vos. 1969. Chlorinated biphenyls in fish, mussels, and birds from the river Rhine and the Netherlands coastal area. Nature 221:1126-1128.

______, H. C. W. Van Velzen-Blad, R. DeVries, and J. G. Vos. 1973. Effects of PCB and DDE in cormorants and evaluation of PCB residues from an experimental study. J. Reprod. Fertil. (Suppl.) 19:353-364.

Koller, L. D., and J. E. Thigpen. 1973. Biphenyl-exposed rabbits. Am. J. Vet. Res. 34:1605-1606.

______, and J. G. Zinkl. 1973. Pathology of polychlorinated biphenyls in rabbits. Am. J. Pathol. 70:363-378.

Lincer, J. L., and D. B. Peakall. 1973. PCB pharmacodynamics in the ring dove and early gas chromatographic peak diminution. Environ. Pollut. 4:59-68.

Lloyd, W., R. M. Moore, Jr., B. S. Woolf, and H. P. Stein. 1976. Polychlorinated biphenyls. J. Occup. Med. 18:109-113.

Merson, M. H., and R. L. Kirkpatrick. 1976. Reproductive performance of captive white-footed mice fed a PCB. Bull. Environ. Contam. Toxicol. 16:392-398.

Nadeau, R. J., and R. A. Davis. 1976. Polychlorinated biphenyls in the Hudson River (Hudson Falls–Fort Edward, New York State). Bull. Environ. Contam. Toxicol. 16:436-444.

Nimmo, D. R., P. D. Wilson, R. R. Blackman, and A. J. Wilson, Jr. 1971. Polychlorinated biphenyl absorbed from sediments by fiddler crabs and pink shrimp. Nature 231:50-52.

Nisbet, I. C. T., and A. F. Sarofim. 1972. Rates and routes of transport of PCBs in the environment. Environ. Health Perspect. 1:21-38.

Parslow, J. L. F., and D. J. Jefferies. 1973. Relationship between organochlorine residues in livers and whole bodies of guillemots. Environ. Pollut. 5: 87–101.

Peakall, D. B. 1975. PCB's and their environmental effects. CRC Crit. Rev. Environ. Control 5:469–508.

______, and M. L. Peakall. 1973. Effect of a polychlorinated biphenyl on the production of artificially and naturally incubated dove eggs. J. Appl. Ecol. 10:863–867.

Pearce, P. A., I. M. Gruchy, and J. A. Keith. 1973. Toxic chemicals in living things in the Gulf of St. Lawrence. Can. Wildl. Serv., Ms. Rep., Pesticide Sect. No. 24.

Platonow, N. S., and L. H. Karstad. 1973. Dietary effects of polychlorinated biphenyls on mink. Can. J. Comp. Med. 37:391–400.

Prestt, I., D. J. Jefferies, and N. W. Moore. 1970. Polychlorinated biphenyls in wild birds in Britain and their avian toxicity. Environ. Pollut. 1:3–26.

Reimold, R. J. 1975. Chlorinated hydrocarbon pesticides and mercury in coastal biota, Puerto Rico and the U.S. Virgin Islands. Pestic Monit. J. 9:39–43.

Ringer, R. K., R. J. Aulerich, and M. Zabik. 1972. Effect of dietary polychlorinated biphenyls on growth and reproduction of mink. Preprints of papers presented, 164th Nat. Meet. Am. Chem. Soc. 12: 149–154.

Risebrough, R. W., P. Rieche, D. B. Peakall, S. G. Herman, and H. N. Kirven. 1968. Polychlorinated biphenyls in the global ecosystem. Nature 220: 1098–1102.

Ryder, J. P. 1974. Organochlorine and mercury residues in gulls' eggs from Western Ontario. Can. Field Natur. 88:349–352.

Stallings, D. L., and F. L. Mayer, Jr. 1972. Toxicities of PCBs to fish and environmental residues. Environ. Health Perspect. 1:159–164.

Stendell, R. C. 1975. Summary of recent information regarding effects of PCB's on birds and mammals. Natl. Conf. Polychlorinated Biphenyls. Nov. 19–21, Chicago, 262–267.

Stickel, W. H. 1975. Some effects of pollutants in terrestrial ecosystems. In A. D. McIntyre and C. E. Mills. Ecological toxicology research. Plenum, New York.

Tucker, R. K., and D. G. Crabtree. 1970. Handbook of toxicity of pesticides to wildlife. U.S. Dept. of Interior, Bureau of Sport Fisheries and Wildlife Service, Res. Publ. No. 84.

Tumasonis, C. F., B. Bush, and F. D. Baker. 1973. PCB levels in egg yolks associated with embryonic mortality and deformity of hatched chicks. Arch. Environ. Contam. Toxicol. 1:312–324.

Veith, G. D. 1975. Baseline concentrations of polychlorinated biphenyls and DDT in Lake Michigan fish, 1971. Pestic. Monit. J. 9:21–29.

Vos, J. G. 1972. Toxicology of PCBs for mammals and for birds. Environ. Health Perspect. 1:105–117.

______, and J. H. Koeman. 1970. Comparative toxicologic study with polychlorinated biphenyls in chickens with special reference to porphyria, edema formation, liver necrosis and tissue residues. Toxicol. Appl. Pharmacol. 17:656–668.

White, R. 1976. U.S. Dept. of Interior, Fish and Wildlife Service, Denver Wildlife Research Center. Personal communication.

Wiemeyer, S. N., P. R. Spitzer, W. C. Krantz, T. G. Lamont, and E. Cromartie. 1975. Effects of environmental pollutants on Connecticut and Maryland ospreys. J. Wildl. Manage. 39:124–139.

Wildish, D. J. 1970. The toxicity of polychlorinated biphenyls (PCB) in sea water to *Gammarus oceanicus*. Bull. Environ. Contam. Toxicol. 5: 202–204.

Zinkl, J. G. 1977. Skin and liver lesions in rats fed a polychlorinated biphenyl mixture. Arch. Environ. Contam. Toxicol. 5:217–228.

5 *Acute Chlorinated Hydrocarbon Pesticide Poisoning*

JOHN W. DAVIS

DDT. DDT, or 1,1,1-trichloro-2,2-bis(*p*-chlorophenyl)ethane, is an organochloride insecticide that has been widely used for prevention and control of insect infestations that occur about the premises of commercial concerns, farms, homes, and on animals. However, in the United States the present use of DDT is restricted. This material has worldwide distribution and persists in the environment to the extent that it may be found as an apparent "naturally" occurring product in animal tissues, especially animal fats.

DDT was first synthesized by Othman Zeidler in 1874 (Taggart, 1946). In 1939, Paul Müller found this compound to be effective against the Colorado potato beetle, *Leptinotarsa decimlineata* (Taggart, 1946). Also, it was found that this compound would kill lice and other insect pests. In 1942, the Bureau of Entomology and Plant Quarantine, U.S. Department of Agriculture conducted a very successful test with this material at their Orlando Experimental Station in Florida. DDT was used vigorously by the armed forces in World War II against typhus-carrying lice. Later DDT was used worldwide in the control of malaria, as well as other insect-borne diseases. With the conclusion of World War II, DDT became available for a wide range of insecticidal applications. DDT is very persistent in the environment, being resistant to chemical or microbial decomposition (Hatch, 1977).

Etiology. DDT is a white crystalline tasteless chemical that has a slight odor and is poorly soluble in water but readily soluble in oils and organic solvents. It has been used as wettable powders, dusts, suspensions, or emulsions.

Transmission. Poisoning of an animal may be accomplished by ingestion of contaminated foods or water, by inhalation, or by absorption of the chemical from the skin after topical application.

Pathogenesis and Signs. The acute clinical signs produced by organochlorine pesticides result from interference with the axonic transmission of nerve impulses, and are about the same in all species. The onset of signs can be different and the number, severity, and duration in individual animals may vary. This depends on the kind and amount of pesticide involved and certain factors encountered, such as illness and environmental changes that enhance toxicity. The presence of other pesticides, poisons, or drugs; size of particles in emulsions used as sprays or dips; age; sex; amount of body fat; species, and factors that alter drug response can influence response to pesticides. The onset of acute signs varies from minutes to hours. Generally, signs develop as hypersensitivity, involuntary contraction, or twitching involving a group of muscle fibers, with twitching and spasms most frequently involving the cervical, forequarter, and hindquarter muscles in that order. This may progress through intermittent or continuous course spasms and jaw clamping to sudden clonic-tonic convulsions that are accompanied by high body temperature. If death does not occur during the first convulsion, depression may result; later convulsions can occur and be precipitated by external stimuli.

Behavior may be unusual and begin with apprehension or apparent anxiety; hostility or aggressiveness often follows. The head may be lowered between the legs, the animal may kneel with the rump in the air, jump over nonexistent objects, try to climb walls, or develop a delirious behavior. Vomiting, diarrhea, urination, profuse salivation, or tachycardia can occur. Sometimes cardiac arrhythmias develop. Locomotor disturbances may include stiff gait, incoordination, ataxia, and circling; all may be accompanied by frenzied behavior or jaw clamping. Hot ears and skin can develop. Rapid and deep respirations may occur, along with fluid sounds in the lungs. Death can follow in minutes, hours, several days, or not at all (Hatch, 1977).

Signs seen in robins, *Turdus migratorius,* after being fed DDT-injected earthworms were tremors (Bernard, 1963). The quantity of DDT in robin tissues was variable, and in a few of the tremoring birds there were low quantities or no DDT at all in breast muscle, heart, liver, and kidney. Levels of DDT in tissues of trembling robins of both sexes averaged 93.3 μg of DDT/gm of brain, 115.7 μg in the breast muscle, 143.8 μg in heart tissues, and 18.71 μg in the liver. The highest number of robins found dying of tremors had concentrations of DDT that ranged from a low of 50 to a high of 120 μg of DDT/gm of brain tissue. Sparrows, *Passer domesticus,* fed DDT developed tremors. Since DDT is stored in fat tissues, this reserve may be utilized in starvation or during migration. The compound may be released and activate areas such as the brain, which results in tremors and is followed by death.

When adult wild mallard, *Anas platyrhynchos,* and pintail, *A. acuta,* ducks were fed DDT in their diets, all levels above 0.025% caused toxicity, as evidenced by tremors, loss of appetite and weight, paralysis, and death (Coburn and Treichler, 1946). When five-week-old bobwhite quail, *Colinis virginianus,* were fed at levels of 0.05 to 0.4% DDT in the diet they all died. There was 50% mortality at 0.025% of DDT in the diet and there were some losses at 0.005%. Signs noted for the quail included nervousness, anorexia, and tremors prior to death.

Coburn and Treichler (1946) found evidence of acute toxicity only after oral dosing of starlings, *Sturnus vulgaris,* for all levels of DDT above 0.025% in the diet. Toxic conditions were observed in birds that received 1,000 mg/kg, but no deaths occurred in any dosed at this level. Stewart et al. (1946) conducted experiments in which DDT was used as an orchard spray at a 1:7 ratio. One pheasant, *Phasianus colchicus,* that had received DDT at 1:1,000 ratio exhibited typical tremors before death, and another bird exposed to the same ratio died on the 23rd day after exposure. A similarly exposed pheasant exhibited severe tremors on the 21st day but recovered. Pheasants receiving a diet containing a normal orchard use ratio of DDT at a concentration of 1:1,000 or 0.909 kg of 50% wettable powder per 264.2 liters of water accumulated relatively large quantities of pesticide. The bird that had stored the largest concentration of DDT in the fat tissue died with typical tremors on the 23rd day. A cock that had stored 94 ppm in liver tissues exhibited severe tremors on the 21st day but recovered 7 days later. A sick hen pheasant found in the orchard was observed for 48 hours, during which time it developed anorexia and slight tremors. Genelly and Rudd (1956) stated that signs of acute poisoning depend on the amount of DDT assimilated. In low amounts the only observable reaction is increased sensitivity and hyperexcitability; at amounts approaching the lethal dose, tremors may appear for a time and then disappear.

Only one of the five cottontail rabbits, *Sylvilagus* sp., that received 0.2% DDT in the diet showed evidence of toxicity (Coburn and Treichler, 1946). Slight tremors were exhibited in only one of the five for a period of more than three days. Three of four rabbits receiving a 0.4% level died by the 21st day after showing severe tremors.

Meadow voles, *Microtus pennsylvanicus,* were fed 0.2% and 0.4% levels of DDT in their diets and chronic toxicity occurred in the voles at the 0.2% level. Tremors occurred in three of five voles and death in two within 28 days. At the 0.4% level all five animals fed DDT died by the 21 st day, whereas all voles fed the 0.2% level survived the 31-day trial period.

White-footed mice, *Peromyscus leucopus,* showed moderate to severe tremors when fed 1,500 mg/kg DDT orally. Five of six of the white-footed mice, after being dosed at 2,000 mg/kg, died within 3 to 49 hours; the other survived following severe tremors. When similar mice were fed diets containing 0.01, 0.02, 0.04, and 0.10% DDT, they did not develop clinical toxicity over a 30-day period, but slight tremors became evident by the 3rd day in all animals fed at 0.2 to 0.4% levels. The tremors disappeared on the 5th day, and did not reappear in the duration of the experiment (Coburn and Treichler, 1946).

Pathology. Rabbits, *Oryctolagus cuniculus,* and Norway rats, *Rattus norvegicus,* that received toxic doses of DDT showed hepatic hyalin degeneration, focal hydropic degeneration, and vacuolation (Kanegis and Roepke, 1946). Striated myocardial necrosis in guinea pigs, *Cavia porcellus,* and rabbits, as well as necrosis in striated muscle, have been recorded (Nelson et al., 1944). Lillie and Smith (1944) observed varying degrees of fatty degeneration in the hepatic cells and areas of coagulation necrosis in rats and rabbits. Coburn and Treichler (1946) recorded multiple areas of focal necrosis in the livers and kidneys of rabbits that had received a 0.4% level of DDT in their diet for 15 to 21 days.

Ring-necked pheasants given DDT at a concentration in the total diet of 90 ppm developed moderate fatty changes, focal damage, margination of cytoplasmic granules, some necrosis, and occasionally peripheral granulation and light vacuolation in the liver over a 74-day experimental period (Genelly and Rudd, 1956). Extreme fatty changes, engorged sinusoids, swollen nuclei, focal damage in streaks radiating from major vessels, and light vacuolation occurred in the liver when 355 ppm concentration of DDT in the total diet was used over a 74-day experimental period. Birds may also lose significant weight.

Diagnosis. Diagnosis is determined by history, clinical signs, and pathological lesions. Since organochlorine pesticide residues are found "normally" in the body fat as a result of exposure to small amounts of pesticide in the environment, a positive laboratory test for these compounds does not always mean the animals were poisoned by them. When animals manifest muscle tremors, apprehension, or salivation, poisoning by an anticholinesterase pesticide, urea, or lead must be considered. Parts per million concentrations in body tissues may be significant for diagnostic purposes if they correlate with the postmortem findings, history, and clinical signs found associated with poisoning by organochlorine pesticides. Brain concentrations of the pesticide are a better indication of poisoning than concentrations in the body fat (Ecobichon and Saschenbrecker, 1968).

Where exposure has been recent and excessive to a pesticide, the liver and kidney of dead animals or milk or blood of live animals should be tested. Other specimens that might be tested are stomach contents, vomitus, stomach washings, bile, and suspected sources of pesticide.

Treatment. Convulsions are treated with anesthetics, such as chloral hydrate or pentobarbital; however, since postconvulsive depression can be additive the animal may become overdosed. If an animal is in a depressed state due to known or suspected pesticide toxicity, an anesthetic is contraindicated. Central nervous system stimulants are also contraindicated as additional stimulation would only worsen the condition.

Usually, sedative doses of chloral hydrate or barbiturate will control most of the nervous, locomotor, and behavioral signs. Atropine is used in small dosage to control parasympathetic signs. Sedation permits the body temperature to drop slowly. Animals exposed by the dermal route must be bathed with soap and water two or three times and rinsed thoroughly. If the pesticide has been consumed orally, a saline purgative or gastric lavage may be necessary.

Calcium borogluconate and glucose in saline given intravenously has been suggested by Clarke and Clarke (1967) to avoid liver damage and neutralize the effects of preconvulsive hyperkalemia, that is, the elevation above normal of potassium in the blood.

Prevention. To prevent free-ranging animals from becoming poisoned with pesticides is difficult, as the environment can be polluted with organochloride pesticides that apparently have longevity and can be stored in body fat over a period of time even with small amounts of exposure. If pesticides are judiciously used and animals are kept in good condition without excessive stresses and starvation, few detrimental effects should be encountered by wildlife populations.

DIELDRIN

Etiology. Dieldrin, or 1,2,3,4,10,10-hexachloro-6,7-epoxy-1,4,4a,5,6,7,8,8a-octahydro-1,4-endo, exo-5,8-dimethanonaphthalene, is an oxidized chlorinated hydrocarbon insecticide that was first introduced in 1948. Fiedler and DuToit (1951) noted dieldrin was lethal to larval stages of the sheep maggot fly, *Lucilia cuprina,* and Downing et al. (1952) observed that it was also effective against the sheep maggot fly, *L. sericata.* Stones et al. (1954) demonstrated that when 0.05% dieldrin was used it gave protection against body "strike" of 16 weeks, which covered the entire period of observation. Dieldrin has been used worldwide.

Signs. Year-old blesbok, *Damaliscus dorcas phillipsi,* after a three-month taming period were fed dietary levels of dieldrin at the rate of 5, 15, 25, 35, and 50 ppm. Signs noted were death in some animals within 24 hours; other antelope demonstrated nervous signs that consisted of hypersensitivity, imbalance, and intermittent clonic convulsions over a 48-hour period prior to death (Wiese et al., 1973).

McEwen and Brown (1966) orally dosed wild sharp-tailed grouse, *Pedioecetes phasianellus,* with dieldrin at the rates of 5.0, 8.0, 12.84, and 20.5 mg/kg. Deaths occurred in some birds and the LD_{50} was calculated at 6.9 mg/kg. In captive sharp-tailed grouse mortality was reported to occur at 6.4 mg/kg, and maximum effect was usually absent until the 3rd to 4th day after administration of the insecticide. Other signs noted were reduced flushing distance, irregular flight, and circular and uncoordinated walking, along with distress calls. There was periodic wing beating and thrashing that was intermixed with periods of apparently normal coordination and alertness. These signs became increasingly severe with frequent convulsive attacks that were followed by death.

One-day-old quail and pheasant chicks were given dieldrin at the rate of 50 ppm in the diet for 40 to 87 days; death occurred in all of them. Signs of acute toxicity occurred by 48 to 72 hours and consisted initially of muscular incoordination with occasional tremors, bedraggled appearance, and a stiff-legged hesitating movement in walking. The birds in the advanced stage made spasmodic leaps and exhibited violent cartwheels that lasted for several minutes; these signs were delayed if dieldrin was fed at lower levels. Growth, however, was depressed, but birds remained in a relatively good condition for the first few days of the experimental period (Dewitt, 1956).

Eight-week-old bobwhite quail and trapped mourning doves, *Zenaidura macroura,* received oral doses of dieldrin; the LD_{50} doses ranged from 12 to 14 mg/kg for quail and 44 to 46 mg/kg for doves (Dahlen and Haugen, 1954). There was a general loss of body weight. Signs observed were convulsions and subsequent depression that preceded death. Birds did not normally respond to external stimuli and motor coordination appeared to be affected. There were tremors with occasional shaking of the head. Birds while in the moribund state often backed into a corner of the enclosed area and were usually found on their backs after death with their necks drawn back and to one side. The wings were partially expanded and the legs were extended. Many times at death there was a milky exudate that flowed from the mouth and nares of birds. Genelly and Rudd (1956) found that ring-necked pheasants had rapid weight loss after the birds consumed 100 to 200 ppm of dieldrin; those that consumed 25 to 70 ppm differed little from the controls. At 100 ppm five males died by the 38th day. Wiese and Basson (1967) noted a spreading of the large tail feathers, seizures, and profuse salivation that preceded death.

Murphy and Korschgen (1970) fed sublethal amounts of dieldrin daily, 5 to 25 ppm, to white-tailed deer, *Odocoileus virginianus,* and their progeny were maintained at these levels for three years. Dieldrin-treated does, which were immature at the initiation of the study, grew more slowly and remained this way. Fawns from dieldrin-fed does were smaller at birth and weight gains were significantly reduced.

Pathology. Wiese and Basson (1967) found on postmortem examination of the crowned guinea fowl, *Numida meleagris,* no obvious abnormalities; however, there was general congestion of the kidneys, liver, pancreas, and brain. Histopathology was inconclusive. Histological findings in ring-necked pheasants are recorded, including light vacuolation around vessels and light fatty change concentrated around the major vessels (Genelly and Rudd, 1956). Dahlen and Haugen (1954) recorded pathology in doves and quail as dilated auricles; discoloration and atrophy of the liver; congestion of the lungs and kidneys; hemorrhages in the pleural cavity, trachea, and neck; petechiation in the breast muscle; and visceral gout.

Wiese et al. (1973) found no major tissue difference in antelope between the changes produced by dieldrin and photodieldrin except that there were more widespread petechial hemorrhages, especially subepicardially, in the photodieldrin-poisoned animals. Serous atrophy of the fat and hydrothorax were observed in the antelope poisoned with dieldrin, while there was atony of the stomach in about one-half of the photodieldrin group. The most consistent findings were general congestion of the lungs, kidneys, and particularly the liver; cyanosis; various degrees of pulmonary edema; mild to moderate localized muscular and subcutaneous hemorrhages; mild subendocardial hemorrhages in either or both ventricles; prominent congestion of the brain; and atrophy and contraction of the spleen. Myocardial and skeletal muscular degeneration was found infrequently in experimental animals; however, this lesion is very striking in natural cases. Other lesions occasionally found were myocardial hemorrhages, hydropericardium, swelling of the optic chiasma, hemorrhages in the lymph nodes, hemorrhages on the pulmonary valves, hepatic degeneration, and nephrosis.

Free-ranging antelope exposed to commercially treated grazing had more traumatic injuries—subepicardial and subendocardial hemorrhages, severe degeneration of the myocardium, and hemorrhages in and degeneration and necrosis of the skeletal muscles—than did captive animals. Histologically, lymph nodes were congested with hemorrhages and some karyorrhexis of follicles. The spleen was usually contracted with a few red and white cells in the red pulp. Splenic corpuscles were usually small with karyorrhexis necrosis of the germinal centers in some cases. Skeletal muscles appeared degenerated and were accompanied by edema and hemorrhages. The myocardium had lesions similar to the muscular lesions but with reduced severity.

The liver was congested and had various gradations of cloudy swelling with hydropic and fatty changes. The kidneys were usually congested and contained varying degrees of nephrosis. Occasionally, tubular necrosis and glomerular edema were noted. The lungs were nearly always congested and frequently edema was observed. The brain usually had moderate to severe congestion with mild hemorrhages and some edema. Murphy and Korschgen (1970) found the pituitary gland somewhat atrophied and the thyroid somewhat hypertrophied in dieldrin-fed deer.

Diagnosis. A diagnosis is usually based on the history, signs, and lesions, along with the finding of significant amounts of pesticide in tissues, especially in the brain tissues.

Treatment and Prevention. Similar to that outlined for DDT.

2,4-D. 2,4-D is a white crystalline substance that is very slightly soluble in water or aliphatic oil. It is somewhat soluble in aromatic oil and highly soluble in ethyl alcohol and other similar organic solvents. The real use of 2,4-D did not emerge until early in World War II. By 1949, the United States was considered to be manufacturing approximately 10,000 tons of the chemical a year. This herbicide has had worldwide distribution and use.

Etiology. 2,4-dichlorophenoxyacetic acid, its amine, or sodium salt.

Transmission. Poisoning is usually acquired by accidental ingestion of concentrates or sprays. Only occasionally would treated forages be hazardous to wildlife.

Signs. Organic herbicides may cause signs of abdominal distress, such as occasional colic, diarrhea, anorexia. In addition, 2,4-D may cause ataxia, weakness and muscle spasms, or rigidity (Hatch, 1977). Acute signs of oral poisoning in mallard ducks, pheasants, quail, and mule deer, *O. hemionus,* presented as tremors, hyperpnea, ataxia, excessive thirst, prostration, drooping of the eyelid, and salivation (Tucker and Crabtree, 1970). All of these animals had undergone a fasting period. The birds were fasted for 20 hours pretreatment, while the mule deer were fasted for 24 hours.

Range-finding doses were initially administered. Two to seven animals at four dosage levels were employed for each LD_{50} determination; a standard 14-day posttreatment observation period was made before final death counts. If toxicity was observed past 14 days, the observation period was extended until death or recovery resulted. This did not have to be extended beyond 30 days. When one mule deer doe was given 2,4-D acid orally for 30 days at 80 mg/kg/day and another received 240 mg/kg/day, they only showed slight signs of toxicity. Combinations orally of 2 gm/kg to mallards were not lethal.

Renzoni (1973) gave Japanese quail, *Coturnix coturnix japonica,* a herbicide preparation containing 36.5% 2,4-D as a part per thousand of drinking water and observed that egg fertility and production were reduced. There was also a delay in the onset of laying.

Diagnosis. Diagnosis may be difficult since many of the herbicides are rapidly excreted; however, suspected poisoning by 2,4-D may be confirmed by laboratory analysis of ruminal contents, plasma, and urine (Milhaud and Alvariza, 1970).

Treatment and Control. There are no specific treatments except for arsenicals. If the various synthetic organic herbicides are used properly and the withholding times observed, they are not considered a great hazard for animals. Buck et al. (1973) should be consulted for clinical and diagnostic veterinary toxicology.

REFERENCES

Bernard, R. F. 1963. Studies on the effects of DDT in birds. Michigan State Univ. Mus. Biol. Ser. 2:155–192.

Buck, W. B., G. D. Osweiler, and G. A. Van Gelder. 1976. Clinical and diagnostic veterinary toxicology. Kendall-Hunt, Dubuque.

Clarke, E. G. C., and M. L. Clarke. 1967. Garner's veterinary toxicology. 3rd ed. Williams & Wilkins, Baltimore.

Coburn, D. R., and R. Treichler. 1946. Experiments on toxicity of DDT to wildlife. J. Wildl. Manage. 10:208–216.

Dahlen, H., and A. O. Haugen. 1954. Acute toxicity of certain insecticides to the bobwhite quail and mourning dove. J. Wildl. Manage. 18:477–481.

Dewitt, J. B. 1956. Chronic toxicity to quail and pheasants of some chlorinated insecticides. Agric. Food Chem. 4:863–866.

Downing, W., H. E. Harbour, and L. C. Stones. 1952. Modern insecticides and ectoparasite control. Vet. Rec. 64(6):787–803.

Ecobichon, D. J., and P. W. Saschenbrecker. 1968. Pharmacodynamic study of DDT in cockerels. Can. J. Physiol. Pharmacol. 46:785.

Fiedler, O. G. H., and R. DuToit. 1951. A new biological method for evaluating the efficiency of insecticides for protection of sheep against blowfly strike. Nature 168:608–609.

Genelly, R. E., and R. L. Rudd. 1956. Chronic toxicity of DDT, toxaphene and dieldrin to ring-necked pheasants. Calif. Fish Game 42:5–14.

Hatch, R. C. 1977. Poisons causing nervous stimulation or depression. In L. Meyer Jones, N. H. Booth, and L. E. McDonald. Veterinary pharmacology and therapeutics. Iowa State Univ. Press, Ames.

Kanegis, L. A., and M. H. Roepke. 1946. DDT: A review with special reference to veterinary medicine. J. Am. Vet. Med. Assoc. 108:316–321.

Lillie, R. D., and M. I. Smith. 1944. Pathology of experimental poisoning in cats, rabbits, and rats with DDT. Public Health Rep. 59:979–984.

McEwen, L. C., and R. L. Brown. 1966. Acute toxicity of dieldrin and malathion to wild sharp-tailed grouse. J. Wildl. Manage. 30:604–611.

Milhaud, G., and F. Alvariza. 1970. Toxicology of hormone weed-killers (2,4-D). Recl. Med. Vet. 146: 345–357.

Murphy, D. A., and L. J. Korschgen. 1970. Reproduction, growth and tissue residues of deer fed dieldrin. J. Wildl. Manage. 34:887–903.

Nelson, A. A., J. H. Draize, G. Woodard, O. Fitzhugh, R. G. Smith, R. Blackwell, Jr., and H. O. Calvery. 1944. Histopathological changes following administration of DDT to several species of animals. Public Health Rep. 59:1009–1020.

Renzoni, A. 1973. The influence of some toxicants on the reproductive activities of the Japanese quail, *Coturnix coturnix japonica.* Biol. Conserv. 181–184.

Stewart, R. E., J. B. Cope, C. S. Robbins, and J. W. Brainerd. 1946. Effects of DDT on birds at the Patuxent Research Refuge. J. Wildl. Manage. 10:195–201.

Stones, L. C., J. C. Wood, and C. B. Hart. 1954. The use of dieldrin for sheep maggot fly control. Vet. Rec. 66:183–187.

Taggart, R. S. 1946. DDT. Cornell Vet. 36:159–169.

Tucker, R. K., and G. D. Crabtree. 1970. Handbook of toxicity of pesticides to wildlife. U.S. Dept of Interior, Fish Wildlife Service, Res. Publ. No. 84:39–40.

Wiese, I. H., and N. C. J. Basson. 1967. The oral toxicity of dieldrin to the crowned guinea-fowl, *Numida meleagris* (L). S. Afr. J. Agric. Sci. 10:697–706. Extracts reproduced under copyright authority G245 of 14-7-1978 of the Government Printer of the Republic of South Africa.

———, ———, P. A. Basson, T. W. Aude, and B. P. Maartnes. 1973. The toxicity and pathology of dieldrin and photodieldrin poisoning in two antelope species. Onderstepoort J. Vet. Res. 40:31–40. Extracts reproduced under copyright authority G245 of 14-7-1978 of the Government Printer of the Republic of South Africa.

6 *Shock*

S. J. PROCTOR

A GREAT DEAL of confusion and controversy exists regarding shock. Frequently any catastrophic syndrome that occurs while wild animals are being captured or transported is indiscriminately attributed to shock; and other syndromes, such as drug overdose, hyperthermia, and so on are not considered. In nature shock probably plays a significant role by allowing an animal to die quickly with less pain after it is captured by a predator. Clinically, shock is defined as severe hypotension or decreased blood pressure due to acute generalized circulatory failure. In normal animals, blood pressure depends on three basic factors: cardiac output, peripheral vascular resistance maintained by capillaries and veins, and a normal blood volume. Disturbance of any one of these factors causes a precipitous decrease in blood pressure, resulting in shock.

The adrenal gland plays a leading role in adaptive adjustment. Removal of the adrenal gland in experimental animals obliterates the capacity to make homeostatic adjustments in response to injury, hemorrhage, metabolic increases, and environmental stress. Acute stress decreases the size of the adrenal gland, while a lower level of chronic stress increases its size. During acute stress the adrenal medulla releases epinephrine, and the cortex releases glucocorticoids, causing the heart to beat faster and stronger, the spleen to contract, the blood to be diverted by selective vasoconstriction to striated muscles, and serum glucose levels to be elevated. These are transient compensatory reactions that allow sudden bursts of muscular power necessary for fleeing or fighting for existence. These compensatory reactions may be detrimental in certain situations. For example, they may hinder heat dissipation by contracting cutaneous vessels or they may potentiate shock.

ETIOLOGY. Shock can be classified in several ways, and each is an arbitrary division for discussion purposes. It is generally accepted that all types of shock have at least one feature in common: failure of the microcirculation. This circulatory failure may be caused by a failure in one of three basic locations of the cardiovascular system: 1) cardiac shock caused by damage to the pump mechanism, the heart; 2) hypovolemic shock that occurs after a sudden decrease in total blood volume; and 3) vasculogenic shock resulting from a change in peripheral arterial resistance or an increase in total venous capacity (Weil and Shubin, 1972). Neurologic shock, a division of vasculogenic shock observed in captured wild animals, will also be discussed.

CARDIAC SHOCK. Cardiac shock is caused by an acute disturbance in the pumping ability of the heart. Myocardial injuries, including gunshot wounds, ruptured chordae tendineae, fluid collection in the pericardial sac or tamponade, air in the thoracic cavity, and severe myocardial depression or heart blockage following administration of an anesthetic or a tranquilizer are all potential initiators of cardiac shock (Shoemaker, 1972). After the initial insult or injury, the heart may stop or it may beat and contract irregularly. If both the right and left sides of the heart are involved, the normal blood flow from the large veins to the heart is hindered and blood pools in the large veins leading to the heart, liver, and intestines. If only the left side of the heart is involved, blood will pool in the vessels of the lungs.

HYPOVOLEMIC SHOCK. Hypovolemic shock is caused by the loss of whole blood or fluids, and may be the most common type of shock in wild animals. Massive volumes of fluid or whole blood may be lost through external skin lacerations, internally into body cavities, or into traumatized and crushed tissues. Blood losses through external wounds are easy to observe, evaluate, and understand clinically.

Loss of blood or fluids into traumatized tissues, body cavities, or the intestinal tract is deceiving and more difficult to evaluate but is just as significant as external hemorrhage (Shoemaker, 1972). For example, if an injured thigh of an average person increases 1 cm in diameter, it will contain an extra 2.0 liters of blood and fluid; and if its diameter is increased 2 cm, it will contain an extra 4.5 liters of blood and fluid. After forest or prairie fires, severely burned animals lose large amounts of fluid through the burned skin. This loss of fluid and pain may initiate shock and result in death. Hemorrhage and loss of plasma may initiate terminal shock in several diseases with severe vascular lesions, such as hemorrhagic disease of deer and simian hemorrhagic fever.

Probably the most common cause of hypovolemic shock in captured wild animals is hemorrhage into a body cavity, into traumatized tissue, or through a skin laceration. The response of wild animals to hemorrhage has not been as well studied as that of the dog. The normal blood volume of most animals is about 10% of the body weight. A normal healthy unexcited dog may lose one-fourth of its blood volume without showing clinical evidence of shock, but loss of one-half may result in terminal shock and death.

After significant blood loss, arterial blood pressure decreases, venous return to the heart decreases, and the heart rate increases. Pressure receptors in the large arteries initiate a compensatory mechanism involving the nervous system and adrenal gland. Peripheral vessels in less essential tissues, such as the skin, contract, while vessels in life-giving organs, such as the heart and brain, dilate. The spleen also contracts, pouring erythrocytes into the circulatory system. If blood loss continues and blood pressure continues to fall, a second more powerful constriction of the vessels in nonessential organs occurs when the oxygen levels in the brain fall below a critical level (Cheville, 1976).

VASCULOGENIC SHOCK. Vasculogenic shock is caused by dilatation of the capillary beds beyond the capacity of the blood to fill them, and, consequently, blood is not returned to the heart. Since only 25 to 30% of the peripheral capillaries in a normal animal are open at any one time, dilatation of all these capillary beds greatly increases the capacity of the cardiovascular system and causes pooling of blood (Stickles, 1976a). For example, when all blood vessels in the abdominal organs of the dog are fully dilated, they have the capacity to hold nearly the entire blood volume. Vascular shock occurs in toxic and septic conditions, allergic reactions, and neurologic stimulation secondary to severe pain, trauma, or fright.

The most studied toxic shock is endotoxin shock, which is produced by lipopolysaccharide in the cell wall of gram-negative bacilli such as *Escherichia coli* (Coalson et al., 1970; Emerson, 1972). In the dog a precipitous decline in arterial blood pressure occurs after the experimental injection of endotoxins. Examination of the canine viscera reveals congestion and pooling of blood in the liver, spleen, and intestines. Blood flow through the kidneys is reduced, and urine production is subsequently reduced. Endotoxin injures vascular endothelium, initiating platelet aggregation and coagulation. This intravascular coagulation is responsible for thrombosis of small pulmonary vessels (Berman, 1972).

Shock secondary to allergic reactions, or anaphylactic shock, follows the binding of an antigen, reagin, to a cell-bound antibody. The cellular bound antigen-antibody complex causes release of massive amounts of histamine, serotonin, and other vasoactive compounds from the cell and causes widespread arteriolar and venous dilatation. Immune complexes also initiate intravascular platelet aggregations that can be trapped in small vessels of the lung. Increased resistance and permeability in pulmonary vessels occurs, particularly in guinea pigs, *Cavia porcellus,* cows, sheep, and other animals in which the lung, or "shock organ," is predominantly involved in shock (Hsu, 1976).

Neurologic Shock. Neurologic shock may occur in animals following severe pain, trauma, or fright. Neurologic stimulation instigates a peripheral vasodilatation that decreases the effective circulating blood volume. The best model of neurologic shock is crush injury. After limbs of an animal have been crushed, the application of tourniquets above the crushed areas will prevent fluid loss into injured tissue but they will not prevent the circulatory collapse of shock. In contrast, cutting the nerves to the limbs will prevent shock even without a tourniquet (Cheville, 1976).

Neurologic shock undoubtedly plays an important role in wild animals by contributing to pain relief in the predator-prey relationship. How fear, pain, sight, stress, or hearing initiate neurologic shock has not been elucidated experimentally. However, certain sounds have been reported to initiate neurologic seizures in mice, *Mus* sp.; rabbits, *Oryctolagus* sp.; and rats, *Rattus* sp. (Collins, 1972; Hohenboken and Nellhaus, 1970). Photogenic stimuli have been demonstrated to cause similar neurologic seizures in baboons, *Papio* sp. (Naquet and Meldrum, 1972).

Stress due to sight, sound, fear, and so on has produced physiological changes of adaptation, for example, the flight-fight syndrome as postulated by Selye, as well as shock in animals (Gronow, 1974). Chronic environmental stress, such as light, sound, and cage oscillation, has been reported to increase the enzymatic activity of monoamine oxidase in the liver, brain, and heart of rats (Maura et al., 1974). Capture and transport of mud fish, *Labeo umbratus,* have been reported to decrease hemoglobin concentrations, blood pH, hematocrits, red and white blood cell counts, and serum protein, while increasing red blood cell fragility and thrombocyte counts (Hattingh and Van Pletzen, 1974). Similar changes have been observed in captured flounder, *Pseudopleuronectes americanus* (Fletcher, 1975). Functional deterioration of olfactory and gustatory receptors is caused by capture and confinement of wild catfish, *Ictalurus* sp. (Tucker, 1973).

The adrenal gland has a prominent role in the adaptation and metabolic changes mentioned above. For example, in captured meadow voles, *Microtus pennsylvanicus,* serum adrenal corticosterone levels are elevated (Churcher et al., 1973). Chronic low levels of stress cause adrenal cortical hyperplasia and increase the size of the adrenal gland (McCarty and Richardson, 1974). In contrast, acute severe stress markedly depletes the adrenal cortex of steroid lipid granules. As a result, the gland is buff colored and many contain scattered hemorrhages. After severe stress, hemorrhages may be present in the adrenal gland. It is unclear whether stress causes shock by overstimulation and depletion of the adrenal gland or if the nervous system directly causes the vasodilatation of shock. Experimental evidence suggests that the adrenal gland has a protective or inhibitory function in shock since its removal makes an animal more susceptible.

Although unexplained death has been reported in several species of captured wild animals and has been attributed to shock, few describe the syndrome. Capture or confinement shock in the snowshoe hare, *Lepus americanus* (Adams, 1959; Green et al., 1939; Iversen et al., 1972), and gray squirrels, *Sciurus carolinensis* (Guthrie et al., 1967; Hoff et al., 1976), has been described. There is considerable variation in the susceptibility of hares to shock. Some have signs the first time they are captured, while other hares never have signs. Hares mildly affected only stop to eat instead of running away after being released. In more severe forms the hares have reduced hunger with some sneezing, and in the most severe form hares convulse and die. Rigor mortis occurs quickly after death. At necropsy the liver is depleted of glycogen, and ulcers are frequently found in the glandular portion of the stomach.

Like the hare, some gray squirrels are extremely susceptible to confinement stress during trapping, while others are quite resistant. Shock in the gray squirrel is characterized by muscular incoordination, loss of orientation, convulsions, and unconsciousness culminating in death. Lymphopenia, hypoglycemia, increased blood urea nitrogen (BUN) levels, and elevated packed red blood cell volumes (PCV) are evident. In one study few lesions were found at necropsy, except for slightly decreased adrenal gland weights in stressed animals (Guthrie et al., 1967).

PATHOGENESIS. Regardless of what causes shock, its principal feature is the reduction of blood flow through tissues, or tissue perfusion. This results in a deficit of essential nutrients, primarily oxygen, and a build-up of toxic metabolites at the tissue and cellular levels. If anoxia, or lack of oxygen, is permitted to persist, the circulatory deficiency is aggravated; and self-perpetuating processes cause shock to progress into a vicious cycle (Fig. 6.1).

Compensatory Mechanisms. Early in shock, compensatory mechanisms occur that attempt to prevent the detrimental effects of reduced tissue perfusion (McDonell, 1974). Neural and hormonal influences produce widespread peripheral vasoconstriction and increase the heart rate in an attempt to stabilize cardiac output and blood pressure. Anoxia and hypotension stimulate chemoreceptors and pressoreceptors respectively in the large arteries. These receptors initiate the release of adrenal hormones. Adrenal hormones, catecholamines, cause widespread vasoconstriction of peripheral vessels in the skin and abdominal viscera and are responsible for the cutaneous coolness of animals in shock.

Peripheral vasoconstriction causes a redistribution of blood flow to vital organs, such as the brain and heart. Widespread arteriolar constriction also lowers the capillary blood pressure and causes tissue fluids to flow into vessels, thus increasing the blood volume. Catecholamines, decreased renal blood flow, and hypovolemia, or decreased volume, initiate the release of antidiuretic hormone from the posterior pituitary. These processes decrease glomerular filtration and increase resorption of fluids from the renal tubules in an attempt to conserve body fluids. Renin is released from ischemic kidney, which in turn activates angiotensin. This substance also causes vasoconstriction in an attempt to increase blood pressure (Blair et al., 1976).

In many animals these compensatory mechanisms may be effective enough to reestablish normal circulation. However, in severe shock the compensatory mechanisms do not prevent circulatory deterioration. In these circumstances, prolonged compensatory vasoconstriction may even aggravate and perpetuate cellular anoxia. If anoxia persists, capillaries and venules throughout the body are injured.

Anoxia. Anoxia is probably one of the most significant factors of shock. In the peripheral microcirculation, prolonged vasoconstriction with subsequent anoxia eventually causes a loss of the integrity of the microvascular smooth muscles, resulting in a decrease in vasomotion, an unrestricted capillary dilatation, and pooling and stasis of blood. Permeability of anoxic vessels is increased, and plasma exudes into tissues.

Vascular stasis and anoxic injury to the vascular walls initiate vascular thrombosis, or formation of blood clots, decreasing plasma concentration of platelets and some clotting factors (Balis et al., 1978; Wilson, 1976). Vascular thrombosis then further hinders circulation by direct vascular occlusion or by forming emboli that occlude small arteries or capillaries of the lung or kidney. Tissues supplied by these vessels become necrotic or infarcted. Vascular degeneration in necrotic tissue results in hemorrhage and fluid exudation into tissue. The net result of direct or indirect anoxic vascular injury is loss of circulating blood volume due to vascular occlusion, loss of blood into tissue by hemorrhage, or loss of plasma due to increased vascular permeability.

The effect of anoxia on body tissues also contributes to the decreased tissue perfusion associated with shock. For example, cardiac anoxia causes a decrease in cardiac output, which leads to a decrease in blood pressure and tissue perfusion. Anoxia in the intestine has been reported to release a myocardial depressant factor that will decrease cardiac output (Lundgren et al., 1976). Cerebral anoxia is associated with depression of the vasomotor centers, with subsequent peripheral vasodilatation and stasis of blood. This further reduces venous return to the heart and decreases cardiac output.

Intestinal anoxia destroys the selective absorption properties of the intestinal wall. Bacterial toxins, especially endotoxins, may be absorbed into the circulation where they both potentiate and initiate shock. The reticuloendothelial system, ordinarily the primary defense system against bacterial infections, is of little help in this case since it is impaired by the toxins.

In canines the intestine appears to be an important organ in the pathogenesis of shock. Intestinal lesions have been attributed to prolonged vasoconstriction and thrombus formation in omental and intestinal mucosal vessels. Blood and serum are lost in the intestinal lumen, resulting in a decrease in total blood volume, venous return, and cardiac output.

In the liver anoxia may cause focal necrosis and hemorrhage, but the loss of detoxifying properties of the liver is an important factor in irreversible shock. The liver is a central focus for gluconeogenesis, glycolysis, destruction or neutralization of vasodepressant factors and endotoxins, and removal of fibrin products from the circulation.

Anoxia is thought to be responsible for injury at the cellular level in shock (Fig. 6.2). A decreased supply of oxygen causes the cell to switch from aerobic or mitochondrial respiration to anaerobic metabolism. Increased anaerobic metabolism increases the cellular utilization of glucose and causes a build-up of lactic and pyruvic acids that decrease the cellular and blood pH leading to acidosis (Wendt and Saunders, 1973; William, 1976). Decreased tissue perfusion potentiates cellular acidosis by depriving the cell of buffering systems in the blood. Cellular acidosis damages nuclear and cellular membranes, causing pyknosis and cellular swelling. Damage to lysosomal membranes due to acidosis allows hydrolytic enzymes to flow into the cytoplasm, resulting in damage to other cellular organelles (Bitensky et al., 1963; Janoff et al., 1962). In mitochondria anaerobic metabolism decreases the production of high-energy adenosine triphosphate (ATP). Mitochondria initially condense and then begin to swell (Trump et al., 1972).

Adenosine triphosphate is also an essential energy source for the cellular ionic pump. Without energy for maintaining physiological ionic equilibrium, sodium and calcium flow from the surrounding fluid into cells; and potassium flows from the cell cytoplasm into the tissue fluids. The osmolality of the cytoplasm increases, and fluids flow into the cytoplasm. Ionic and fluid changes in the cytoplasm cause cell swelling, dilatation of the endoplasmic reticulum, detachment of ribosomes from rough endoplasmic reticulum, and polysome dispersion. Calcium influx into mitochondria causes the formation of electron dense deposits. In anoxic skeletal muscle cells a calcium influx causes muscle tremors that increase energy needs and potentiate cellular acidosis.

Hormones. Hormones also apparently play a role in cellular energy metabolism in shock (Shoemaker, 1972). Adrenal glucocorticoids increase hepatic glycolysis and gluconeogenesis and are responsible for the elevated blood glucose levels and for the decrease in hepatic glycogen in early shock. As shock progresses, blood glucose levels decline, and hypoglycemia occurs (Filkins and Cornell, 1974; Green et al., 1939; Parratt and Sturgess 1975). Serum insulin levels are increased in shock, but for some reason skeletal muscles in shock are refractory to insulin (Blackard et al., 1976; Wolfe et al., 1976). It has been conjectured that this may be a physiological mechanism to conserve glucose for vital organs such as the brain.

SIGNS, PATHOLOGY, AND DIAGNOSIS. Classical clinical signs of shock are similar in most species of animals and consist of increased heart rate, increased respiratory rate, reduction or absence of pulse pressure, pale mucous membranes, decreased body temperature, dilated pupils, muscular weakness, mental depression, and decreased urine production (McDonnell, 1974). Detailed clinical signs of shock vary with the stage of shock, type of shock, species involved, and

SELF-PERPETUATING AND COMPENSATORY VASCULAR FEATURES OF SHOCK

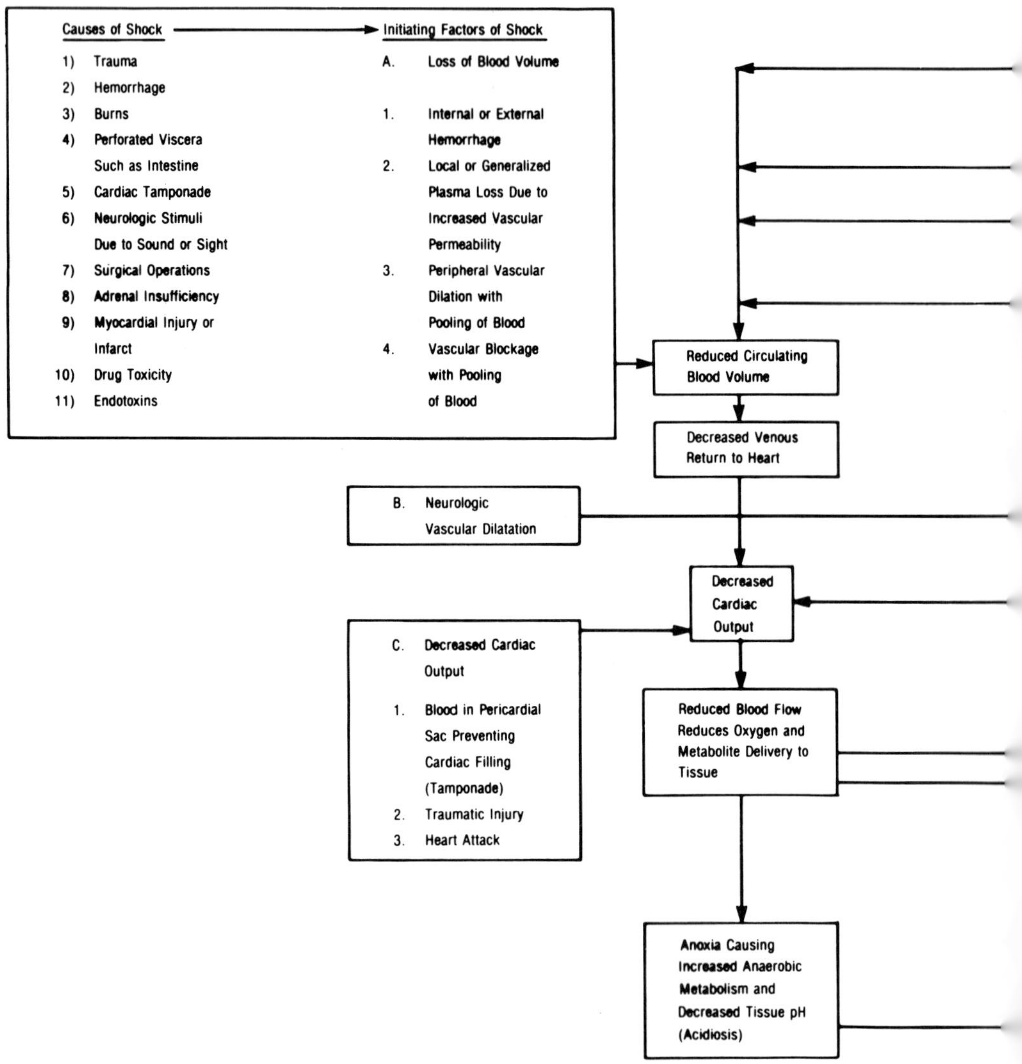

Fig. 6.1.

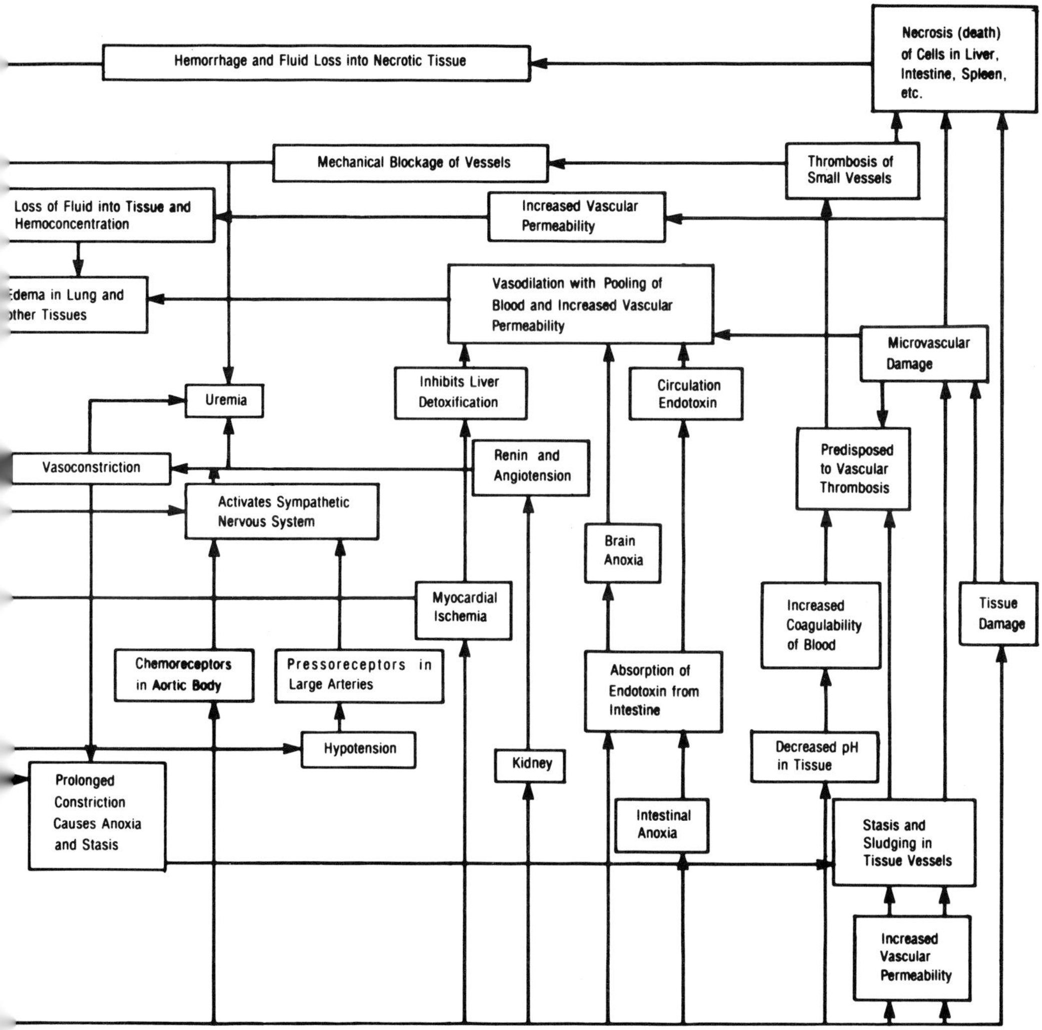
Necrosis (death) of Cells in Liver, Intestine, Spleen, etc.
Hemorrhage and Fluid Loss into Necrotic Tissue
Mechanical Blockage of Vessels
Thrombosis of Small Vessels
Loss of Fluid into Tissue and Hemoconcentration
Increased Vascular Permeability
Edema in Lung and other Tissues
Vasodilation with Pooling of Blood and Increased Vascular Permeability
Microvascular Damage
Uremia
Inhibits Liver Detoxification
Circulation Endotoxin
Vasoconstriction
Renin and Angiotension
Predisposed to Vascular Thrombosis
Activates Sympathetic Nervous System
Brain Anoxia
Myocardial Ischemia
Increased Coagulability of Blood
Tissue Damage
Chemoreceptors in Aortic Body
Pressoreceptors in Large Arteries
Absorption of Endotoxin from Intestine
Hypotension
Kidney
Decreased pH in Tissue
Prolonged Constriction Causes Anoxia and Stasis
Intestinal Anoxia
Stasis and Sludging in Tissue Vessels
Increased Vascular Permeability

PATHOGENIC SEQUENCE OF SHOCK AT THE CELLULAR AND BIOCHEMICAL LEVELS

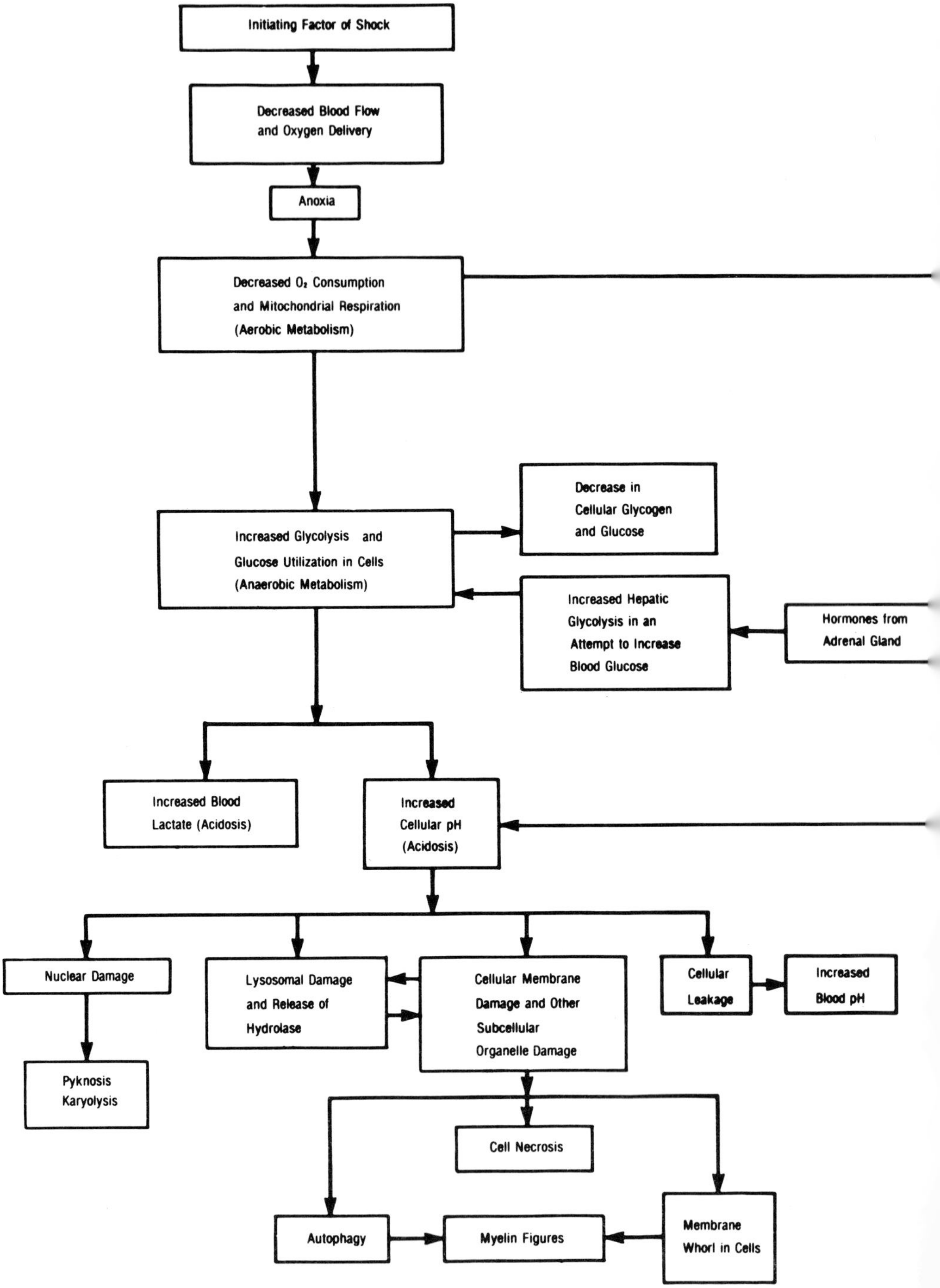

Fig. 6.2.

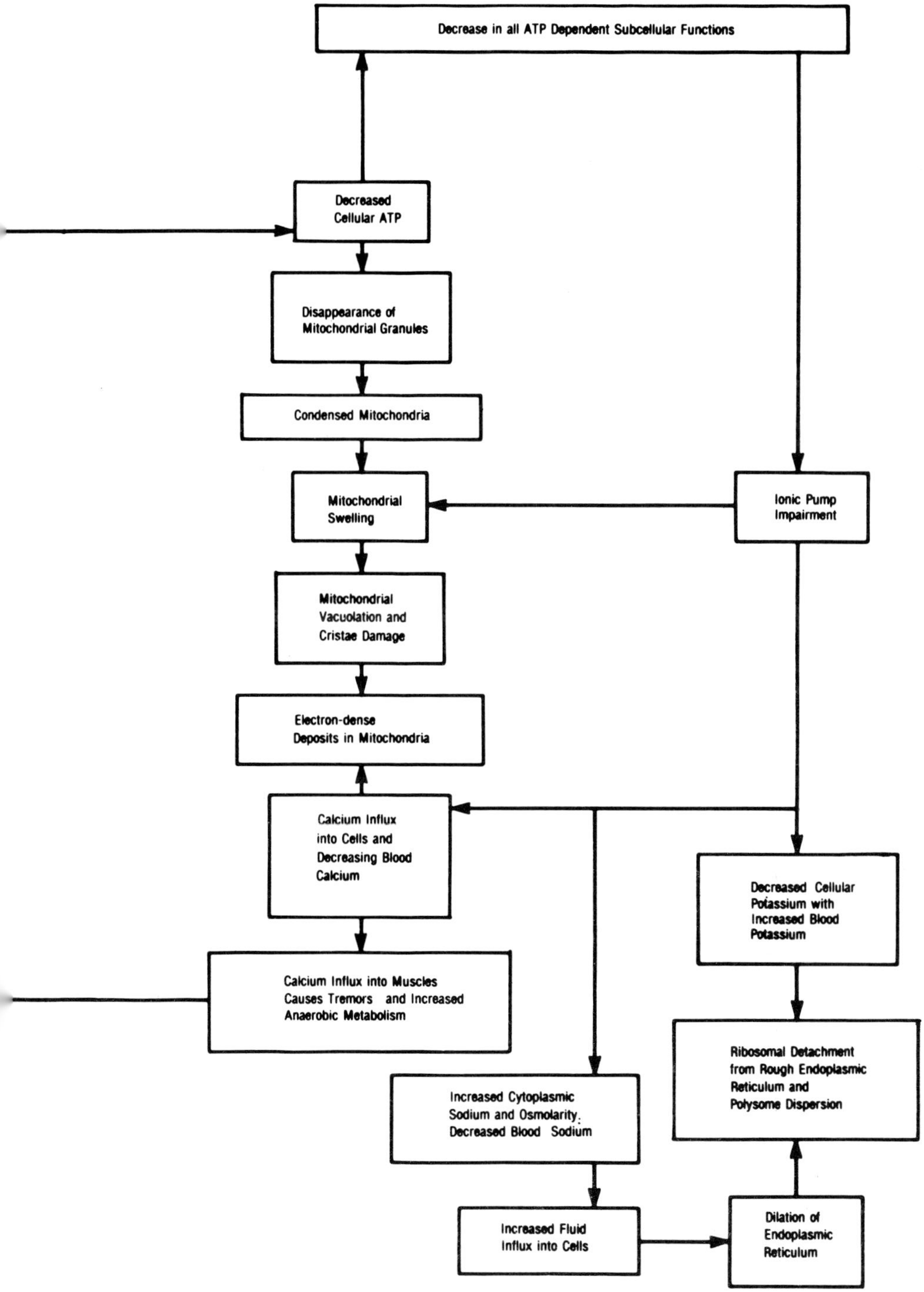
Decrease in all ATP Dependent Subcellular Functions
Decreased Cellular ATP
Disappearance of Mitochondrial Granules
Condensed Mitochondria
Mitochondrial Swelling
Ionic Pump Impairment
Mitochondrial Vacuolation and Cristae Damage
Electron-dense Deposits in Mitochondria
Calcium Influx into Cells and Decreasing Blood Calcium
Decreased Cellular Potassium with Increased Blood Potassium
Calcium Influx into Muscles Causes Tremors and Increased Anaerobic Metabolism
Ribosomal Detachment from Rough Endoplasmic Reticulum and Polysome Dispersion
Increased Cytoplasmic Sodium and Osmolarity. Decreased Blood Sodium
Increased Fluid Influx into Cells
Dilation of Endoplasmic Reticulum

other contributing or initiating factors. For example, in domestic ruminants atony of the rumen may be the first indication of shock. In wild animals muscular weakness, which is manifested by incoordination and/or inability to fight or flee effectively, may be the first indication of shock. In other animals, such as the snowshoe hare, abnormal behavior may be the first indication of impending shock, for example, stopping to eat instead of running when released or increased appetite with reduced wariness (Adams, 1959).

As shock progresses, the animal's response to such external stimuli as noise becomes sluggish, and somnolence occurs. Although an animal does not respond to noises, it probably hears them (if it is like a human in shock); and loud noises or other neurologic stimuli may potentiate the condition of shock. In terminal shock, brain anoxia depresses the vital respiratory and cardiac centers, and death ensues.

During and after capture, trauma, hemorrhage, and loss of body fluids are important indicators, initiators, and potentiators of shock. Hemorrhage from lacerations is relatively easy to evaluate or even overestimate in some situations. Hemorrhage into body cavities following traumatic rupture of the spleen, liver, or aorta is difficult and sometimes impossible to assess. Centesis of a body cavity to substantiate internal hemorrhage may be impractical, especially in larger wild animals. Even more difficult to evaluate clinically is the amount of blood or fluid loss into traumatized or burned tissues.

Although external clinical signs may suggest shock, the cardiovascular system must be evaluated before shock can be diagnosed. Heart and pulse rates are increased in shock, but in wild animals the stress of capture or handling also increases the heart rate. Decreased blood pressure is the primary decisive factor in human and experimental shock evaluation. But in wild animals blood pressure measurements are usually impractical or even impossible, although some newer cuff techniques for measuring blood pressure are being used on dogs (Spangler et al., 1977; Weiser et al., 1977).

The rate and quality of pulses in the major arteries of the head, neck, and legs are the best indices of blood pressure in wild animals. For example, in dogs a strong full femoral pulse indicates the blood pressure is greater than 100 mm of mercury. A weak, thready, nonfull pulse or decreased difference between systolic and diastolic pressure suggests hypotension and shock. If the femoral pulse is not palpable in the dog, the blood pressure is less than 60 mm of mercury and inadequate blood is flowing through body organs to sustain the animal (Stickles, 1976a).

Other clinical indices of shock are pallor of the mucous membranes, decreased blood flow through small peripheral vessels, decreased urine and tear production, and decreased body and skin temperature. Skin and especially the mucous membranes of animals in shock are pale, cold, and somewhat moist; however, if an animal has been chased, the skin may be warm and moist. If digital pressure is applied temporarily to the oral mucous membranes, the blanched area disappears slowly in shocked animals due to decreased blood pressure and the action of adrenal hormones that decrease blood flow through these vessels. In normal animals color returns to digitally induced blanched areas on the mucous membranes within two to three seconds. In severe shock the tongue will be pale and shriveled due to reduced peripheral blood pressure and a concomitant shift of tissue fluids into vessels. Tear production is decreased in severe shock, and the eyes appear dry and sunken. Urine production is decreased because blood is shunted to more vital organs, such as the heart and brain (Stickles, 1976a).

In hemorrhagic shock the PCV may be decreased. Several hours after hemorrhage, tissue fluids shift into the vascular system and decrease the PCV as the body attempts to compensate for the loss of total blood volume. In shock initiated by burns, fluids move from vessels into damaged tissues and the PCV increases. Arterial oxygen tension is usually near normal unless the lungs are traumatized. Blood acid-base and carbon dioxide analyses usually reveal a moderate metabolic acidosis, which is caused by increased anaerobic metabolism and decreased renal circulation. This is partially compensated by a mild respiratory alkalosis of hyperventilation. Serum sodium and chloride levels are decreased, while potassium levels are elevated. Hypoglycemia and elevated BUN are common in shocked animals (Adams, 1959; Guthrie et al., 1967; Hoff et al., 1976; Iversen et al., 1972).

Specific factors associated with the general condition of the animal, such as malnutrition, dehydration, or exhaustion, and environmental factors, such as heat, cold, or high humidity, are not essential features of shock; but they may potentiate mechanisms causing circulatory collapse in shock and must be considered when capturing a wild animal. Tranquilizers or anesthetics, barbiturates particularly, used for capture may cause pooling of blood and hypotension; may depress respiration, especially in prolonged usage or when an animal is overdosed; and may secondarily potentiate shock in captured animals (Stickles, 1976b).

Gross lesions at necropsy are usually not specific enough to make a diagnosis, but they may contribute to a diagnosis if clinical evidence is considered in the overall evaluation. Diffuse congestion, multiple focal hemorrhages, and edema accompanied by ischemia of the peripheral parts of the body, such as the skin, are the predominant lesions observed. Organs containing the majority of these lesions depend upon initiating factors, that is, hemorrhage, trauma, endotoxin, and so on, and the species involved in shock. For example, in the dog the liver and intestines are the "shock organs." The liver is diffusely congested, and the intestines are congested and hemorrhagic. In sheep, monkey, cow, cat, rabbit, guinea pig, and mouse the lung is the predominant organ grossly involved in shock, while the intestine is the "shock organ" in the rat (Hsu, 1976). Scattered subepicardial hemorrhages are present in most animals in shock, and multiple hemorrhages may be present in the adrenal gland.

Focal areas of cellular necrosis and degeneration, organelle degeneration, and hemorrhage have been described histologically and ultrastructurally in several tissues. Myocardial zonal lesions have been described in the myocardial fibers of cats, pigs, dogs, and human hearts (Chang and Hackel, 1973).

In acute shock, capillary congestion, atelectasis, and intraalveolar hemorrhage and edema are present in histological sections of the lung. In animals surviving for two or three days, focal areas of alveolar cell hyperplasia, interstitial edema, and early fibrosis are apparent (Ratliff et al., 1971). Focal areas of cellular degeneration and hemorrhage have been described in the liver, kidney, intestine, and central nervous system (Chang and Hackel, 1973; Russo and Conforti, 1977). Thrombosed vessels can frequently be detected in the small capillaries of most organs (Garner et al., 1974).

SIMILAR CLINICAL DISEASES. Several diseases should be considered before making a diagnosis of shock: overdose of capture drug, capture myopathy, heat stress, porcine stress–like syndrome, hypoglycemia, and water deprivation or salt toxicity. Determining that an animal has been given too much drug due to an error in calculation or in estimating the animal's weight may be difficult in some instances. Capture myopathy is described in Chapter 9.

Heatstroke. Heatstroke or heat stress is a very poorly characterized syndrome in wild and domestic animals (Hickey and Kelly, 1972; Krum and Osborne, 1977). Although some animals have unique ways of tolerating increased body temperatures (Dawson, 1977), most animals cannot tolerate an increase of a few degrees in body temperature. It has been estimated that for every 1° C increase in body temperature the animal's basal metabolism increases by 10 to 20% (Andersson, 1970).

Clinical signs of heatstroke include elevated body temperature, panting and/or sweating, congested mucous membranes, vomiting, stupor, lack of response to stimuli such as noise, coma, and even death. Dilatation of cutaneous vessels decreases venous return to the heart; the pulse is weak, similar to that observed in shock (Krum and Osborne, 1977). The increased body temperature causes necrosis of cells throughout the body, that is, liver, kidney, and muscle. Release of enzymes from necrotic muscle elevates serum enzymes in a manner similar to that observed in capture myopathy. Hemorrhages occur throughout the bodies of some animals, and blood coagulates in the vascular system as reported in shock.

Porcine Stress-like Syndrome. Porcine stress syndrome, or malignant hyperthermia, is a disease of pigs prominent in Poland China, Landrace, and Pietrain breeds (Johansson and Jönsson, 1977; Nelson et al., 1976). Susceptibility appears to be controlled by a dominant gene and has been reported in cats, dogs, and horses (Bagshaw et al., 1978). The syndrome occurs in susceptible pigs after exposure to a variety of stresses, such as crowding during transport, high humidity, fighting, emotional excitement, and physical exertion, and is clinically similar in many ways to shock and capture myopathy observed in wild animals. General anesthetic agents such as halothane and muscle relaxants such as succinylcholine also will induce the syndrome.

Initial clinical signs of an impending stress syndrome are rapid muscular tremors that progress into muscular rigidity. Body temperature rises rapidly after muscle tremors begin, and the heart beats rapidly and irregularly. Alternating blanched and hyperemic areas are present on the skin. Affected pigs frequently die quickly with clinical evidence of heart failure, and rigor mortis develops rapidly. At necropsy the muscular pH may drop as low as 5. Carcass temperature is increased and falls slowly. Cardiac muscles and skeletal muscles throughout the body, particularly those in the hindlimb, are pale and soft.

Evidence suggests the primary lesion may be due to a metabolic defect in skeletal muscles. Colorimeter studies indicate that metabolism in susceptible resting pigs may be five times normal and may be even higher in exercised animals. Serum lactic acid, potassium, and creatine phosphokinase levels are elevated. Muscle pH and ATP content are decreased, and lactate content is increased.

Multiple foci of degenerate myofibers are present histologically. Fibers are homogeneous with intervening granular myolytic areas. Ultrastructurally, glycogen granules are decreased in the muscle fiber, and cross-striations are absent. Similar myocardial lesions have been observed in baboons after short periods in captivity (Groover et al., 1963).

Although the significance of a porcine stress–like syndrome as observed in pigs has not been documented in wild animals, capture myopathy and shock are recognized syndromes. Creatine phosphokinase, an enzyme liberated from damaged muscle, may be elevated in all three conditions; and all three may be initiated by forced exercise, stress of capture, and/or transportation. The high incidence of myopathy and shock in some captured species, such as the blackbuck, *Antilope cervicapra,* and snowshoe hare, suggests a genetic predisposition, a similarity to porcine stress syndrome. Differentiation between porcine stress syndrome, shock, and capture myopathy would be difficult or impossible under field conditions. Capture myopathy and a porcine stress–like syndrome could be differentiated in the laboratory on the basis of susceptibility to halothane anesthetics.

Hypoglycemia and Water Deprivation. Hypoglycemia is a condition reported in animals during exercise. Because of poor nutrition, these animals are apparently not able to mobilize their glycogen stores or lack sufficient stored glycogen. When blood glucose levels fall below 30 to 40 mg/100 ml of blood, clonic and tonic convulsions occur. In crocodilians put under stress, hypoglycemia is manifested by pupillary dilatation, followed by muscular tremors, terminating in cataleptic seizures (Wallach, 1971).

Water deprivation or salt toxicity is a syndrome that occurs after an animal has been given access to water following a long period without. Animals may die suddenly or exhibit periods of convulsions.

TREATMENT. The initial therapeutic approach to shock in any animal should include the three following basic procedures: ensure adequate ventilation by establishing a patent air pathway, control all observable hemorrhage, and initiate fluid replacement to ensure an adequate blood volume (Stickles, 1976b). There is no one simple routine to manage all cases of shock encountered in wild animals; therefore, therapy must be modified and tailored to meet the animal's needs and responses to therapy.

Ventilation. During capture and shock inadequate ventilation may result from airway blockage or from injury or trauma to respiratory centers in the brain, thoracic wall, diaphragm, or pulmonary tissue. Good ventilation is essential to promote oxygen and carbon dioxide exchange, to prevent acidosis, and to facilitate heat dissipation. One of the initial signs of an oxygen deficiency may be restlessness and delirium.

An estimation of pulmonary ventilation can be made by observing the rate, depth, sound, and force of respiration. Very rapid, shallow respiration is not an efficient means of moving air in and out of alveoli where oxygen exchange occurs. Abnormal sound caused by air entering and leaving the respiratory system is indicative of an airway blockage. Extensive use of abdominal muscles during expiration may indicate that the diaphragm is injured or ruptured.

Restoring adequate ventilation in delirious wild animals during shock may be dangerous or even impractical and must be approached with caution. A tracheotomy may be a useful procedure in small animals but is impractical in large animals unless they are tranquilized or anesthetized.

Another means of respiratory therapy is oxygen administered via a small tube placed in the nasal cavity. A soft flexible rubber tube coated with a topical anesthetic agent is passed into the nasal cavity and taped to the nose. Oxygen is then administered into the nasal cavity at the rate of 2 to 5 liters per minute, depending on the size of the animal, to meet the animal's need. Oxygen can be humidified by bubbling it through a water-filled container, but this is not necessary under field conditions.

Fluid Therapy. The primary goal of fluid therapy is to restore blood volume and secondarily to correct electrolyte, acid-base, and glucose imbalance. One of the most common errors in shock fluid therapy is to administer too little fluid in the early phases when it is the most beneficial. Transfusion of whole blood is probably the best therapy, especially in hemorrhagic shock; but animals can survive extensive fluid therapy, even though their erythrocyte PCV falls to 16%, if an adequate circulatory volume is maintained (Stickles, 1976b). Several isotonic sterile electrolyte solutions, such as 0.9% sodium chloride, 2.5% dextrose and 0.45% sodium chloride solution, 5% dextrose, Ringer's solution, Ringer's lactate solution, 2.5% dextrose in half strength Ringer's lactate, or 2.5% dextran 40 in Ringer's solution may be used in shock therapy (Benjamin, 1978).

An isotonic, balanced electrolyte solution, such as Ringer's lactate, is usually the fluid of choice. Circulatory support from balanced electrolyte solutions lasts 40 to 60 minutes, and only about 17% of the fluid is still in the circulation after 2 hours. The addition of 2.5% dextran 40 to the fluid will prolong vascular retention. Sodium bicarbonate can be incorporated into the solutions to combat acidosis, although the best way to correct acidosis in shock is to improve tissue perfusion so the lungs and kidneys can function.

Other drugs frequently included in shock therapy are steroids, antibiotics, glucose, heparin, vasodilators, vasoconstrictors, and cardiac stimulators. Although the use of steroids in shock is controversial (Wilson, 1976), most animals appear to respond better when pharmacologic doses of corticosteroids are used during therapy (Balis et al., 1978; Corwin et al., 1973; Schuler et al., 1976). Two steroids used intravenously are methylprednisolone sodium succinate at 30 mg/kg of body weight and prednisolone sodium succinate at 40 mg/kg of body weight. Glucose or dextrose are beneficial ingredients of shock fluid therapy, especially in the snowshoe hare and gray squirrel (Archer et al., 1976).

Antibiotics are added to prevent secondary infections. Heparin helps prevent vascular thrombosis in shock, but it also may increase the amount of blood lost by hemorrhage into injured tissues. Vasodilators such as chlorpromazine, vasoconstrictors such as norepinephrine, and cardiac stimulants such as dopamine are used only when the animal's response can be monitored closely.

Anesthetic agents, narcotics, and tranquilizers should never be given to animals in shock. Most drugs depress cardiovascular and respiratory function and should be used only after a risk-benefit assessment has been made. For example, the vasodilatory activity of phenothiazine tranquilizers (adrenergic blocking agents) may cause severe and rapid decline in blood pressure, especially in shocked patients who have a minimal or nonexistent cardiovascular reserve.

PREVENTION. Prevention is the best means of shock therapy in wild animals and begins with a well-planned capture and continues through acclimatization of the animal in its new environment. Capture, restraint, and transport techniques for individual species of animals are scattered throughout the literature (Braker, 1974; Fowler, 1974a,b; Lubbock, 1974; Van Den Sande, 1974; Young, 1973). The primary goal of good capture techniques is to minimize stress. Tranquilizers administered by a blowgun (Haigh and Hopf, 1976) have their maximum effect if given to undisturbed animals, and the drug used depends upon the species being captured (Custer et al., 1977; King et al., 1977; Roughton, 1975; Smuts, 1973; Young, 1973). After the animal has been captured, sight and noise stimuli can be minimized by blindfolding the animal, putting cotton in its ears, and working quietly. Animals should be transported with a minimum of handling to nearby holding facilities where they can be acclimatized prior to shipment (Seago, 1974).

Great care should be taken to prepare a shipping cage. The floor surface should support the animal when standing, but it should be smooth enough for it to be comfortable when lying down. Cages must protect the animals from the heat of the sun and drafts and have adequate ventilation but be constructed in such a way that the animal cannot injure itself. The International Air Transport Association (1970) has published a guide describing a variety of transportation cages and crates.

Requirements for food and water for animals in transit vary and can be supplied by an attendant traveling with them (Fowler, 1974a,b). For example, hummingbirds require a constant food supply, while some ungulates do not need food on a trip less than 24 hours long. All animals need water at least every 12 hours, and many will refuse to eat or drink from a strange container. After an animal has been placed in its new environment, the shipping cage should be left with the animal. If the animal has been shipped for a long distance over an extended time, the cage may serve as a source of refuge for a few days.

REFERENCES

Adams, L. 1959. An analysis of a population of snowshoe hares in northwestern Montana. Ecol. Monogr. 29:141–170.

Andersson, B. E. 1970. Temperature regulation and environmental physiology. In M. J. Swenson. Dukes' physiology of domestic animals. 8th ed. Cornell Univ. Press, Ithaca.

Archer, L. T., B. Benjamin, M. M. Lane, and L. B. Hinshaw. 1976. Renal gluconeogenesis and increased glucose utilization in shock. Am. J. Physiol. 231:872–879.

Bagshaw, R. J., R. H. Cox, D. H. Knight, and D. K. Detweiler. 1978. Malignant hyperthermia in a greyhound. J. Am. Vet. Med. Assoc. 172:61–62.

Balis, J. V., E. S. Rappaport, L. Gerber, J. Fareed, F. Buddingh, and H. L. Messmore. 1978. A primate model for prolonged endotoxin shock: Blood-vascular reactions and effects of glucocorticoid treatment. Lab. Invest. 38:511–523.

Benjamin, M. M. 1978. Outline of veterinary clinical pathology. 3rd ed. Iowa State Univ. Press, Ames.

Berman, I. R. 1972. The lung lesion in shock. In L. B. Hinshaw and B. G. Cox. The fundamental mechanisms of shock. Plenum Press, New York.

Bitensky, L., J. Chayen, G. J. Cunningham, and J. Fine. 1963. Behaviour of lysosomes in haemorrhagic shock. Nature 199:493–494.

Blackard, W. G., J. H. Anderson, and J. J. Spitzer. 1976. Hyperinsulinism in endotoxin shock in dogs. Metabolism 25:675–684.

Blair, M. L., E. O. Feigl, and O. A. Smith. 1976. Elevation of plasma renin activity during avoidance performance in baboons. Am. J. Physiol. 231:772–776.

Braker, W. P. 1974. Collection and transport of Caribbean marine fishes. Int. Zoo Yearbook 14:40–43.

Chang, J., and D. B. Hackel. 1973. Comparative study of myocardial lesions in hemorrhagic shock. Lab. Invest. 28:641–647.

Cheville, N. F. 1976. Cell pathology. Iowa State Univ. Press, Ames.

Churcher, C. S., C. R. Harington, B. Lawrence, and J. L. Paradiso. 1973. Adrenocortical response to captivity in *Microtus pennsylvanicus.* J. Mammal. 54: 779–781.

Coalson, J. J., L. B. Hinshaw, and C. A. Guenter. 1970. The pulmonary ultrastructure in septic shock. Exp. Mol. Pathol. 12:84–103.

Collins, R. L. 1972. Auditory seizures. In D. P. Purpura, J. K. Penry, D. B. Tower, D. M. Woodbury, and R. D. Walter. Experimental models of epilepsy: A manual for the laboratory worker. Raven Press, New York.

Corwin, D. S., G. D. Bottoms, and O. F. Roesel. 1973. Distribution of 3H-hydrocortisone in dogs with hemorrhagic shock. Am. J. Vet. Res. 34:1015–1019.

Custer, R., L. Kramer, S. Kennedy, and M. Bush. 1977. Hematologic effects of xylazine when used for restraint of Bactrian camels. J. Am. Vet. Med. Assoc. 171:899–901.

Dawson, T. J. 1977. Kangaroos. Sci. Am. 237:78–89.

Emerson, T. E., Jr. 1972. Participation of endogenous vasoactive agents in the pathogenesis of endotoxin shock. In L. B. Hinshaw and B. G. Cox. The fundamental mechanisms of shock. Plenum Press, New York.

Filkins J. P., and R. P. Cornell. 1974. Depression of hepatic gluconeogenesis and the hypoglycemia of endotoxin shock. Am. J. Physiol. 227:778–781.

Fletcher, G. L. 1975. The effect of capture, "stress," and storage of whole blood on the red blood cells, plasma proteins, glucose and electrolytes of the winter flounder (*Pseudopleuronectes americanus*). Can. J. Zool. 53:197–206.

Fowler, M. E. 1974a. Restraint and anesthesia in zoo animal practice. J. Am. Vet. Med. Assoc. 164:706–711.

______. 1974b. Veterinary aspects of restraint and transport of wild animals. Int. Zoo Yearbook 14:28–33.

Garner, R., B. V. Chater, and D. L. Brown. 1974. The role of complement in endotoxin shock and disseminated intravascular coagulation: Experimental observations in the dog. Br. J. Haematol. 28:393–401.

Green, R. G., C. L. Larson, and J. F. Bell. 1939. Shock disease as the cause of the periodic decimation of the snowshoe hare. Am. J. Hyg. 30:83–102.

Gronow, V. G. 1974. Uber die Belastung von *Idus idus* L., Teleostei, durch Fang Narkose und experimentelle Umgelring. [Stress in *Idus idus* L., Teleostei, due to capture, anesthesia, and experimental environment.] Zool. Anz Jena 193:17–34.

Groover, M. E., E. L. Seljeskog, J. T. Haglin, and C. R. Hitchcock. 1963. Myocardial infarction in Kenya baboons without demonstrable atherosclerosis. Angiology 14:409–416.

Guthrie, D. R., J. C. Osborne, and H. S. Mosby. 1967. Physiological changes associated with shock in confined gray squirrels. J. Wildl. Manage. 31:102–108.

Haigh, J. C., and H. C. Hopf. 1976. The blowgun in veterinary practice: Its uses and preparation. J. Am. Vet. Med. Assoc. 169:881–883.

Hattingh, J., and A. J. J. Van Pletzen. 1974. The influence of capture and transportation on some blood parameters of fresh water fish. Comp. Biochem. Physiol. 49A:607–609.

Hickey, T. E., and W. A. Kelly. 1972. Heatstroke in a colony of squirrel monkeys. J. Am. Vet. Med. Assoc. 161:700–702.

Hoff, G. L., L. E. McEldowny, W. J. Bigler, L. J. Kuhns, and J. A. Tomas. 1976. Blood and urinary values in the gray squirrel. J. Wildl. Dis. 12:349–352.

Hohenboken, W. D., and G. Nellhaus. 1970. Inheritance of audiogenic seizures in the rabbit. J. Hered. 61: 107–112.

Hsu, C. K. 1976. Immunology. In E. C. Melby, Jr., and N. H. Altaman. Handbook of laboratory animal science. Vol. 3. CRC Press, Inc., Cleveland.

International Air Transport Association. 1970. International live animal manual. 2nd ed. Int. Air Transport Assoc., 1155 Mansfield Street, Montreal, 113 P. Q., Canada.

Iversen, J. O., G. L. Hoff, T. M. Yuill, and R. P. Hanson. 1972. Gastric lesions in the snowshoe hare. J. Wildl. Dis. 8:7–9.

Janoff, A., G. Weissmann, B. W. Zweifoch, and L. Thomas. 1962. Pathogenesis of experimental shock. IV. Studies of lysosomes in normal and tolerant animals subjected to lethal trauma and endotoxemia. J. Exp. Med. 16:451–466.

Johansson, G., and L. Jönsson. 1977. Myocardial cell damage in the porcine stress syndrome. J. Comp. Pathol. 87:67–74.

King, J. M., C. R. Brian, M. A. Bertram, and P. H. Hamilton. 1977. Tiletamine and zolazepam for immobilization of wild lions and leopards. J. Am. Vet. Med. Assoc. 171:894–898.

Krum, S. H., and C. A. Osborne. 1977. Heatstroke in the dog: A polysystemic disorder. J. Am. Vet. Med. Assoc. 170:531–535.

Lubbock, M. R. 1974. Capture and transport of waterfowl. Int. Zoo Yearbook 14:61–63.

Lundgren, O., V. Haglung, O. Isaksson, and A. Tetsuo. 1976. Effects on myocardial contractility of bloodborne material released from the feline small intestine in simulated shock. Circ. Res. 38:307–315.

Maura, G., A. G. Vaccari, A. Gemignani, and F. Cugurra. 1974. Development of monoamine oxidase activity after chronic environmental stress in the rat. Environ. Physiol. Biochem. 4:64–79.

McCarty, R., and J. Richardson. 1974. Adrenal response of male mice to variations in living space. Physiol. Rep. 34:787–790.

McDonnell, W. 1974. The clinical diagnosis of shock. J. Small Anim. Pract. 15:293–301.

Naquet, R., and B. S. Meldrum. 1972. Photogenic seizures in baboons. In D. P. Purpura, J. K. Penry, D. B. Tower, D. M. Woodbury, and R. D. Walter.

Experimental models of epilepsy: A manual for the laboratory worker. Raven Press, New York.

Nelson, T. E., E. W. Jones, and I. L. Anderson. 1976. Porcine malignant hyperthermia. Am. J. Pathol. 84:197–199.

Parratt, J. R., and R. M. E. Sturgess. 1975. *E. coli* endotoxin shock in the cat: Treatment with indomethacin. Br. J. Pharm. 53:485–488.

Ratliff, N. B., J. W. Wilson, E. Mikat, D. B. Hackel, and T. C. Graham. 1971. The lung in hemorrhagic shock. IV. The role of neutrophilic polymorphonuclear leukocytes. Am. J. Pathol. 65:325–334.

Roughton, R. D. 1975. Xylazine as an immobilizing agent for captive white-tailed deer. J. Am. Vet. Med. Assoc. 167:574–576.

Russo, M. A., and A. Conforti. 1977. Subcellular reactions to injury. I. Ultrastructural and biochemical investigations on the hepatic cellular damage produced by hemorrhagic shock in dogs. J. Pathol. 121:107–113.

Schuler, J. J., P. R. Erve, and W. Schumer. 1976. Effect of glucocorticoids on carbohydrate metabolism and survival of endotoxin-shocked monkeys. Ann. Surg. 183:345–354.

Seago, J. 1974. Responsibilities of an animal catcher. Int. Zoo Yearbook 14:39–40.

Shoemaker, W. C. 1972. Physiological mechanisms in clinical shock. In L. B. Hinshaw and B. G. Cox. The fundamental mechanisms of shock. Plenum Press, New York.

Smuts, G. L. 1973. Xylazine hydrochloride (Rompun) and the new retractable-barbed dart ("drop-out" dart) for the capture of some nervous and aggressive antelope species. Koedoe 16:159–178.

Stickles, L. E., Jr. 1976a. Shock: Part 2—Assessment and monitoring of the shock patient. Canine Pract. 3(1):43–49.

______. 1976b. Shock: Part 3—Treatment of the shock patient. Canine Pract. 3(2):12–42.

Trump, B. F., B. P. Croker, and W. J. Mergner. 1972. The role of energy metabolism, ion and water shift in the pathogenesis of cell injury. In G. W. Richter and D. G. Scarpelli. Cell membrane. Williams & Wilkins, Baltimore.

Tucker, D. 1973. Rapid decline of olfactory and gustatory receptor sensitivity of wild catfish (Ictaluridae), after capture. J. Fish Res. Board Can. 30:1243–1245.

Van Den Sande, A. P. 1974. The long-distance transport of fishes and aquatic invertebrates. Int. Zoo Yearbook 14:43–44.

Wallach, J. D. 1971. Diseases of reptiles and their clinical management. In R. W. Kirk. Current veterinary therapy. IV. Small animal practice. W. B. Saunders, Philadelphia.

Weil, M. H., and H. Shubin. 1972. Proposed reclassification of shock states with special reference to distributive effects. In L. B. Hinshaw and B. G. Cox. The fundamental mechanisms of shock. Plenum Press, New York.

Weiser, M. G., W. L. Spangler, and D. H. Gribble. 1977. Blood pressure measurement in the dog. J. Am. Vet. Med. Assoc. 171:364–368.

Wendt, C. A. G., and R. L. Saunders. 1973. Changes in carbohydrate metabolism in young Atlantic salmon in response to various forms of stress. Int. Atlantic Salmon Found. Spec. Pub. Ser. 4:55–82.

William, S. 1976. Metabolism during shock and sepsis. Heart Lung 5:416–421.

Wilson R. F. 1976. The diagnosis and management of severe sepsis and septic shock. Heart Lung 5:422–429.

Wolfe, R. K., J. J. Spitzer, H. L. Miller, and D. Elahi. 1976. Effect of insulin infusion on glucose kinetics in normal and burned guinea pigs. Life Sci. 19:147–155.

Young, E., ed. 1973. The capture and care of wild animals. Human and Rousseau, Pretoria.

7 Stress and Diseases of the Cardiovascular System

R. N. T. W. FIENNES

ECOLOGISTS are in general agreement that there are fewer deaths from disease among wild populations than among captive animals, except at times when population numbers become excessive. At such times, epidemics may occur. Normally inactive commensal organisms or parasites may come to induce disease in stress circumstances. On such occasions, the underlying cause of the increased susceptibility is stress acting on the endocrine, circulatory, and other systems, especially the reproductive and immune mechanisms. Apart from accidents to young animals and predation, stress acting on the cardiovascular system is possibly the most important mechanism for population control, and in this sense, is a natural phenomenon.

The social structure of a population can influence the degree of stress to which an individual is subjected. Animals at the lower end of the pecking order, the subordinates, tend to be permanently stressed as revealed by enlarged adrenal glands, whereas the dominant individuals live in a relatively unstressed state. This means that when stress conditions prevail, the first to succumb to predation, malnutrition, or disease will be the subordinates. A high proportion of animals trapped by collectors probably are subordinates. This may explain why so many newly captured animals, more than 50% in many cases, fail to survive. Once animals have become accustomed to new surroundings, their high susceptibility to stress seems to diminish, but it is easily resurrected. Signs of stress may recur if animals are moved to new quarters, even ones with improved conditions. The den or cage represents security, and its removal represents a threat and a new stressing factor. Much is known of the circumstances and results of stress, but little of its mechanisms, though reasons are given below for supposing it to be a state of chronic hypotension.

ETIOLOGY. Selye (1950) has characterized stress as the general adaptation syndrome (GAS). He likens stress to inflammation, regarding inflammation as a local reaction to trauma and stress as a general reaction. The forms of trauma involved may be psychological, physical injury, disease, or exposure to adverse conditions. The three stages of the general adaptation syndrome are defined below.

The Alarm Reaction (AR). In its uncomplicated forms, the AR is purely physiological and corresponds to the fear/flight reaction. Ultimately it can cause death from circulatory failure. The primary stimulus to the hypothalamic area of the brain is transmitted by way of the sympathetic nervous system. Epinephrine secretion is increased and this enhances the direct sympathetic effect. The heart rate is increased and digestive processes are reduced. Arteries become constricted, except to the heart and muscles where they are dilated. The respiratory rate increases, hairs become erected, and sugar is mobilized from reserves.

At the same time, impulses from the hypothalamus shift the emphasis in production of pituitary hormones. The hormones acting on the sex glands are diminished in favor of production of adrenocorticotropic hormone (ACTH), which stimulates the adrenal cortex to produce increased amounts of glucocorticoids. If the adrenergic response is frustrated, the response of the glucocorticoids becomes preponderant with results that may be unfavorable. The adrenal cortex may become exhausted and death will ensue because these hormones are essential to life. Such failure may occur in case of extreme fear, as may happen at a time of danger when the escape route is blocked.

The Stage of Resistance (SR). In the SR the adrenergic responses of the AR disappear. As the system adapts to the stressor, the adrenal cortex becomes hypertrophied, maintaining a high output of glucocorticoids and storing greater reserves. In this way, the deleterious action of the stressor is countered and the animal may be seemingly normal. It is, however, in a stressed condition, lacking reserves with which to respond to any enhancement of the stress, whether arising from intensification of the preexisting situation or from superimposition of further stress. In this case, the final, or third, stage of the reaction will occur, the stage of exhaustion. On the other hand, if the stressor is removed, the condition of the animal returns to normal and the adrenal cortex resumes its normal size and appearance. During the SR, behavior patterns tend to be altered, leading to aggressiveness and intraspecific fighting.

The Stage of Exhaustion (SE). When the SE occurs, the adrenal cortex becomes exhausted and the output of corticoids ceases. Death occurs either as a sudden event or following a period of torpor that may last up to five days.

PATHOGENESIS, SIGNS, AND PATHOLOGY.

If death occurs in the AR, it is sudden and due to hypotensive shock. The main feature is a sudden fall of blood pressure accompanied by abdominal hyperemia and a failure of blood return to the heart. The condition appears to be the same as sudden death from anaphylactic shock. This situation is believed to arise because of a sudden relaxation of the powerful muscle present in the tunica adventitia of the abdominal vena cava. The vein becomes so distended that forward movement of the blood no longer occurs. At autopsy, the vessel is seen to be widely distended and filled with blood as far forward as the diaphragm. The thoracic cava, which is elastic and nonmuscular, is empty and the lungs anemic. Pressures of blood in the abdomen lead to hemorrhages in the adrenal cortex, sometimes hemorrhage into the small intestine, and dilatation of the hepatic sinusoids giving a pseudo-nutmeg appearance to the liver, pseudo because it is not due to congestive heart failure.

During the SR the animal is not only at risk from an increase or long duration of the stressor or the introduction of a fresh stressor, it is a sick animal, although temporarily adjusted to the stressing situation. It is during this stage that ulceration of the pylorus often occurs and death may result from this cause. The condition, as with shock, appears to be one of chronic hypotension. It is recognized at autopsy by the great enlargement of the adrenal glands with the cortical cells being packed with secretory granules. The wall of the pylorus may be ulcerated to a greater or lesser extent. Whether ulcerated or not, the wall is covered with viscid mucus.

During this stage there are a number of other changes in metabolism, none of which has been fully studied. The blood is hypercoagulable and intravascular clotting is more likely to occur. There is interference with the production of immunologically competent cells from the bone marrow, lymphatic tissue, and thymus, and the animal is more liable to contract infectious disease or be exposed to flare-up of its own resident pathogens. Thus, the direct cause of death may vary and may not indicate the underlying nature of the condition. This is observed best in herds of animals under stress.

In the SE stage, death may occur as soon as the animal is exposed to the stressor, or the animal may linger in a state of torpor for days. Again, the condition appears to be mainly hypotensive, although hypoglycemia is also described and may be the major or a contributory factor. The condition of animals that survive for days is intriguing. They lie torpid and listless, occasionally stirring themselves to take food or water. If attempts are made to arouse them, the animals become aggressive and then revert to the previous torpid condition. No treatment appears to revive them, although no thorough studies of this aspect have been made. After some days the animals are found dead without any external signs. At autopsy the adrenal glands are found to be small, shrunken, and flaccid, and the cells of the cortex are depleted of secretory material. Other signs are those of hypotension as described above.

Initially the adrenergic reaction is clearly hypertensive, under the influence of catecholamines and the sympathetic nervous system. If escape from the stressor is not achieved, the opposite condition of hypotension results. The acute manifestation of hypotension is known as shock, and rapid death may result. The stages of the stress reaction succeeding the adrenergic reaction have not hitherto been recognized as hypotensive, although postulated by the author and his collaborators as a result of detailed studies of flow mechanisms through the abdominal vena cava.

The anatomy of the posterior vena cava has been studied in detail in relation to structures such as the liver and diaphragm, and the movement of the blood through it has been studied in relation to respiratory movements and intra-abdominal pressures. The key factor that has so far been overlooked is found in the structure of the abdominal section of the posterior vena cava from its origin in the pelvis to the caval foramen, where diaphragmatic muscle and tendon are inserted in the wall (Fig. 7.1).

Throughout this section, there is found in the tunica adventitia a powerful coat of longitudinal smooth muscle (Fig. 7.2). This muscle is normally in tone. During inspiration this section of the vena cava is shortened because of the backward movement of the diaphragm, but without diminution of tension in the vessel because of the shortening of the longitudinal muscle. At the same time, the flow of blood to the thorax is blocked by the closure of the vessel at the caval foramen, which occurs because the vessel passes obliquely through the diaphragm. Thus, in most animals, though not in man, blood flows from abdomen to thorax during expiration and not during inspiration.

The flow depends on two factors: increased abdominal, particularly intrahepatic, pressure during inspiration; and maintenance of muscular

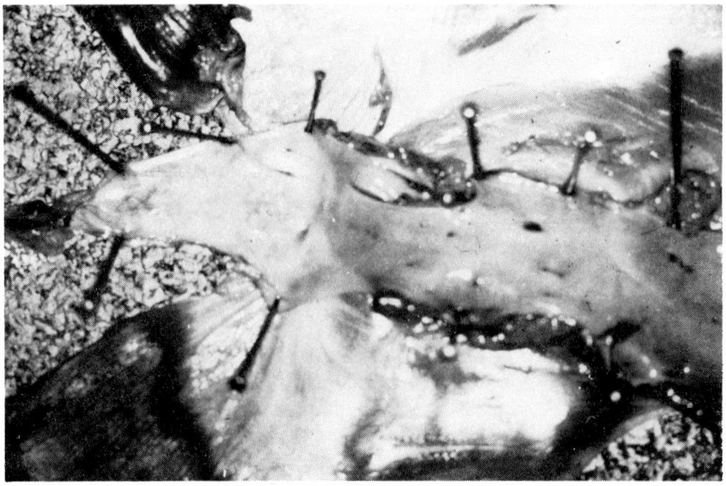

Fig. 7.1. Dissection of the abdominal vena cava of a coati, *Nasua narica.* Note the fleshy nature of the cava wall due to the presence of longitudinal muscle in the tunica adventitia and the insertion of the tendon of the diaphragm into the cava wall.

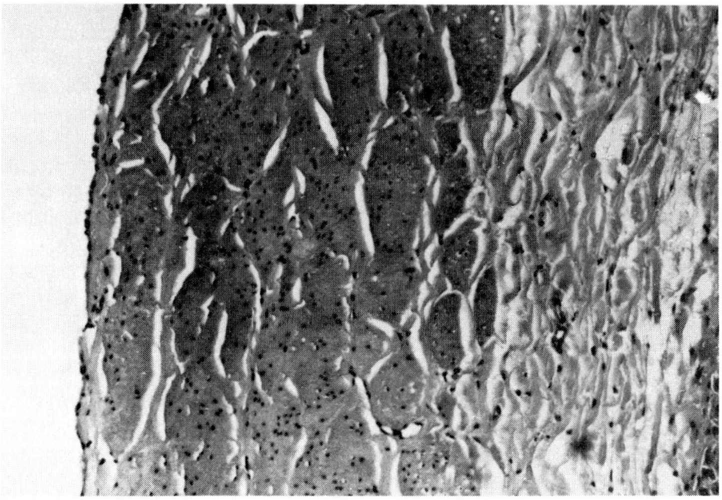

Fig. 7.2. Transverse section of the abdominal vena cava of a chimpanzee, *Pan troglodytes,* showing the interlacing bundles of longitudinal smooth muscle in the tunica adventitia.

tone in the vena cava. Given a constant volume of blood, if the vena cava is narrowed, pressure will decrease but flow velocity will increase. Conversely, if the vena cava is widened, pressure will increase but flow velocity will diminish. In shock, whether due to histamine or anaphylaxis, it was found that the caval muscle was relaxed to such an extent that flow ceased, although cardiac action, as determined by the electrocardiogram, was for a time unimpaired. The action of epinephrine increases the caliber of the vena cava physiologically to admit the flow of a greater volume of blood. Between the extreme of shock and a variable normal function, there can plainly be degrees of dysfunction, and it is this which is believed to occur during the various stages of the stress reaction.

CARDIAC INCOMPETENCE WITHOUT ORGANIC DISEASE OF THE HEART. Sudden death associated with stress or fright is probably commonplace in nature. A large predator, such as a lion, kills its prey quickly and cleanly. On the other hand, small predators are unable to kill large prey in any other way than by eating it alive. By a merciful dispensation the prey will usually die from shock or first-stage stress once escape is hopeless.

A specific study of this point with respect to predation of stoats, *Mustela erminea,* on rabbits, *Oryctolagus cuniculus,* was made (Hewson and Healing, 1971). The mean adult weight of the stoat is 0.2 kg, that of the rabbit 1.4 to 2.0 kg, giving a prey/predator weight ratio of 8:1. Furthermore, the stoat, although it attacks the rabbit very accurately at the base of the neck at the junction of the atlas and axis vertebrae, is unable to inflict mortal wounds on it. Stoats cannot damage the major blood vessels of rabbits in the same way as they do with birds, and it takes them a long time to kill rabbits. This is done by repeated attacks until the victims die of shock brought on by an accumulation of injuries.

The same phenomenon is found in the attacks of canids on large prey, though the reaction of the prey may differ. A bison, *Bison bison,* attacked by a pack of wolves, *Canis lupus,* will fight to the end, unless it manages to escape. The end is the gory and painful fate of being torn to pieces. Other prey, less well equipped to resist, will submit once escape is hopeless. In such cases, death is believed to occur, as with the rabbit attacked by a stoat, from heart failure resulting from shock. A striking instance of this was shown in a film of the Cape hunting dog, *Lycaon pictus,* taken by Jane and Hugo Lawick-Goodall. In this, the dogs were shown attacking Burchell's zebra, *Equus burchelli.* First, the selected victim was isolated from the herd and surrounded by the dogs, one of which succeeded in seizing it by the upper lip. At this point, the zebra continued to fight, lashing out with its hindlimbs and attempting to escape. The other dogs then attacked from the rear attempting to seize the waving tail. When a second dog was successful, the zebra, pulled from front and rear by tail and nose, gave up the fight and subsided to the ground on its flank. It appeared then to succumb to shock.

Immediate or rapid death also commonly occurs in wild animals brought into captivity, though some species are much more susceptible to shock than others. Hares, *Lepus europaeus,* are notoriously difficult to keep alive when captured, since they usually die from shock within two to three days. Bennett's wallabies, *Protemnodon bennetti,* are another highly susceptible group, even when accustomed to captive life. Often catching them and picking them up or removing them to a new enclosure proves fatal.

Instances of deaths from primary shock have been reported by this author in a variety of animals in the Pathologists' Reports published in the Proceedings of the Zoological Society of London between 1960 and 1966. The animals involved have been wallaby; kangaroo, *Macropus* sp.; galago, *Galago* sp.; Burchell's zebra; tiger, *Panthera tigris* (Fig. 7.3); lion, *P. leo;* marmoset, *Callithrix* sp.; and loris, *Nycticebus coucang.* In one instance, some short-tailed wallabies, *P. brachyura,* which had been newly imported became involved in a fight. When the fight was over, all had wounds except for one small wallaby, which was unscathed but had died of fright cowering in a corner away from the fight.

The chinchilla, *Chinchilla laniger,* is another animal that is very susceptible to stress of all kinds and may die if roughly handled (Fig. 7.4). Breeders are well aware of the necessity of careful handling of these animals, even when the time has come to kill them for the pelts. If scared, the animal sheds its fur and the pelt becomes useless. An untrained attendant can cause the animals to become stressed and to show all stages of the syndrome.

Long-term Stress. Deaths from long-term stress arise from two main factors. First, long continuation of the stressing situation or imposition of an additional stressor may lead to failure of the com-

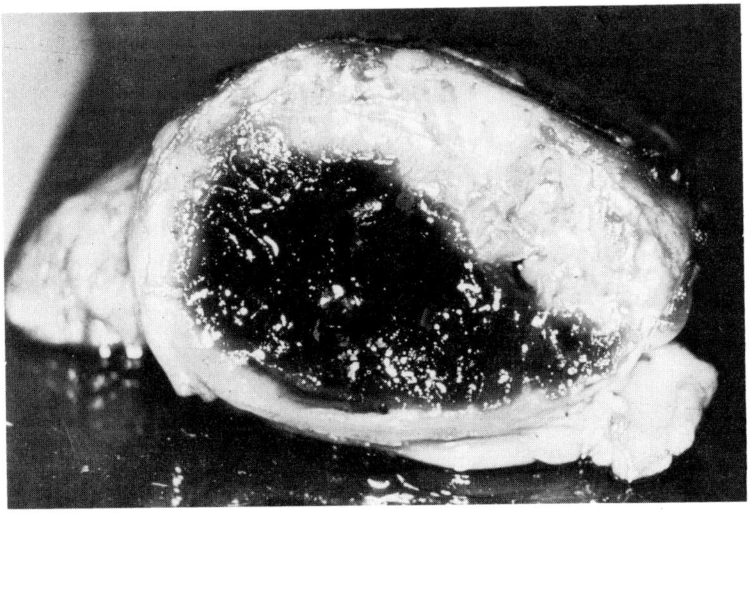

Fig. 7.3. Massive hemorrhage in the adrenal gland of a tiger, *Panthera tigris,* that died of acute shock.

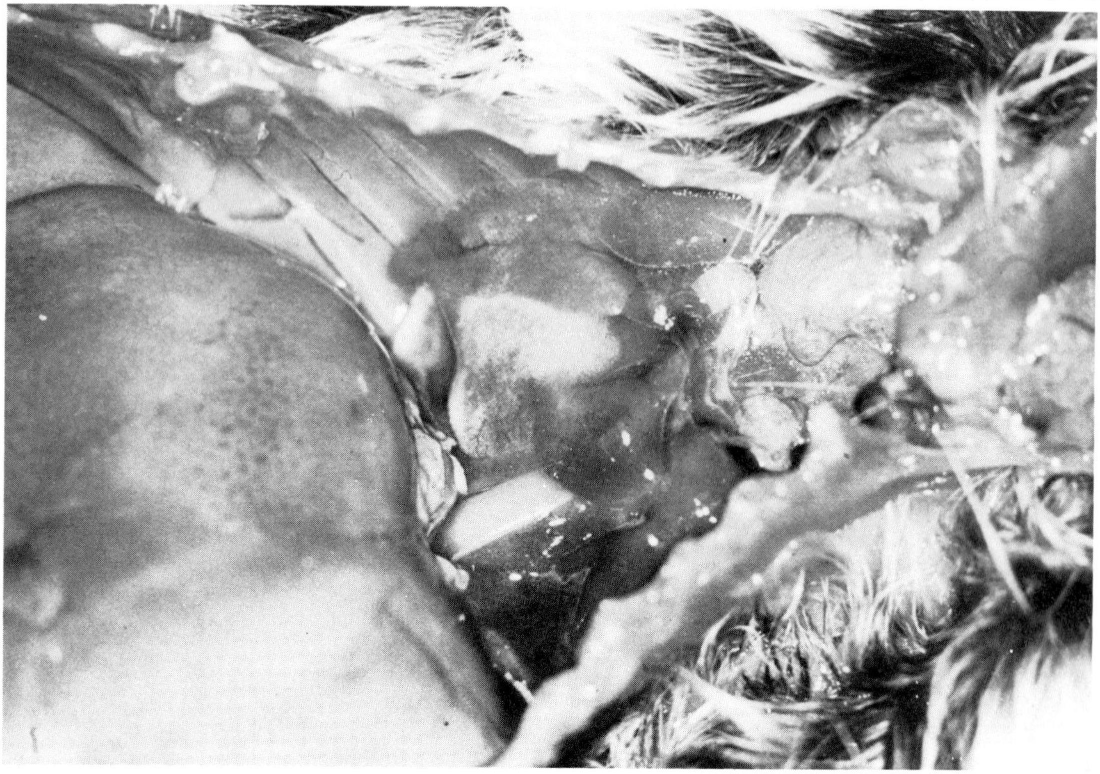

Fig. 7.4. Dissection of the thorax of a chinchilla, *Chinchilla laniger,* that died of acute shock. The lungs are collapsed and anhydremic and the liver is swollen with a pseudo-nutmeg appearance due to distension of the sinusoids with blood.

pensated adrenal glands and the development of the SE. Second, although the adrenals are in a state of compensation, the affected animal is hypotensive and apprehensive. The pituitary, under influence of the hypothalamus, is producing more ACTH and less hormone directed to thyroid and reproductive organs. Many bodily systems are functioning subnormally, including that concerned with immunity.

The situation arising from the SR is seen most commonly in herds or communities of animals, whether in the wild or in captivity. In single animals it manifests itself most commonly in the development of ulceration of the pylorus (Fig. 7.5). The development of the SE from the SR will be encountered most commonly in captive single animals. The SR acts on the herd in two ways: it limits reproductive activity and efficiency, and it removes the weaker and subordinate animals of the herd. Deaths are due to a variety of causes, for example, infection, predation, fighting, killing of surplus young animals, abortion, and development of the SE in any emergency. When such a situation arises in captive herds, it is often some time before the basic cause of the trouble is realized. The animals begin to die, but no coherent pattern of deaths emerges. One such instance occurred some years ago at the London Zoo (Fiennes, 1964b).

The animals involved were a herd of blackbuck, *Antilope cervicapra,* that were thriving and bred regularly. It became necessary during rebuilding operations to move them to a new paddock that was slightly smaller and near noisy machinery. After some months, they were again moved to a different area with newly constructed sheds for their accommodation. During a period of 18 months, the size of the herd was reduced from 26 animals to 16. Deaths were due to fighting and injury, killing of the young, infection, abortion, and metritis. After 12 months in their final quarters, the herd began to recover and their numbers were quickly reconstituted.

In such instances, deaths are only indirectly associated with cardiac incompetence because of the hypotensive state. Where single animals are involved, the connection may or may not be more direct, and it certainly is when the SE develops from the SR. A typical instance of this was described by Fiennes (1964a). Two otters, *Lutra*

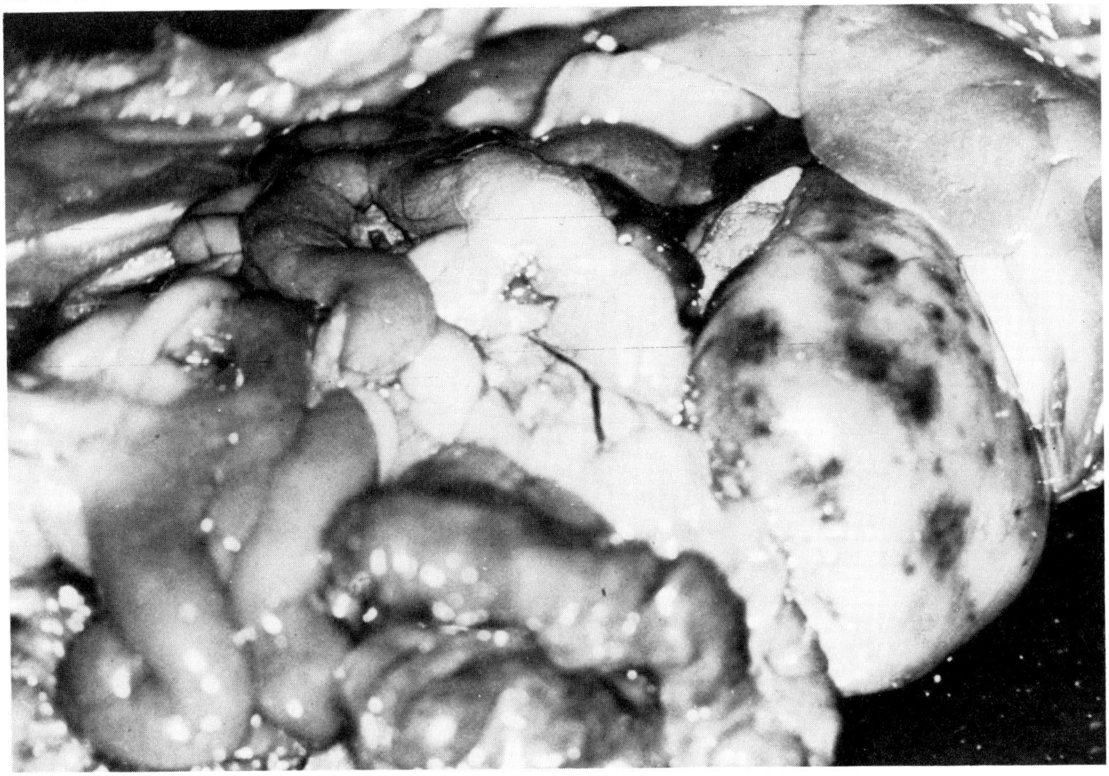

Fig. 7.5. Severe ulceration of the stomach in a chinchilla, *C. laniger,* that died during the SR stage of stress.

perspicillata, imported to England from India were conveyed by air in an adequate crate and appeared to be in good health. When the crate was opened and the otters removed, both died within minutes. Autopsy revealed the typical picture of cardiac failure from stress. During shipment the animals were in SR. The crate had come to represent security to them, so that when they were taken from it the further element of stress converted the SR to the SE.

Animals vary greatly in their response to stress, and the type of injury or trauma to which they will succumb is also greatly variable. The importance to importers of the stress risk is undoubted, since as many as 50% of the imported animals may be lost from various manifestations of stress within the first two to three months. Sometimes they may be found dead with no clue as to what had disturbed them.

Climate-related Factors. In wild herds, there are always stressed individuals, the subordinates. Throughout the year adrenal weights vary seasonally, but those of the subordinates are always greater than those of the dominants. In some species, there is also a more subtle influence at work, as exemplified by the studies of Cowan et al. (1962) in mule deer, *Odocoileus hemionus columbianus,* and white-tailed deer, *O. virginianus.* In these deer there is, throughout the year, a feeding cycle. At the beginning of winter, they are fat and well nourished, but refuse to feed for as long as 60 days even if abundant food is available. The result is that the weaker and older die and herd numbers are reduced. Weight loss in adult deer in Canada continues for as long as 220 days, but not as long in more southerly areas. No cause has been suggested for this phenomenon, but it it is evidently a climate-related manifestation of the SR, that is, another hypotensive state. Another climatically related rhythm is the phenomenon of hibernation, in which profound modifications of blood flow and other physiological phenomena occur. Apart from these naturally occurring states, two main environmental factors commonly affect wild animals in captivity: hyperthermia and hypothermia.

Environmental Factors. Wild animals in hot countries do not spend all their time in the sun; rather, they take shelter from it. Some species are inactive during the day, being crepuscular or noc-

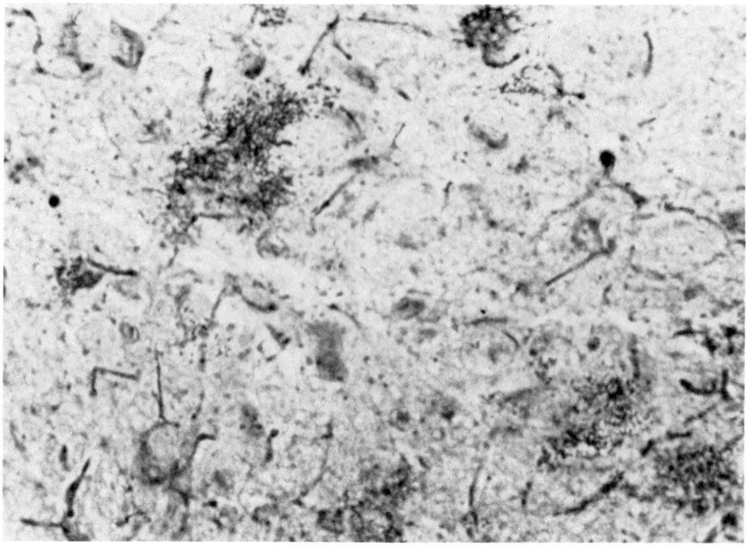

Fig. 7.6. Hemorrhages in the medulla of a bear, *Ursus* sp., as the result of heatstroke.

turnal in their habits. In zoos, animals are often excluded from their houses during the daytime so that they may be on view to the visiting public. When the sun is strong, the animals may be subjected to considerable distress if there is no shade. Deaths from heatstroke are not uncommon, especially if there is a tendency to obesity, as is common in captive animals that get little exercise (Fig. 7.6). The body temperature rises and death occurs from heart failure.

The opposite of heatstroke, hypothermia, can also easily occur in old or badly constructed houses, again especially in countries with a temperate climate where blizzards and arctic conditions occur with extreme rarity. It is the usual practice with captive wild animals to provide minimum heat in houses, compatible with health and comfort. In inadequately constructed houses, heated in this manner, sudden blizzard conditions may result in icy drafts. An animal thus exposed may be found in a state of hypothermia, and it may be impossible to revive it. Death occurs from heart failure associated with the fall of body temperature.

A wild animal may conceal the fact of morbidity by continuing to feed and behave apparently normally, although it is extremely sick. Often, the first indication of an animal's sickness, even to a keeper who is observing it every day, is when it collapses and dies from heart failure. Birds fall dead from their perch or even when on the wing. The reason is probably two-fold: sick animals tend to be attacked and killed by their mates, and predators, such as wolves, seek out the sick and weak to attack.

Special signs are seen in birds, notably rupture of the right auricle or hemorrhage into the calvarium on the upper part of the skull. When such are found at autopsy, they should be regarded as terminal events and other underlying causes of death should be sought (Fiennes, 1969).

Animals dying unexpectedly are often found to have shot or other missiles in the chest, sometimes penetrating the pericardium. This may have occurred during capture or have been caused maliciously. Small lead shot are easily overlooked. If suspected, the body may be X-rayed. Alternatively, the skin should be carefully examined on the inner surface where the missile track will be found. Parrots, particularly African grey parrots, *Psittacus erithacus,* are often captured when trees are felled. As a result, they frequently suffer from internal injuries from which they ultimately die.

ORGANIC DISEASE OF THE HEART. In captive wild animals, dilatation of the heart is usually a sequel to some infectious condition or to pneumonia. An inactive life makes it improbable that such could occur as a result of overexertion. It is unnecessary to dwell on the subject, but an account may be given of a typical case in an elderly female black rhinoceros, *Diceros bicornis,* at the London Zoo, which developed pneumonia. She became recumbent and unable to rise to her feet, and there was little hope that she could survive. However, she was propped on hay bales, turned over from time to time, and given antibiotic treatment. As a result, she eventually recovered and appeared to regain full health. Twelve months later she died suddenly of cardiac failure, and it was found at autopsy that the right side of the heart was grossly dilated and that there was stenosis of the mitral valve.

Myocardial Degeneration. Far more common are various forms of cardiac degeneration. These regrettably are a hazard of the captive way of life. Not only are opportunities for captive animals to exercise adequately denied to them, but many species become very lazy and do not avail themselves of opportunities that are available. They have no need to seek or capture their food nor are they required to flee from predators. Table 7.1 shows the numbers of deaths for various orders of mammals from different forms of noninfectious cardiac disease. It is probable that a great many cases of myocardial degeneration are overlooked when there is another more obvious cause of death.

A typical case of myocardial degeneration occurred at the London Zoo, when two elephant seals, *Mirounga leonina,* were lost. In their confined pool, little activity was possible and the seals spent most of their time on the land. They ate voraciously and became grossly obese. Both died after about two years from myocardial degeneration.

Endocarditis is rarely seen in zoos, except in a few Primates and mostly in Carnivora. It usually takes the form of a myxomatous enlargement of the tricuspid valve, though the mitral is sometimes involved. The condition is in all probability postinfectious, though the characteristic features of rheumatic endocarditis in man are lacking and no specific organism has been associated with it.

Atherosclerosis. While atherosclerosis is not uncommon in certain animals in the wild and in captivity, its complications, thrombosis, aneurysm, and myocardial infarction, are rare. Lapin and Cherkovich (1972) and Miminoshvili et al. (1960) succeeded in inducing hypertension, coronary insufficiency, and myocardial infarction in baboons, *Papio cynocephalus,* subjected to neurogenic stress, in the absence of both thrombosis and atheroma. This work is of importance because it shows that psychological trauma may induce coronary spasm and could be an important factor in the stressed herd in the wild. However, the work has not been repeated nor extended to other species. The subject has been reviewed by Fiennes (1965), who concluded that myocardial infarction and degeneration is associated in almost all cases with obstruction of the artery and only rarely with thrombosis.

Myocardial infarction has been reported mostly in Primates (Fig. 7.7), and only occasionally in birds and other animals (Blair, 1916; Fiennes, 1972; Fox, 1923; Ratcliffe and Cronin, 1958; Vastersaeger et al., 1965). It had been supposed that man's susceptibility to this condition was associated with increased coagulability of the blood or alternatively reduced fibrinolytic factors. However, Hawkey (1972) and Hawkey and Symons (1969) have shown that the opposite is the case, and indeed that the blood of man has to some extent compensated for a tendency to intravascular clotting by reduced coagulability, though fibrinolytic activity is about the same.

Table 7.1. Summary of Reported Cases of Heart Disease in Captive Wild Mammals

Order	Degeneration/ Dilatation	Myo- carditis	Peri- carditis	Endo- carditis
Artiodactyla	9	7	10	—
Carnivora	5	3	3	7
Chiroptera	—	—	1	—
Edentata	3	—	—	1
Marsupialia	—	—	—	1
Perissodactyla	1	1	—	—
Pinnipedia	—	—	1	—
Primates	6	—	9	4
Proboscidea	2	1	—	—
Rodentia	2	—	2	1

Aneurysms. Aneurysms of arteries are reported more frequently in the literature: *Cercopithecus* sp. (Fox, 1929); *Vulpes vulpes* (Hamerton, 1933); *Felis onca* (Hamerton, 1934); *Uncia uncia* (Kelly, 1949); *P. tigris* (Seligman, 1906); *P. leo* (Crisp, 1860); *Cuon alpinus* (Lucas, 1921); *Nasua narica* (Plimmer, 1916); *Viverra* sp. (Scott, 1926); *Thalarctos maritimus* (Salaman, 1903); *Hydrochoerus hydrochoeris* (Crisp, 1860); *Arvicanthis abyssinica* (Fiennes, 1964b); *D. bicornis* (Blair, 1919); *Rangifer arcticus* (Brooks and Blair, 1904; *Bibos sondaicus* (Noback, 1931); and *Gazella* sp. (Urbain et al., 1944).

The cases quoted must be taken as a sample of what undoubtedly occurs quite frequently both in the wild and in captivity. Systematic examination of the arteries of almost any wild animal will reveal scars due to the migration of helminth larvae. In some cases, damage to the arterial wall will be sufficient to result in the development of an aneurysm in time. Lesions are most extensive in zebras due to *Oxyuris equi.* In horses, this worm causes the well-known aneurysms of the mesenteric arteries; in zebras the reaction is somewhat different. Great tumorlike masses, verminous cavernomata, are developed and canalized by numerous small arteries that restore the circulation at least partially. Fatalities from this cause are frequent and may result in serious losses in newly imported zebras.

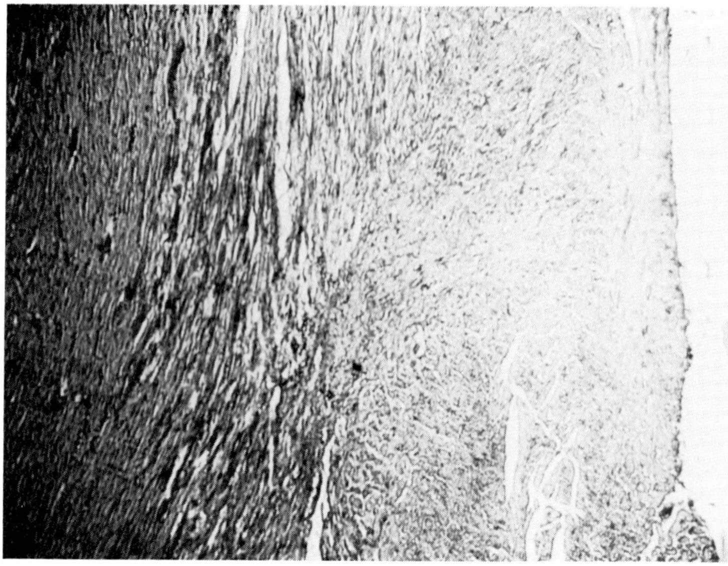

Fig. 7.7. Transverse section of cardiac muscle from an owl monkey, *Aotus trivirgatus,* showing a small myocardial infarction due to thrombosis of a small branch of a coronary artery.

Tumors. Tumors of the heart are rare. In a complete review of all recorded primate tumors, O'Gara and Adamson (1972) list no tumors of the heart. Other records are carcinoma of the pericardium in a Siberian tiger (Fox, 1934); round cell sarcoma of the left ventricle in an opossum, *Didelphis marsupialis* (Hamerton, 1933); sarcoma of the heart in a black rhinoceros (Scott, 1927).

Genetic and Developmental Defects. The incidence of genetic and developmental defects of the heart in wild animals cannot even be guessed at. Animals born with such defects would be most unlikely to survive under wild conditions, and until recently breeding records in zoos have been very poor. The following few samples taken from the literature serve to show that they do occur and that their incidence in different genera is widespread: pericardial patency and a partial ectocardia in a newborn orangutan, *Pongo pygmaeus* (de Garis, 1934); persistent foramen ovale in *Ammatragus lervia* (Fox, 1926); patent foramen ovale in a seal (Garrod, 1877); widely patent ductus arteriosus in two-day-old lion cubs (Rewell, 1948/1949); patent foramen ovale in a wallaby (Scott, 1928); and duplication of the mitral valve and a rare apical interventricular foramen in the heart of a yak calf, *Poephagus grunniens* (Wimsatt and Lewis, 1948).

DISEASES OF THE ARTERIES. Intravascular clotting is rare in wild animal species. Myocardial infarction is usually associated with obstruction of the artery, for instance by spasm, and only rarely with thrombus formation (Fiennes, 1965). On the other hand, arterial diseases are commonly encountered in captive animals (Fiennes, 1965), and these diseases have been studied in fishes and reptiles (Vastersaeger et al., 1965), whales (Roberts et al., 1965), hippopotamus, *Hippopotamus amphibius* (Thurlbeck, 1965), and Primates (Clarkson, 1965). A general review is given by Fox (1933). These and other studies have shown that arterial lesions are not confined to animals in captivity. Studies by Sikes (1969) have shown that, if anything, the incidence in animals in the wild was higher than in captivity, though there were various complicating factors, which will be discussed below.

Arterial diseases have in recent years been studied extensively in wild and laboratory animals, both naturally occurring lesions and lesions experimentally induced by dietary and other means. They have, however, been studied to the greatest extent in man, and the question of whether naturally occurring or experimentally induced lesions in animals are homologous with those of man has still not been fully answered. It would appear that the naturally occurring lesions of animals are comparable with those in man and arise from similar causes, though they may take somewhat different forms in different species.

The term arteriosclerosis simply means hardening of an artery and was used for many years to describe any type of degenerative arterial disease. Today, it is realized that at least three distinct conditions are involved: hypertensive arteriosclerosis; medial sclerosis (Monckeberg's sclerosis); and atherosclerosis.

Hypertensive Arteriosclerosis. According to Simonson and Brozen (1959), spontaneous arterial hypertension occurs in monkeys. Three hundred monkeys, including baboons, *Papio* sp., rhesus, *Macaca mulatta,* and others were studied, among which 20 were found to be hypertensive, 6 transiently and 14 permanently. The authors claimed that the condition was identical with hypertension in man. However, results with monkeys must be accepted with reserve, because of the known rise of blood pressure that occurs when they are restrained. Ratcliffe and Cronin (1958) and Ratcliffe et al. (1960) have also associated changes in the incidence of arterial lesions in animals at the Philadelphia Zoo with hypertensive conditions. Christian (1958) has postulated an incidence of hypertension in a crowded population of wild woodchucks, *Marmota monax,* associated with glomerulosclerosis.

No precise experimental evidence exists, though it appears likely that hypertensive disease occasionally occurs in wild animals with effects on the small arteries of thc kidneys and sometimes of other organs also. In monkeys, fibrous, internal thickenings of the small renal arteries are quite commonly encountered.

Medial Sclerosis. Degeneration of the tunica media of the aorta and small arteries, including the renal, are found quite frequently in some animals, especially wallabies (Fig. 7.8) (Rigg et al., 1960). These degenerations are mucoid or fibrotic and may become calcified. They have been described in wild animals, especially by Sikes (1969). The etiology is unknown, though Sikes's studies suggest environmental relationships.

The inner linings of arteries may show a fatty

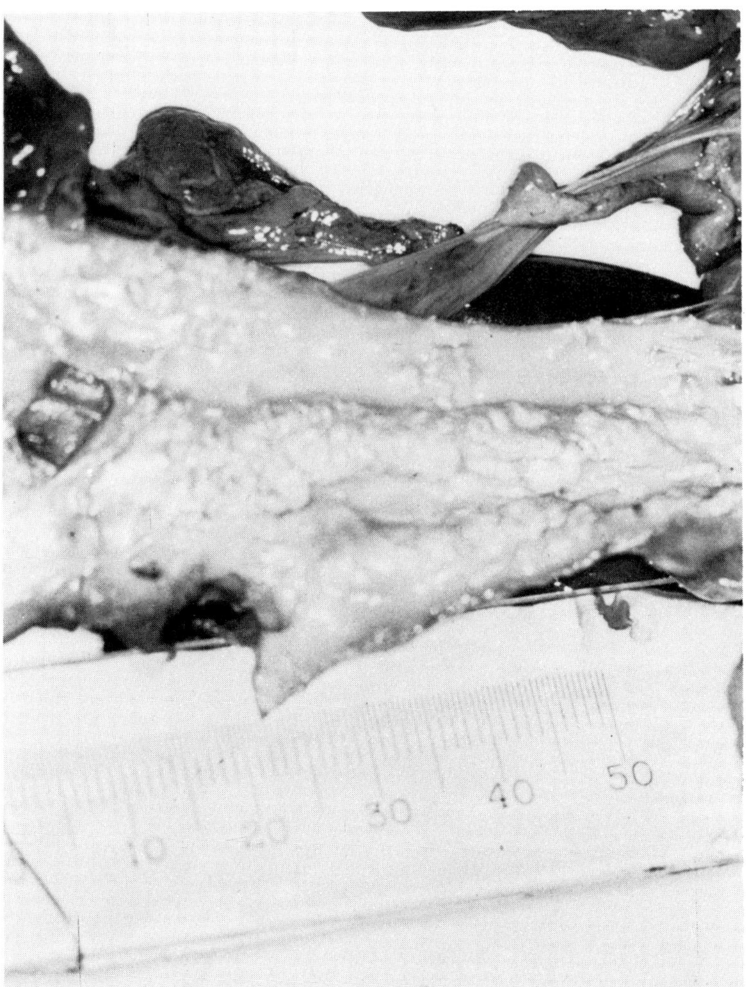

Fig. 7.8. Aorta of a Bennett's wallaby, *Protemnodon bennetti,* showing medial sclerosis.

streak as a barely elevated streak or spot that is stained distinctly by Sudan IV or other fat-soluble dyes. These streaks are commonly found in the arteries of wild animals, usually in the aorta, and may be extensive. They are to be seen regularly in the aortae of newly hatched chickens, but disappear in a week or two. In older animals, the streaks are believed to be reversible, but may well be the forerunner of the advanced lesions of atherosclerosis. As such, fatty streaks have no pathological significance.

Atherosclerosis. Atherosclerosis is a type of arteriosclerosis characterized by a variable combination of intimal changes of arteries consisting of the focal accumulation of cholesterol and other lipids, complex carbohydrates, blood and blood products, fibrous tissue, and calcium deposits. If the internal elastic lamina is breached, elastosis, the tunica media also becomes involved in the process. This type of lesion gives rise to the atheromatous plaque upon which the mural thrombus develops, in time possibly occluding the whole vessel. Such thrombi are serious if they occur in the coronary or cerebral arteries, giving rise to cardiac infarction or stroke. These may occur in wild animals but are rare. Ulceration of such a plaque may give rise to aneurysm, although aneurysms in wild animals are usually associated with other causes.

In wild animals, atheromatous lesions mostly occur in the aorta, except in birds in which the brachiocephalic arteries are also commonly involved. Small lipid-containing thickenings are often seen at the junctions of smaller arteries, such as the intercostals. Today it is generally accepted that these lesions can regress, as long as only lipids and carbohydrates have accumulated in them. However, calcification, chondrification, and even ossification are long-term sequelae, from which there is no return. Unless thrombosis occurs, the course of the disease is long-term. Death occurs in old age when the vessels become inelastic and totally occluded. In old parrots, arteries may become so impregnated with calcium salts and so brittle that they snap like dry twigs.

Arterial Diseases in Free-living Animals. As a contrast to studies on captive animals, it is necessary to review the work by Sikes (1969) on free-living wild animals in East Africa. The research falls into two parts: that on wild animals and birds generally, and that on elephants, which were found to be a particularly rewarding object of study. Before this work was undertaken, it was fully realized that wild animals in Africa, owing to the presence of human populations, were not always living in fully wild or natural habitats. The truly wild animal is one living in a habitat untampered with by man. Where man has interfered with the habitat, even by creation of game reserves, there could be interference both with amenities, such as shade, and with the types of food available. Furthermore, interference with the seasonal migratory movements of some groups of animals might introduce a stressing factor, which would be revealed in their condition. These surmises were amply justified, as is seen especially from the work on elephants.

The findings of Sikes (1969) in relation to the comparative incidence of arterial changes in birds strikingly confirms the incidence shown by Fiennes (1965) in captive specimens. In mammals other than elephants, the position was obscured by the extensive arterial damage caused by migrating worm larvae; however, lesions were found affecting intima and media, frequently containing lipid and sometimes calcium. Among Primates, cercopithecid monkeys showed little arterial damage, and examination of chimpanzees, *Pan troglodytes,* was restricted for reasons of conservation. However, one very old male chimpanzee was shot and showed a condition of the arteries comparable to that which might be expected in an elderly man. There were extensive, partially occlusive, atheromatous plaques in the aorta, coronaries, and other muscular arteries. This was one of a population of forest chimpanzees from the Kigezi Game Reserve in Uganda. The habitat had been much disturbed by human activities and encroachment into the forest and by overspill of the elephant population from the Queen Elizabeth National Park. This was, therefore, a stressed habitat, a point of importance in relation to the work on elephants.

The clearest pictures came from Sikes's work on elephants, *Loxodonta africana,* which were studied from three different habitats. One was a normal, unstressed montane habitat. The other two were scrubland and grassland, both stressed in the following ways: 1) prolonged exposure of the animals to unmitigated sunlight, because of removal of tree cover; 2) overpopulation; 3) restricted diet; and 4) frustration of the migratory habit and a breakdown of environmental conditions suited to the birth and nurture of young calves, coupled with boredom and lack of exercise for the adults and overcrowding.

In the unstressed montane habitat, extremes of temperature and altitude and irregular hunting evidently did not act as stressors, and no elephants showed arterial lesions, although as in all habitats the elephants shot for study were aging or aged.

Elephants from the stressed habitats showed the following changes of the cardiovascular system in varying degree: 1) fenestration of one or

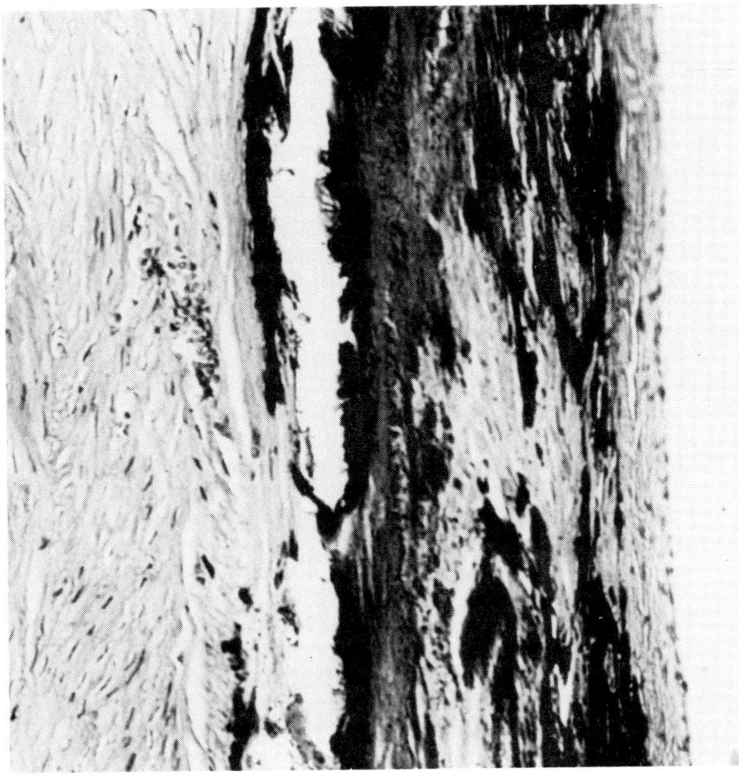

Fig. 7.9. Transverse section of the aorta of an elephant, *Loxodonta africana,* showing extensive calcification of the tunica adventitia and media, with elastosis.

more cusps of the aortic valve and of the semilunar valves of the pulmonary arch; 2) calcium flecks in the media of the extramural coronary arteries; 3) lipid streaks and plaques in the intima of the coronaries; 4) roughness and soft white plaques in the intima of the coronaries, in two cases causing slight occlusion of the right coronary; 5) in the aorta, invariable atheroma and/or calcification of the media in certain of Sikes's five defined segments, together with fibrous intimal buttons (Fig. 7.9); 6) in the iliacs and femorals, the lumina of branch ostia were partially occluded with lipid plaques (in one case, the lumina of the entire right common iliac and femoral were affected with intimal plaque formation and medial calcification, the corresponding foot was much swollen, and the veins varicose); and 7) the carotids were similarly affected, which may have accounted for an abnormal head posture of some elephants.

In marsupials, medial sclerosis of the aorta is commonly found but only a few references to this condition appear in the literature (Fox, 1923).

In Primates, Lindsay and Chaikoff (1966) made a limited survey of animals in the wild, but concluded that atheroma only occurred in spider monkeys, *Ateles* sp., chimpanzees, and some species of *Macaca.* Blair (1916) described a case of coronary thrombosis in an orangutan and Burlingame (1945) in a chimpanzee. Fox (1923) described a case of sclerosis of the coronary arteries in a baboon and of medial sclerosis in a monkey, *Macaca* sp. Hamerton (1931, 1941/1942) diagnosed a case of myocardial infarction and atheroma in a lemur, *Lemur mongoz,* and in a monkey, *Cercopithecus* sp., and myocarditis, sclerosis of the cardiac valves, atheroma of the coronaries, and ulceration of the aorta in a baboon.

In Edentata, Hamerton (1930) found fibrofatty degeneration of the myocardium and atheroma in an anteater, *Myrmecophaga* sp. In Rodentia, there are no reports of atheroma in captive collections, except for Dieterich (1969) who described medial sclerosis in a crowded population of captive beavers, *Castor canadensis.* In Carnivora, Hamerton (1930, 1941/1942) described calcareous atheroma in a badger, *Meles meles,* and fatty degeneration of the myocardium and extensive arterial disease in a bear, *Ursus* sp. Plimmer (1916) found diffuse atheroma of the aorta in a lion and Seligman (1907) of the aorta in a tiger. Vastersaeger et al. (1959) found coronary atheroma and myocardial infarction in a red panda, *Ailurus fulgens.* In Proboscidea, Zvetaeva (1940) described senile sclerosis in an Indian elephant, *Elephas maximus.* In Perissodactyla, Fox (1923) described a case of atherosclerosis in the thoracic aorta of a zebra, *E. burchelli.* In the Artiodactyla, Cameron (1923) found arteriosclerosis of the posterior aorta in a buffalo, *Syncerus caffer.* Fox (1923) found degenerative sclerosis of the coronaries in a nilgai, *Boselaphus tragocamelus.* Hamerton (1934) found atheroma of the coronaries in a peccary, *Pecari angulatus,* and atheroma of the aorta in a yak. In addition Hamerton (1938/1939, 1945/1946) found degeneration of the heart and arteriosclerosis in a European bison, *B. bonasus,* and senile arteriosclerosis and myocardial degeneration in a gazelle, *Gazella* sp. Noback (1926) found calcareous plaques in the aorta, and axillary and iliac arteries of a nilgai. Finally, Scott (1928) found atheroma in the aorta and pulmonary artery of a tahr, *Hemitragus* sp. Atheroma is common in some groups of birds (Fiennes, 1965, 1969).

DISEASES OF THE VEINS. The most important condition affecting the veins of wild animals in captivity is probably frostbite. This is comparatively common in animals in temperate climates, where sudden cold snaps are unexpected. Tropical birds fare well during winter in outside flight cages, but when the weather becomes very cold, they suffer frostbite of the toes, one or more of which may be completely lost. The same has been seen in agoutis, *Dasyprocta aguti;* when the ground has been frozen they suffer frostbite of the digits, which may be lost. A further hazard occurs in monkeys and apes, such as gibbons. Such animals are well able to tolerate external temperatures below freezing if warm refuges or sleeping quarters are provided. If, however, the swinging rails are of iron, instead of wood or plastic, the animals will suffer from frostbite of the fingers when the weather becomes very cold.

A specialized form of frostbite that affects the tail was at one time common in monkeys. Although the body of the monkey might be warm, the tail hanging down from the perch might be exposed to an icy draft. The result was a progressive, dry gangrene, from which segments of the tail would be lost. The monkey would bite and worry at the tail, until it became a raw and bleeding stump. Efforts to amputate the tail above the site of injury and so halt the process were not always successful and eventually many monkeys have had to be destroyed because of this lesion. This accident will not occur if the monkeys are kept in houses that are properly heated and ventilated.

Phlebitis often occurs in long-legged birds following comparatively minor injuries to the legs. Treatment is rarely successful. The author has observed one case of typical corded mesenteric veins (Fig. 7.10), arising from portal hypertension, and knows of no reference in the literature. This was in a genet, *Genetta genetta.*

CONTROL. The greatest problem facing the animal importer lies in the serious losses that occur during the first six months of life in captivity. A death rate of 50% to 60% is common, and not infrequently a whole consignment of animals may be lost. Sometimes, the cause is easily determined, such as an epidemic of dysentery or the occurrence of tuberculosis in a batch of monkeys, clearly contracted from the animals' captors and exacerbated by poor conditions of housing prior to shipment and overcrowding during transit. Even when such diseases are absent, the death rate among newly imported animals may be unacceptably high and the cause is often difficult to discover. The apparent causes of death are multifarious and appear to be unconnected. Some animals die from no readily apparent cause, though the investigator will come in time to recognize the characteristic clinical signs and appearances at autopsy of the hypotensive state associated with the stress syndrome.

A great deal of work has been done in recent years on the stress syndrome and much has been written about its nervous and endocrine origins. The most important feature, that of hypotension, has been ignored by most workers and no textbook on animal pathology describes this feature or suggests what lines of treatment are necessary to overcome it. Indeed, there appear to have been no systematic studies on the management and treatment of animals in states of stress. It is initially important to understand the nature and cause of the condition, namely, that stress is primarily a physiological rather than a pathological state and that it operates in wild communities to regulate the birth rate and to determine which animals will fail to survive when conditions are unfavorable. Animals captured in the wild are likely to be already ecologically stressed. The imposition of the additional stressing factors of capture, change of environment, and transit could prove fatal. The use of sedatives and tranquilizing drugs following capture and during transit is clearly indicated and experience shows that they have a beneficial effect.

It should also be realized that to a stressed animal its cage comes to represent security, and removal to new quarters, however ample, is an additional stress. An animal should not be forcibly removed from its transit cage. Where possible, this should be placed in the new den with the door open, so that the animal can cautiously emerge to explore its new surroundings and find food. Where an animal is in the final stage of

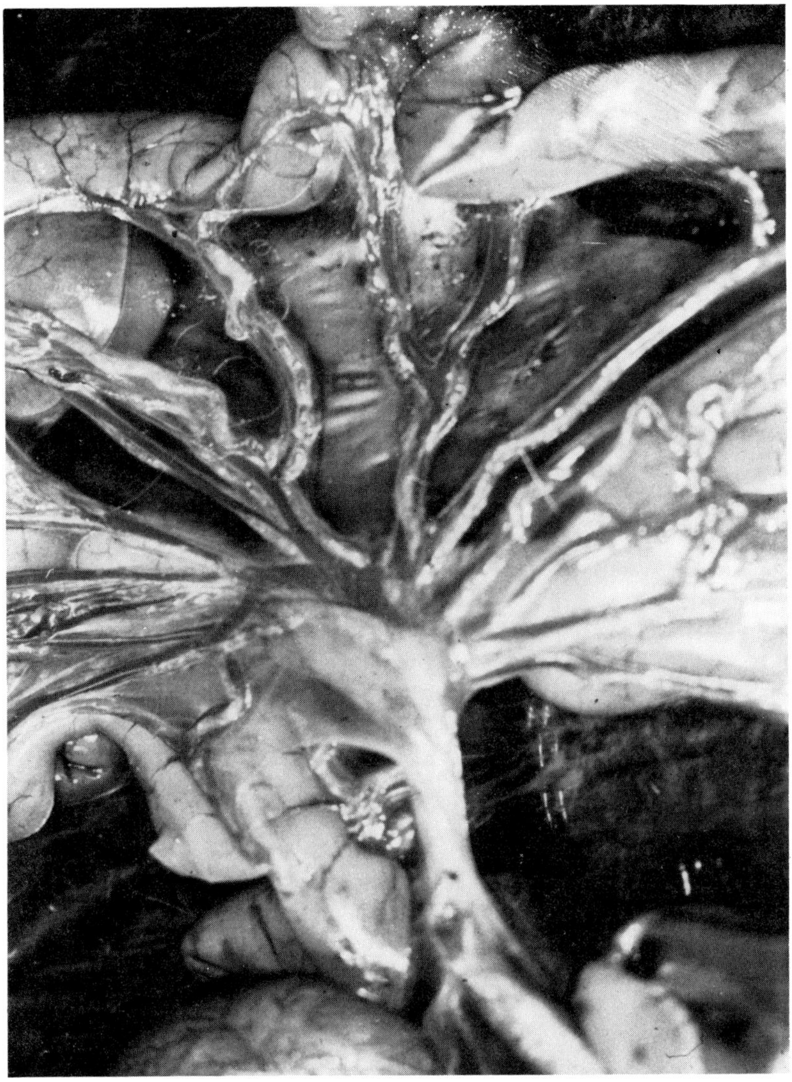

Fig. 7.10. Corded mesenteric veins in a genet, *Genetta genetta*, resulting from portal hypertension.

stress and will evidently die within a day or two from adrenal exhaustion, administration of corticosteroid is obviously sensible, though alone it appears to have little effect. On the assumption that the condition is hypotensive, epinephrine should be administered, though there is no information as to whether this has been tried or as to its effects. Glucose should also be administered to combat the hypoglycemia.

Morbid conditions of the cardiovascular system fall into three categories: postinfectious, namely, valvular endocarditis and cardiac dilatation; traumatic, namely, aneurysms associated with wandering helminth larvae; and degenerative. Only the latter requires comment.

Animals of all kinds, laboratory, domestic and wild, have been used extensively as models in the study of atherosclerosis as it occurs in human populations. Such studies have shown that virtually all groups of animals and birds fed large quantities of saturated fat and cholesterol develop arterial lesions that bear some resemblance to human atheroma. It would be surprising if they did not do so, and it is difficult to see what this proves. Naturally occurring atheroma does, however, occur in some groups of wild animals, being more common in certain species than in others. Among Mammalia, Primates are especially susceptible whereas it is rare in Rodentia, Marsupialia, and Pinnipedia. It is common in some groups of birds, especially those that feed on insects, meat, fruit, vegetable foods, or are mixed feeders. It is rarely found in birds that feed on fish or seeds.

Intravascular clotting is a rare phenomenon in any wild animals, though it occasionally occurs in Hominoidea. The evidence suggests the involvement of dietary factors in the development of degenerative conditions of arteries, although Sikes's work on elephants indicates that stressing conditions are also of importance. The etiology of intravascular clotting is likely to be unrelated to that of atheroma.

REFERENCES

Blair, W. R. 1916. Report of the veterinarian for the year 1915. Annu. Rep. NY Zool. Soc. 20:71.

______. 1919. Deaths for 1918. Annu. Rep. NY Zool. Soc. 23:65.

Brooks, H., and W. R. Blair. 1904. Annual report of the medical department of the zoological park for 1903. Annu. Rep. NY Zool. Soc. 8:111.

Burlingame, E. 1945. Zoonooz 17(8).

Cameron, A. E. 1923. Notes on buffalo: Anatomy, pathological conditions, and parasites. Vet. J. 30:331–336.

Christian, J. J. 1958. A diffuse glomerulo-sclerosis of unknown etiology in woodchucks. Fed. Proc. 17: 432.

Clarkson, T. B. 1965. Spontaneous atherosclerosis in subhuman primates. In J. C. Roberts and R. Strauss. Comparative atherosclerosis. Harper & Row, New York.

Cowan, I. McT., A. J. Wood, Jr., and H. C. Nordan. 1962. Growth and nutrition of deer. Proc. 1st Int. Conf. Wildl. Dis. Wildl. Dis. Assoc., Patuxent, Maryland.

Crisp, E. 1860. On the causes of death of the animals in the Society's gardens, from 1851 to the present time, 1860. Proc. Zool. Soc. Lond. 33:178.

Dieterich, R. A. 1969. Medial arterial sclerosis in captive beavers, *Castor canadensis,* Kuhl. Bull. Wildl. Dis. Assoc. 5:115–116.

Fiennes, R. N. T. W. 1964a. Man, nature and disease. Weidenfeld and Nicolson, London.

______. 1964b. Report of the society's pathologist for the year 1962. Proc. Zool. Soc. Lond. 143 (Part 1):53–78.

______. 1965. Atherosclerosis in wild animals. In J. C. Roberts and R. Strauss. Comparative atherosclerosis. Harper & Row, New York.

______. 1969. Diseases of the cardiovascular system, blood, and lymphatic system. In M. L. Petrak. Diseases of cage and aviary birds. Lea & Febiger, Philadelphia.

______. 1972. The owl monkey, *Aotus trivirgatus,* in research. Med. Primatol. 1972 (Part 1):93–94.

Fox, H. 1923. Disease in captive wild animals and birds. J. B. Lippincott Company, Philadelphia.

______. 1926. Report of the Laboratory and Museum of Comparative Pathology of the Zoological Society of Philadelphia.

______. 1929. Report of the Laboratory and Museum of Comparative Pathology of the Zoological Society of Philadelphia.

______. 1933. Arteriosclerosis. In E. W. Cowdry. Arteriosclerosis: A survey of the problem. Josiah Macy Foundation, New York.

______. 1934. Report of the International Conference of Pathology, Philadelphia.

de Garis, C. F. 1934. Pericardial patency and partial ectocardia in a newborn orangutan. Anat. Rec. 59:69–82.

Garrod, A. H. 1877. Note on the possible cause of death in a young seal. Proc. Zool. Soc. Lond. 1877:369.

Hamerton, A. E. 1930. Report on the deaths occurring in the Society's Gardens during the year 1929. Proc. Zool. Soc. Lond. 1930:369.

______. 1931. Report on the deaths occurring in the Society's Gardens during the year 1930. Proc. Zool. Soc. Lond. 1931:541.

______. 1933. Report on the deaths occurring in the Society's Gardens during 1932. Proc. Zool. Soc. Lond. 1933:463.

______. 1934. Report on the deaths occurring in the Society's Gardens during the year 1933. Proc. Zool. Soc. Lond. 1934:403.

______. 1938/1939. Report on the deaths occurring in the Society's Gardens during the year 1937. Proc. Zool. Soc. Lond. 108 (Ser. B):504.

______. 1941/1942. Report on the deaths occurring in the Society's Gardens during the years 1939–1940. Proc. Zool. Soc. Lond. 111 (Ser. B):158.

______. 1945/1946. Report on the deaths occurring in the Society's Gardens during the year 1944. Proc. Zool. Soc. Lond. 115:378.

Hawkey, C. 1972. Coagulation, fibrinolysis and platelet function. In R. N. T. W. Fiennes. Pathology of simian primates. Part 1. Karger, Basel.

______, and C. Symons. 1969. A comparative study of blood coagulation in human and non-human primates. Proc. 2nd Int. Congr. Primatol. Karger, Basel.

Hewson, R., and T. D. Healing. 1971. The stoat, *Mustela erminea,* and its prey. J. Zool. (Lond.) 164:239–244.

Kelly, A. L. 1949. Hospital report. Zoonooz 22(9):6.

Lapin, B. A., and G. M. Cherkovich. 1972. Biological normals. In R. N. T. W. Fiennes. Pathology of simian primates. Part 1. Karger, Basel.

Lindsay, S., and I. L. Chaikoff. 1966. Naturally occurring arteriosclerosis in non-human primates. J. Atheroscl. Res. 6:36–51.

Lucas, N. F. 1921. Report on the deaths which occurred in the Zoological Gardens during 1920. Proc. Zool. Soc. Lond. 1921:180–181.

Miminoshvili, D. I., G. O. Magakian, and G. Kokaia. 1960. Attempts to obtain a model of hypertension and coronary insufficiency in monkeys. In I. A. Utkin. Theoretical and practical problems of medicine and biology in experiments on monkeys. Pergamon Press, London.

Noback, C. V. 1926. Report of the veterinarian. Annu. Rep. NY Zool. Soc. 31:52–62.

______. 1931. Report of the veterinarian. Annu. Rep. NY Zool. Soc. 36:49.

O'Gara, R. W., and R. H. Adamson. 1972. Spontaneous and induced neoplasms in non-human primates. In R. N. T. W. Fiennes. Pathology of simian primates. Part I. Karger, Basel.

Plimmer, H. 1916. Report on the deaths which occurred in the Zoological Gardens during 1915. Proc. Zool. Soc. Lond. 1916:83.

Ratcliffe, H. L., and M. T. I. Cronin. 1958. Changing frequency of arteriosclerosis in mammals and birds at the Philadelphia Zoological Gardens. Circulation 18:41–52.

______, T. G. Yerasimides, and G. A. Elliot. 1960. Changes in the character and location of arterial lesions in mammals and birds in the Philadelphia Zoological Gardens. Circulation 21:730–738.

Rewell, R. E. 1948/1949. Report of the pathologist for the year 1947. Proc. Zool. Soc. Lond. 118:509.

Rigg, K. J., R. Finlayson, K. R. Hill, and R. N. T. W. Fiennes. 1960. Degenerative arterial disease of animals in captivity with special reference to the comparative pathology of atherosclerosis. Proc. Zool. Soc. Lond. 135 (Part 2):157–164.

Roberts, J. C., R. C. Boice, R. L. Brownell, and D. H. Brown. 1965. Spontaneous atherosclerosis in Pacific toothed and baleen whales. In J. C. Roberts and R. Strauss. Comparative atherosclerosis. Harper & Row, New York.

Salaman, R. N. 1903. On the cause of death of a polar bear recently living in the Society's Gardens. Proc. Zool. Soc. Lond 1903:348–349.

Scott, H. H. 1926. Report on the deaths occurring in the Society's Gardens during the year 1925. Proc. Zool. Soc. Lond. 1926:241–242.

______. 1927. Report on the deaths occurring in the Society's Gardens during the year 1926. Proc. Zool. Soc. Lond. 1927:197.

______. 1928. Report on the deaths occurring in the Society's Gardens during the year 1927. Proc. Zool. Soc. Lond. 1928:108–111.

Seligman, G. C. 1906. Note on deaths occurring in the Society's Gardens during 1905. Proc. Zool. Soc. Lond. 1906:235.

______. 1907. Report on deaths occurring in the Society's menagerie during 1906. Proc. Zool. Soc. Lond. 1907: 171–172.

Selye, H. 1950. The physiology and pathology of exposure to stress. Acta Inc., Montreal.

Sikes, S. K. 1969. Habitat and cardiovascular disease: Observations made on elephants, *Loxodonta africana,* and other free-living animals, in East Africa. Trans. Zool. Soc. Lond. 32:1–103.

Simonson, E., and J. Brozen. 1959. Russian research on arterial hypertension. Ann. Intern. Med. 50:129–193.

Thurlbeck, W. M. 1965. Arteriosclerosis in hippopotami. In J. C. Roberts and R. Strauss. Comparative atherosclerosis. Harper & Row, New York.

Urbain, A., P. Bullier, and J. Nouvel. 1944. Rapport sur la mortalite et la natalite enregistrees au parc zoologique du bois de Vincennes 1943. Bull. Mus. Hist. Natur. Paris 16:58.

Vastersaeger, M. M., R. Delcourt, and P. M. Gilbert. 1965. Spontaneous atherosclerosis in fishes and reptiles. In J. C. Roberts and R. Strauss. Comparative atherosclerosis. Harper & Row, New York.

______, P. Gilbert, and J. Mortelmans. 1959. Thrombose coronarienne ayant entraine la mort chez un panda, *Ailurus fulgens.* J. Bull. Soc. Royal Zool. Anvers. 14:47–51.

Wimsatt, W. A., and P. T. Lewis. 1948. Duplication of the mitral valve and a rare interventricular foramen in the heart of a yak calf. Am. J. Anat. 83:67–107.

Zvetaeva, M. P. 1940. The pathology of the elephant "Djindan." Proc. Moscow Zool. Park 1:375.

8 *Physical Injury*

JOHN E. COOPER

CERTAIN PHYSICAL FACTORS that may cause or influence the course of disease in wild animals are difficult to define, since frequently they are only one contributory factor and their full significance is often not easy to elucidate. Trauma will be discussed in some detail, as it is a common cause of death or injury in both free-living and captive mammals and birds. Despite the importance of trauma in these animals, there is not a great deal of information on its pathogenesis, pathology, and diagnosis in wild species. The incidence and significance of the injuries discussed depend upon management factors or upon the environment (Stout and Cornwell, 1976). For example overheating by the sun is most prevalent in the tropics, but burns from electrical heaters are more common in zoological collections in temperate climates where such artificial aids are necessary. Electrocution from power lines is a greater hazard to birds in places where high-voltage lines stretch for long distances across country that is rich in avifauna, Africa for instance.

INJURIES CAUSED BY ACCIDENTS

Etiology. The etiology of these injuries is quite varied. Important and common examples are trauma, electrocution, burning (heat, friction, or chemicals), and drowning. It is possible to give only a few examples of how these factors can affect wild animal populations.

TRAUMA. A traumatic injury is produced by a sudden, violent force that results in a crushing or separation of the tissues. For example, collisions between wild species and motor vehicles, trains, or aircraft result in injury or death to the animal and occasionally to people. It has been estimated that one million animals a day are killed in this manner in the United States. In some species such deaths may possibly contribute to a reduction in population numbers (Gordon, 1932; Sargeant and Forbes, 1973), although there is controversy over this. Considerable attention has been focused on the European hedgehog, *Erinaceus europaeus* (Brockie, 1960; Davies, 1957) and white-tailed deer, *Odocoileus virginianus* (Allen and McCullough, 1976). Collisions between birds and aircraft have resulted in the instigation of bird control programs on many large airfields in Europe and North America and have affected plans for a new London airport in Great Britain (Wright, 1972). Wildlife may also strike buildings, towers, fences, and so on (Fig. 8.1), and game birds may be traumatized by mowing machines or other agricultural machinery.

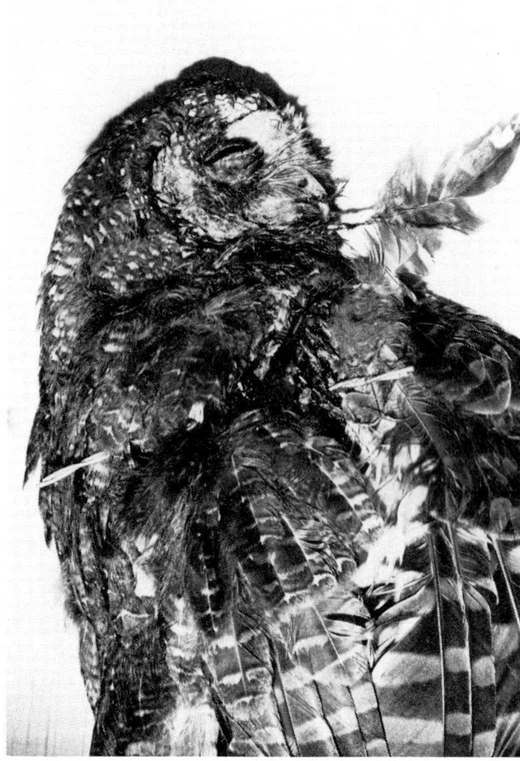

Fig. 8.1. Free-living African wood owl, *Ciccaba woodfordi,* that became transfixed on a barbed wire fence. The owl was removed together with a portion of the wire. The wing was severely lacerated.

Trauma associated with animal population control procedures and capture methods cannot be ignored. Arrows, bullets, explosives, syringes, nets, and traps have their own particular methods of causing injury. Millions of wild animals are killed, crippled, or otherwise injured each year by individuals engaged in scientific, recreational, or other activities.

Interspecific and intraspecific interactions can

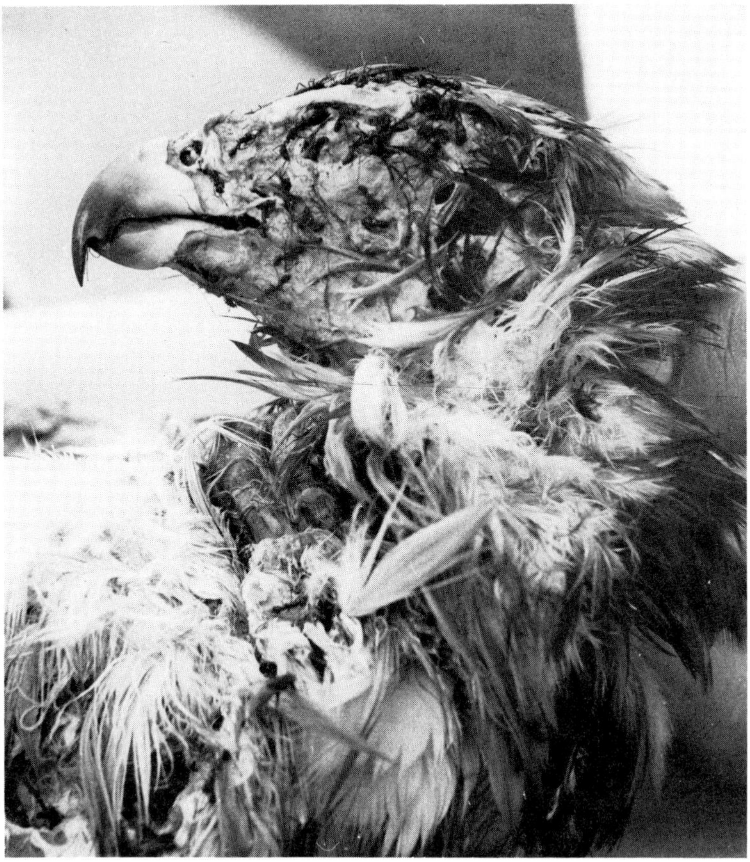

Fig. 8.2. Head of captive lanner falcon, *Falco biarmicus,* showing extensive soft tissue damage by safari ants, *Dorylus* sp. Individual ants can be seen attached to the head.

result in traumatic injury. Predation, territorial defense, mating-related activities, and fratricide are examples (Fig. 8.2) (Wynne-Edwards, 1962). The importance of self-mutilation or injury by other animals in captivity has been emphasized (Fox, 1923).

ELECTROCUTION. The likely sources of electrocution to free-living animals are lightning and electrocution from power lines. Deaths due to lightning occur occasionally among free-living animals (Sugden, 1930), and the significance is usually not great. A recent report (Shaw and Neiland, 1973) described an incident among Alaskan caribou, *Rangifer tarandus,* in which 53 individuals were killed at one time. Power lines are possibly of even more ecological importance. Markus (1972) considered them to play a positive role in the regulation of vulture, *Gyps coprotheres,* numbers in South Africa. Harrison (1963) described a very high mortality (30%) in a flock of swans, *Cygnus olor,* caused by collision or electrocution along a quarter-mile stretch of power line in Great Britain. Electrocution is of far more concern in captive animals since electrical heaters and other appliances are commonly used in their cages and enclosures.

BURNING. Burns can be caused by heat, chemicals or friction. Fires are an important cause of death from burning and suffocation in free-living populations. Chemical burns can also occur as a result of contact with either manmade or natural areas of acid or alkali. The naturally occurring alkaline lakes of East Africa are the home of algae-feeding flamingoes, *Phoeniconaias minor* and *Phoenicopterus ruber roseus,* and it is not uncommon, when the lakes are drying, for groups of birds to be found with soda plastered on their feet. Such birds are quickly killed by predators and some die as a result of the skin damage produced by the soda. Burning by friction is probably of little significance. In captive animals it may occur as a result of a leash or collar that rubs the skin.

DROWNING. Considerable numbers of wild animals drown, but it is unlikely that this plays any significant role in population control except, possibly, in the case of small rodents. Contrary to legend, the Norwegian lemming, *Lemmus lemmus,* does not make a suicidal rush for the sea, but like many other rodents, when its numbers become excessive, a mass movement or "migration" can occur from densely populated areas. A percentage of these animals drown in lakes, rivers, and the sea, but more are killed by predators or starvation.

In a small area drowning can have significant effects on populations. If a new pond is dug, many small rodents may fall into the water and drown; the local population can thus suffer a temporary decline in numbers. Likewise, the construction of steep ditches may result in young gamebirds falling in and drowning, while larger animals may break through ice on lakes and drown. More dramatic examples of drowning are seen when flooding is carried out on a large scale; the closing of the Zambesi River dam to create Lake Kariba in Africa is probably the best known. Here, in the absence of human intervention, the flooding, which finally created 2,500 square miles of lake, would have resulted in the death of many thousands of animals. Another hazard is natural flooding, during which large numbers of animals in a given area may drown. An example was the extensive flooding in Europe in 1953 when in coastal areas many thousands of small mammals died overnight.

Drowning can also occur in aquatic birds during bad weather or, more important, if their plumage becomes waterlogged as a result of oil pollution. Waterlogging in birds may also occur if their preen glands are not functioning properly.

Pathogenesis and Pathology

TRAUMA. Pathogenesis is due to damage of essential epithelial, connective, muscular and nervous tissues coupled with secondary effects, such as anemia caused by loss of blood. The direct effect of a physical blow will depend on the area of the body involved and the tissues damaged. Secondary effects may also include infection, since physical damage can result in the production of wounds through which pathogens may enter; examples are many and varied but include the infection of fight wounds in wild carnivores and the multiplication of *Clostridium* spp. in bruised areas of the body.

External wounds and fractures may be present and subcutaneous hemorrhage is usually detectable if the carcass is skinned. In the case of birds, subcutaneous emphysema may be present due to air-sac damage. Internal lesions may be severe, especially if the trauma has resulted in a ruptured organ. A useful paper on the neuropathology of head injuries described lesions in northern fur seals, *Callorhinus ursinus,* stunned with hardwood clubs (Jortner, 1974). There is a useful review on the pathology of trauma (Sevitt and Stoner, 1970) and one on the metabolic consequences in animals (Michell, 1974).

In other cases signs may be minimal. The author, for example, examined a captive chimpanzee, *Pan troglodytes,* which had died following a severe blow to the head. At postmortem examination the only gross lesions were some subcutaneous hemorrhage and congestion of the meninges. No significant lesion could be detected histologically. The same type of negative picture may be seen in the case of birds, especially long-legged species such as flamingoes and storks, which sometimes become paralyzed during or after capture (Young, 1967). Although in a number of cases lesions can be detected, for example, hemorrhage, especially affecting the muscles, often no pathological lesions are found. Further work is needed on this topic. The pathological findings in animals that die following various trapping techniques were discussed by Basson and Hofmeyr (1973), Harthoorn and Young (1974), and Young and Bronkhorst (1971).

ELECTROCUTION AND BURNING. Electrocution can damage tissues by burning, but the electrical current involved can also produce effects; for example, respiration can cease completely. Ventricular fibrillation is a common sequel to electrocution and is usually the cause of death in fatal cases. Burning or charring of the feathers or hair is usually apparent and in severe cases much of the carcass may be burned to the bone giving a "fossilized" appearance (Fig. 8.3). Lymph nodes are often hemorrhagic and there may be free blood in the respiratory tract. There may be discoloration and rigor of muscles and black unclotted blood. In less severe cases lesions may be few, other than slight burns and petechiae. The distribution of lesions in electrocution depends on the area affected; for example, the current may have passed only through the legs or from a wing tip to a foot, and so on. Therefore, great care must be taken when carrying out the postmortem examination. The pathology of electrocution in domestic mammals was discussed by Giles and Simmons (1975).

The effects of burning are associated with tissue damage. Cells that are burned become desiccated (dry heat) or their protoplasm coagulates (moist heat). As a result there are local lesions, dehydration, pyrexia due to pyrogens, and often secondary infection by such resilient organisms as *Pseudomonas* spp.

Distinct lesions are usually apparent, and these burns may vary in severity from first- to fourth-degree burns. It is sometimes necessary to pluck feathers or to shave hair in order to reveal superficial burns. Dehydration and other secondary effects are often present, and if the animal survives over 48 hours after burning, toxic

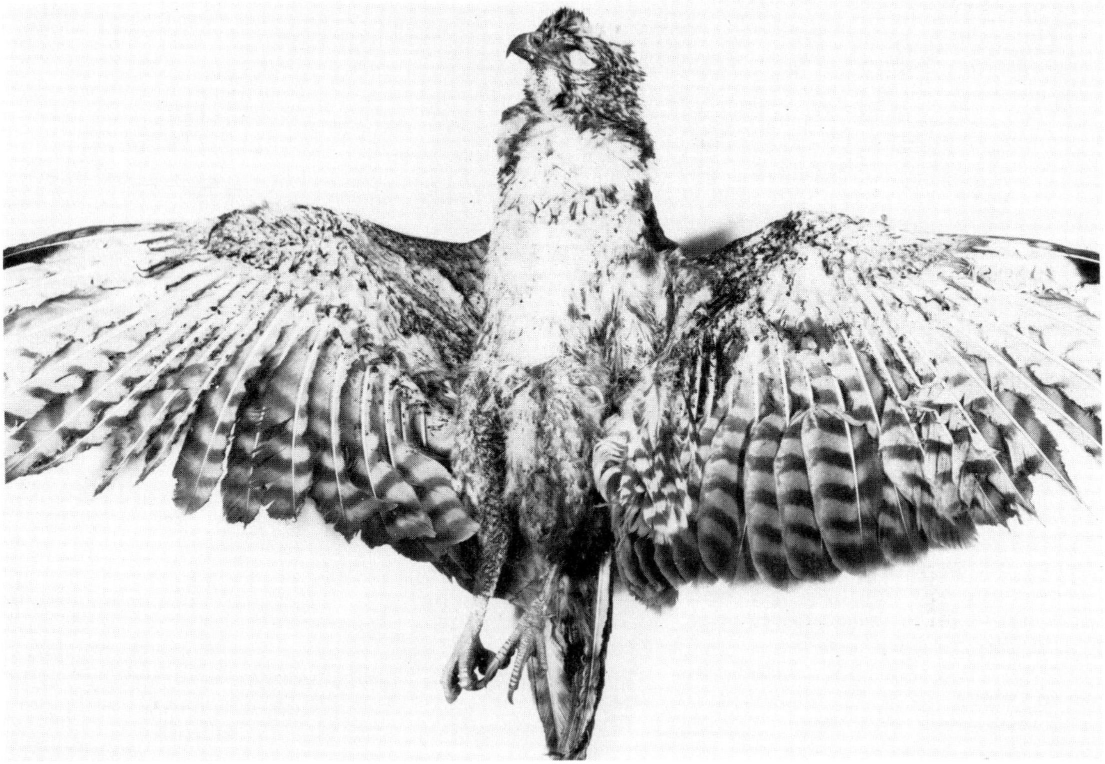

Fig. 8.3. Free-living common buzzard, *Buteo buteo*, that was electrocuted on a power line. Note the severely charred appearance of the feathers.

changes may be detectable in the liver and kidneys. The pathology of burns in animals is described by Jubb and Kennedy (1963).

DROWNING. This results in the intake of water into the respiratory and alimentary tracts. In the case of the latter, little harm may result, though vomiting may occur, especially in the case of sea water. However, in the former the surface area for gaseous exchange is reduced and bronchioles may become blocked, resulting in anoxia. In addition, an osmotic effect is produced that can result in hemolysis in fresh water, or dehydration and pulmonary edema in hypertonic sea water. The pathogenesis of drowning in humans is well understood largely because of experimental work using dogs, and details of the pathological processes involved are summarized by Camps and Cameron (1971). Inflammatory responses may also occur in the lungs in drowning (Modell, 1975).

Clinical Signs and Diagnosis. Diagnosis is based on a combination of clinical signs, postmortem findings, and to a large extent, history. Careful clinical examination is of the greatest importance. Animals should be observed carefully before being handled, and palpation and other diagnostic tests must be carried out quickly and efficiently. In some cases an accident kills the animal outright and clinical signs are not observed. Often, however, the animal is still alive and fairly distinct signs may be seen.

TRAUMA. Clinical signs can range from coma to an almost complete absence of signs. Affected animals usually show pain and often external injuries are visible or palpable. There may be evidence of blood loss and shock. Nervous signs frequently predominate, particularly when the animal has struck its head, and thus a careful differential diagnosis between infectious and metabolic diseases is necessary. There may be difficulty in standing and paralysis can also occur. In extreme cases, limbs or appendages may be completely lost. Other signs may be more subtle, such as subcutaneous emphysema in a bird, which is suggestive of air-sac damage, while an unexplained drop in hematocrit or certain other blood values may reflect internal hemorrhage. Small birds and mammals may also show severe diarrhea, often blood-stained, while internal damage to the respiratory tract can result in the coughing up of blood.

ELECTROCUTION AND BURNING. Again the animal may be comatose or show nervous signs. There may be apnea and ventricular fibrillation. Burning may be apparent and hemorrhages may be visible. The clinical history is often very valuable in diagnosis.

Distinct first-degree burns, painful to the touch, are usually visible, especially on exposed parts of the body. There may be edema and distinct vesicles or, in severe cases, sloughing of the skin. There is dehydration and the animal is often drowsy and depressed as a result of circulatory shock.

DROWNING. The hair or feathers are usually very wet and there may be water in the buccal or nasal cavities. If water has been inhaled, respiratory signs predominate and careful examination and manipulation of the animal may result in fluid sounds being heard and excess water being passed out of the trachea or esophagus. The carcass is usually wet, or if it has dried out, the hair or feathers are matted. Excess frothy fluid is found in the respiratory tract, including air sacs in the case of birds, and often in the esophagus and stomach. The lungs are usually distended and slightly congested, and subpleural petechiae may be present.

Postmortem diagnosis of accidents may not always be easy, since in many cases gross lesions are few and histological changes nonspecific. Very little research has been performed on this subject in domestic animals, let alone wild species, and often the diagnosis must be tentative. This contrasts with human medicine, in which forensic science permits accurate and specific diagnosis of many types of trauma. In certain cases, that is, where legal action is involved, a detailed diagnosis of the cause of death of an animal may be necessary and the investigator may find reference to forensic pathology literature of value. A number of the techniques described there can prove useful. Radiography will assist in the diagnosis of certain types of trauma (Fig. 8.4) while laboratory tests may be valuable. Examples of the latter are hematology and the examination of urine and feces for the presence of free blood. When trauma is suspected, the carcass should always be carefully examined externally and then skinned. In cases of paralysis, careful dissection of the cranium and spinal cord may be necessary to detect localized damage to the central nervous system.

Treatment. Treatment can only be discussed in general terms. In all cases of accidental injury attention must be paid to supportive treatment, since it is frequently the sequelae, rather than the injury itself, that can result in death.

TRAUMA. The usual rules for the treatment of injuries apply here. It is particularly important to nurse the animal, to minimize effects of shock and hemorrhage by administering fluids and analgesics, to clean and treat wounds, by suturing if necessary, and to give systemic antibiotics or corticosteroids where indicated. Internal damage may necessitate surgery, such as the removal of a ruptured spleen or internal fixation of fractures. There is a useful paper on orthopedic procedures in nondomestic species (Rickards et al., 1972). There are a number of publications on the anesthesia of wild animals in texts in both English (Harthoorn, 1971, 1976) and French (Mortelmans, 1971). Care should be taken to prevent self-mutilation, especially in the case of carnivores and primates who will quickly remove sutures or break down a wound. Captive wild animals may need prolonged sedation for this reason. The loss of a limb or a portion of one need not prove fatal to a wild animal, and passerine birds, in particular, seem to survive well with one leg.

ELECTROCUTION AND BURNING. Burns should be treated topically and secondary effects, such as dehydration, dealt with symptomatically. In the case of chemical burns the application of a suitable chemical to neutralize the irritant is important. In addition to fluids, antibiotics can be given to prevent or control infection, and corticosteroids and analgesics may prove valuable to counteract shock. It is important to give artificial respiration if normal breathing has ceased and cardiac massage if there is circulatory arrest. Recent work with human volunteers, following animal experiments, suggests that vaccination against *Pseudomonas aeruginosa* may prove useful in the prevention of secondary infection with this organism (Jones et al., 1976).

DROWNING. As with electrocution, if breathing has ceased, the first priority must be to restore respiration by artificial means. Endotracheal intubation is desirable. Holding the animal upside down will help to remove fluid from the respiratory tract. This accomplished, artificial respiration or oxygen must be administered until spontaneous breathing commences. The animal should be kept warm and nursed with antibiotics given routinely in order to reduce the dangers of pulmonary infection. If other effects are present, for example, anemia due to hemodilution and

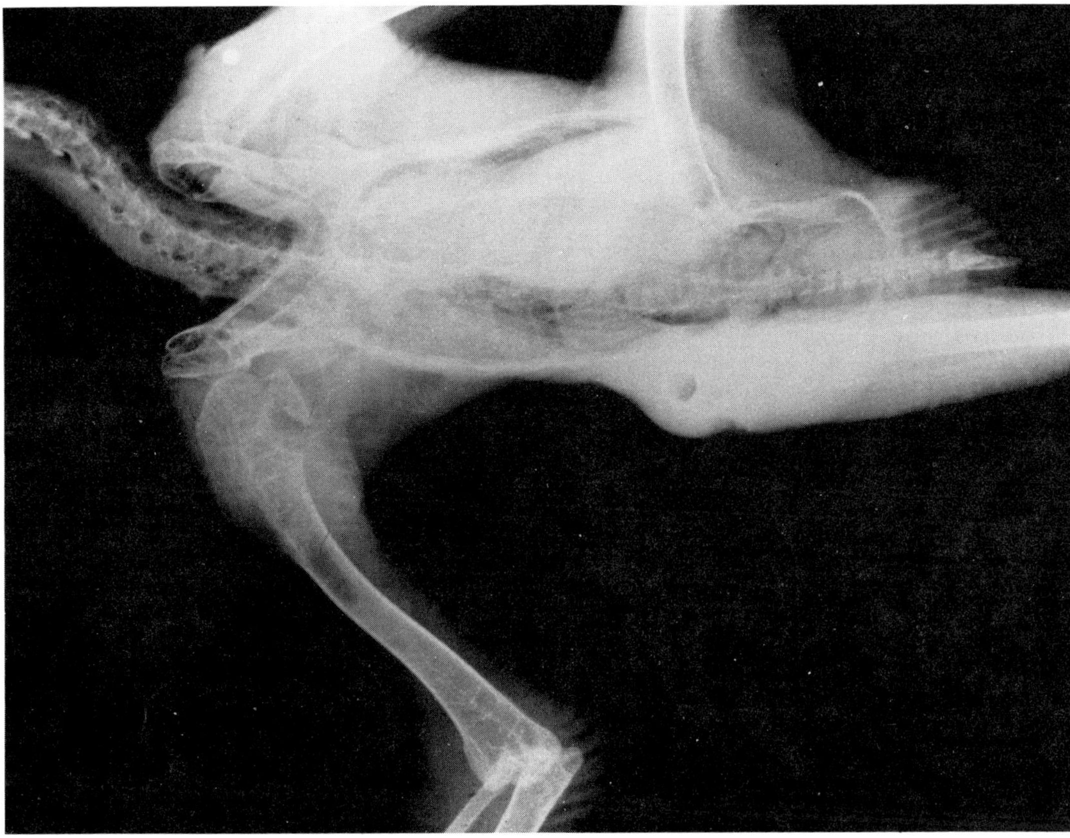

Fig. 8.4. Radiograph of a free-living common buzzard, *B. buteo,* showing dislocation of the left elbow joint and a particle of lead shot near the right shoulder.

erythrocyte hemolysis, symptomatic treatment must be carried out.

Control. Control of the conditions described above hinges mainly on good management techniques. Even in the case of free-living species, injuries can be reduced by careful planning of buildings and construction of power lines. Such measures can prove beneficial in saving lives. In Great Britain, for example, a number of lighthouses have special perches fixed to them so that small migratory birds, which are attracted to the light and may die in thousands, can perch and rest. When captive animals are uncrated, care should be taken to minimize injury (Siegmund, 1967). The design and the construction of enclosures for captive animals is of importance. For example, a moated barrier, rather than fences, may prove more satisfactory for containing wild ruminants and other large species and can reduce traumatic damage. On the other hand, too steep moats or ditches may predispose to drowning. Design of cages is of paramount importance while careful positioning of heaters, electric wires, and water containers will help reduce dangers. Such aspects can only be mentioned briefly here. All too often an aspect of poor design is not appreciated until an animal has been injured. It then becomes imperative to benefit from the experience and redesign or remove the structure as necessary. Preliminary consultations with others working with the same species will often pay dividends; for example, advice can be obtained on the size of fences and wire netting recommended for enclosures, on the strength and correct positioning of lamps for heating, and the like. Useful information can also be gained from the International Zoo Yearbook and journals such as the Journal of Zoo Animal Medicine.

Traumatic injuries inflicted by other animals can be prevented or reduced in captivity by careful management. All too often fighting or aggression is the result of undesirable social interaction, and this can frequently be remedied by careful selection of cage mates and prompt removal of aggressive individuals. This will require intensive knowledge of the animals involved and factors such as their optimal sex ratio and their reaction to other species. With species that show a pecking order, isolation of particularly persecuted individuals may prove useful (Cooper, 1968). The whole question of the psychology and behavior of captive wild animals is complex but one that is increasingly attracting interest. Knowledge of it can be of value in the prevention of boredom and, consequently, a reduction in the incidence of self-inflicted injuries and other wounds. This subject was first touched upon, albeit briefly, by Fox (1923) while Hediger (1955) studied it in some detail in zoo and circus animals. More recent studies include those of Walls and Fox (1973).

INJURIES CAUSED BY IONIZING RADIATION

Etiology. Radiation is probably of no great importance to wildlife in the free-living state. Wild animals rarely encounter high dosages of radiation unless specifically exposed to it by man. Exceptions are animals within the fallout zone of an atomic explosion, but little work seems to have been done in this area, even in Nagasaki and Hiroshima. In recent years, there has been interest in radioactive marking of animals for ecological studies, and this has yielded information on the susceptibility of some species to radiation (Bailey et al., 1973). One interesting group inhabits areas where the background radiation levels, because of radioactive rocks, are high or where reactor effluent elevates the environmental levels. Such a long-term effect may be significant and it is of interest that snakes have been suggested as suitable monitor species for such situations (Brisbin et al., 1974). Animals in captivity may be exposed to radiation either intentionally or by accident. A considerable amount of work on the effects of radiation has been carried out in experimental animals of many species and here extensive information is available (Bond et al., 1965). Of particular interest is the fact that hibernating animals are very resistant to radiation and massive doses are needed to kill them; however, when the animals are awake they will succumb quickly (Alexander, 1957).

The ultraviolet fraction of sunlight may act as a source of irradiation, and dermatitis, neoplasia, and photosensitization have been associated with it in domestic animals (Jubb and Kennedy, 1963). No such relationship appears to have been demonstrated in wild species.

Pathogenesis and Pathology. Pathogenesis is due to damage of tissues, particularly those with a high rate of mitosis, by either particulate or electromagnetic radiation. Pathogenesis has been described by Mole (1960) and pathology by Bond et al. (1965). The actual effect of the radiation will depend on the dose received and the organs affected. As a general rule doses of 200 rads or over are likely to prove fatal, but species vary in susceptibility. At doses of over 50 rads, many cells die and the multiplication of other cells is inhibited. In particular, the hemopoietic tissues are severely damaged so that within one to three weeks of exposure the animal shows leukopenia, thrombocytopenia, and anemia. Bacterial infection is a common sequela. The epithelium of the intestine is usually affected, resulting in diarrhea and severe loss of fluids and electrolytes. The germinal cells of testes or ovaries may also be badly damaged, producing infertility and possibly genetic changes, but the severity and duration of this depends upon the dosage. Fetal tissues can be similarly affected and even low doses, 25 rads, may produce developmental effects in the fetus. The nervous system is usually only slightly damaged unless massive doses, 2,500 to 12,000 rads, are involved but there are exceptions, for example, the burro, *Equus asinus* (Kuhn and Brown, 1962). Work on free-living pocket mice, *Perognathus parvus,* showed evidence of synergism between radiation-induced and environmental sources of mortality (O'Farrell et al., 1973).

Lesions depend on the dose of radiation and the area affected. Petechial hemorrhages are common and enteritis may be present. Lymphoid tissues show aplasia and there is destruction of bone marrow. In certain species, or if the dose of radiation is high, central nervous system changes may be apparent, especially cerebral edema.

Clinical Signs and Diagnosis. Clinical signs depend on whether the exposure to radiation is severe but brief or more chronic, with prolonged exposure to lower doses. Little is known of the significance of the latter in wild animals, but there are data on experimental animals, including monkeys, *Macaca* sp., and various rodents (Bond et al., 1965). A behavioral change noted in deer mice, *Peromyscus* sp., given deuterium oxide in their drinking water, was disturbance of the circadian rhythm (Suter and Rawson, 1968).

In acute exposure, immediate clinical signs may be slight, but vomiting usually occurs within minutes or hours of exposure. Later, cellular changes begin to take effect, and such signs as diarrhea, severe anemia, petechiation, and alopecia occur. A "radiation shock" syndrome was described by Allen et al. (1960) while Bond et al. (1965) discussed clinical signs in man in considerable detail.

Diagnosis is based largely upon clinical history. Clinical signs will assist diagnosis, especially if coupled with laboratory tests such as hematology, and in the case of postmortem material, histopathology.

TREATMENT AND CONTROL. The control of injuries caused by ionizing radiation hinges on prevention, by reducing unnecessary exposure where practicable, and treatment. The latter must be symptomatic. Blood transfusions will help maintain the animal until hemopoiesis begins again. Fluids should be given to replace those lost and antibiotics are necessary to counteract infection. Bond et al. (1965) discussed the modification of irradiation damage by replacement and functional or substitution therapy and, in addition to the points made above, drew attention to the possible role of such techniques as granulocyte and bone-marrow transfusions. They emphasized the control of secondary clinical consequences was usually satisfactory but that the final prognosis depended largely on the original radiation dose.

INJURIES CAUSED BY TEMPERATURE CHANGES

Etiology. Free-living animals can very easily become overheated by the sun in the tropics and morbidity or mortality may result. On the Island of Cousin in the Seychelles, for example, overheating by the sun is a significant cause of death among the young of the fairy tern, *Gygis alba* (Diamond, 1973). Excess cold is of importance in both free-living and captive animal populations. Extreme examples are in the polar and subpolar regions where the ambient temperature may regularly fall below the freezing point. Many species in these localities are adapted to such extremes. Frostbite is a common cause of disease in captive animals (Wallach and Flieg, 1969) and has been recorded as a cause of tail-tip loss in free-living opossums, *Didelphis marsupialis,* in the United States (Siegmund, 1967). Excess cold is recognized as an important cause of death in game management, and ducks and other birds have been recorded as freezing to the ice by their feet and feathers. Leopold (1933) discussed the significance of freezing in game animals and concluded that mortality on a large scale may occur through imprisonment of ground roosting birds and rabbits by sleet or crusted snow.

Chilling is of ubiquitous significance since even a slight drop in temperature can exert a stress effect on animals, especially when they are young. A sudden drop in temperature in the spring in temperate countries can kill large numbers of small birds, especially migrants, both directly and by reducing the quantities of available food. The effect on wild animal populations of periodic frosts and other climatic factors, such as exceptionally hot or cold summers, is discussed in some detail in a number of ecology books.

Pathogenesis and Pathology. Tissues are affected in a number of ways. Overheating has been covered previously under burning; in addition to superficial effects, however, it can cause largely irreversible damage to kidneys, liver, heart, and brain and changes in serum enzymes and electrolytes (Ellis, 1976a). Work on rhabdomyolysis in dogs has shown that, while often a feature of heat stress, it can also occur under cool conditions (Knochel and Schlein, 1972). Exposure to high temperatures also affects spermatogenesis and may cause fetal abnormalities; the latter was reviewed by Edwards (1976). In the case of chilling, the lowered temperature can result in a drop in the body temperature, especially in young animals where homoiothermy is often poorly developed. As a result body metabolism is reduced and the animal becomes weak and unable to feed; hypoglycemia may become a feature as carbohydrate reserves are exhausted. More severe exposure to cold can result in frostbite. Pathogenesis is due mainly to dehydration, disruption of cells by ice crystals, and disturbed metabolic activity. As a result there is ischemia of the superficial tissues that can progress to gangrene and sloughing. Prolonged exposure to cold may predispose wild animals to diseases associated with stress. Karstad and Sileo (1971) found gout, amyloidosis, and myocardial infarction most prevalent in waterfowl in cold weather. Cold injury in newborn lambs was investigated by Haughey (1973) who drew attention to the presence of edema of the subcutaneous tissues and, depending on the ambient temperature and nutritional status of the animal, changes in the adrenal cortex and varying degrees of fat catabolism.

There may be only mild, fairly nonspecific changes in cases of chilling. The lungs are often congested and an excess of clear fluid may be present in the body cavities. The liver is often pale and the stomach is usually empty.

In the case of freezing there may be areas where there is a loss of hair or feathers and specific lesions, such as edema. Tissues may appear avascular or necrotic and, in severe cases, have been sloughed or removed by the animal. Blindness due to corneal epithelial damage in deer exposed to a violent and cold blizzard was reported by Richards (1975a, 1975b) who also described damage to the skin, muscles, and fascia of these animals.

Clinical Signs and Diagnosis. Overheating by the sun falls under the same category as physical burning, but often no lesions are seen. There may be panting or other signs of overheating and in some cases a degree of hyperthermia may be detectable. In some severe cases of sunburn, cutaneous erythema and other skin lesions are present. The animal is frequently prostrate, in a stupor or coma, and very dehydrated; it tends to seek cool or sheltered places. Birds show similar panting respiration and their wings hang loosely. There is a valuable section on heat stress in one publication (Anon., 1968), and although it deals primarily with domestic animals, the clinical and therapeutic data given are equally applicable to wild species.

In mild chilling, the animal may appear cold to the touch, depressed in appearance, and to shiver, but often no other clinical signs are present. In the case of freezing, the body surface feels cold and appears pale; later it may become erythematous and edematous and the animal shows severe pain. As with burns, pruritis may accompany healing. In severe cases the affected area may become ischemic and slough; this has been reported in free-living opossums and in captive mammals and birds in many zoos. Lesions in deer were described in detail (Richards, 1975a, 1975b).

Treatment and Control. If the animal has been overheated, it should be moved to a sheltered place and slowly cooled, if necessary using a cool damp cloth or ice packs applied to the head, ears, or other exposed areas of the body. Fluids can also be given by mouth. Clipping of the hair will improve heat loss but may later make the animal more susceptible to overheating in the sun. In mild cases of sunburn a soothing powder, such as boric acid, may reduce discomfort. If heatstroke is severe, indicated by collapse and severe hyperthermia, rapid immersion in cold water is necessary and intravenous administration of 5% sodium chloride will prove valuable. If respiration has ceased, the priority is to give artificial respiration immediately and to delay treatment of wounds or secondary signs.

Chilled animals should be warmed gradually to a temperature of 24 to 30° C for a mammal or 32 to 38° C for a bird. They should be encouraged to feed by offering small amounts of readily digested food at frequent intervals and glucose should be given. In the case of freezing, the same principles apply, but it is important to treat local lesions with antibiotics or a liniment, and analgesics may also be necessary. Necrotic lesions of the appendages necessitate amputation. Corneal damage should be treated by irrigation and local application of antibiotics.

In some cases control of thermal injuries may be a matter of opinion and no hard and fast rules can be made. For example, the logical way to prevent chilling and frostbite in captive flamingoes in temperate countries in winter is to house them indoors in heated quarters. However, a number of experienced aviculturists and veterinarians disapprove of this since it can so easily result in other disease problems; they recommend instead that the birds should be kept outdoors in the winter but have access to warm quarters if they require them.

Captive wild animals will often adapt to extremely different temperatures from those to which they are accustomed in the wild but acclimatization must be gradual and every effort made to ensure that the animal receives an adequate diet. There is little information available on this, but Beer (1964) discussed practical methods of reducing mortality in captive waterfowl due to adverse cold weather and Vaneysinga (1969) described the dietary requirements of wild felids kept outdoors during winter. This is in contradistinction to the medical situation in which data are available on acclimatization of humans, especially to high temperatures (Ellis, 1976b). Similar work is needed on wild animals.

REFERENCES

Alexander, P. 1957. Atomic radiation and life. Penguin Books, Middlesex.

Allen, R. E., and D. R. McCullough. 1976. Deer-car accidents in southern Michigan. J. Wildl. Manage. 40:317–325.

Allen, R. G., F. A. Brown, L. C. Logie, D. R. Rovner, S. G. Wilson, and R. W. Zellmer. 1960. Acute effects of gamma radiation in primates. Radiat. Res. 12:532–539.

Anon. 1968. Handbook on animal disease in the tropics. Br. Vet. Assoc., London.

Bailey, G. N. A., I. J. Linn, and P. J. Walker. 1973. Radioactive marking of small mammals. Mammal Rev. 3:11–23.

Basson, P. A., and J. M. Hofmeyr. 1973. Mortalities associated with wildlife capture operations. In E. Young. The capture and care of wild animals. Human and Rousseau, Cape Town.

Beer, J. 1964. Wildfowl mortality in the Slimbridge collection during the winters of 1961–62 and 1962–63. Wildfowl Trust Annu. Rep. 15:50–56.

Bond, V. P., T. M. Fliedner, and J. O. Archambeau. 1965. Mammalian radiation lethality. Academic Press, New York.

Brisbin, I. L., M. A. Staton, J. E. Pinder, and R. A. Geiger. 1974. Radio-cesium concentrations of snakes from contaminated and noncontaminated habitats of the AEC Savannah River Plant. Copeia 2:501–506.

Brockie, R. E. 1960. Road mortality of the hedgehog, *Erinaceus europeaeus* L. in New Zealand. Proc. Zool. Soc. Lond. 134:505–508.

Camps, F. E., and J. M. Cameron. 1971. Practical forensic medicine. Hutchinson Medical Publications, London.

Cooper, J. E. 1968. Veterinary examination of exotic animals prior to export. J. Small Anim. Pract. 9:237–243.

Davies, J. L. 1957. A hedgehog road mortality index. Proc. Zool. Soc. Lond. 128:606–608.

Diamond, A. 1973. Warden, Cousin Island, Seychelles. Personal communication.

Edwards, M. J. 1976. The influence of heat stress on the developing fetus. Vet. Ann. 16:227–231.

Ellis, F. P. 1976a. Heat illness. II. Pathogenesis. Trans. Royal Soc. Trop. Med. Hyg. 70:412–418.

______. 1976b. Heat illness. III. Acclimatisation. Trans. Royal Soc. Trop. Med. Hyg. 70:419–423.

Fox, H. 1923. Disease in captive wild mammals and birds. J. B. Lippincott, Philadelphia.

Giles, N., and J. R. Simmons. 1975. Electrocution of pigs. Vet. Rec. 97:305–306.

Gordon, K. 1932. Rabbits killed on an Idaho highway. J. Mammal. 13:169.

Harrison, J. G. 1963. Heavy mortality of mute swans from electrocution. Wildfowl Trust Annu. Rep. 14:164–165.

Harthoorn, A. M. 1971. Advances in anaesthesiology in zoo and wild animals (A review of recent advances). Proc. XIX World Vet. Congr., Mexico 2:509–514.

______. 1976. The chemical capture of animals. Ralph Curtis Books, Hollywood.

______, and E. Young. 1974. A relationship between acid-base balance and capture myopathy in zebra, *Equus burchelli,* and an apparent therapy. Vet. Rec. 95:337–342.

Haughey, K. G. 1973. Cold injury in newborn lambs. Aust. Vet. J. 49:554–563.

Hediger, H. 1955. Studies of the psychology and behaviour of captive animals in zoos and circuses. Butterworths, London.

Jones, R. J., E. A. Roe, E. J. L. Rowbury, J. J. Miler, and J. F. Spilsbury. 1976. A new *Pseudomonas* vaccine: Preliminary trial on human volunteers. J. Hyg. (Camb.) 76:429–439.

Jortner, B. S. 1974. Neuropathologic observations of head trauma in the northern fur seal. J. Wildl. Dis. 10:121–129.

Jubb, K. V. J., and P. C. Kennedy. 1963. Pathology of domestic animals. Academic Press, New York.

Karstad, L. H., and L. Sileo. 1971. Causes of death in captive wild waterfowl in the Kortright Waterfowl Park, 1969–1970. J. Wildl. Dis. 7:236–241.

Knochel, J. P., and E. M. Schlein. 1972. On the mechanisms of rhabdomyolysis in potassium depletion. J. Clin. Invest. 51:1750–1758.

Kuhn, U. S. G., and D. G. Brown. 1962. Head irradiation of the burro with cobalt-60. JAMA 180:671–675.

Leopold, A. 1933. Game management. Charles Scribner and Sons, New York.

Markus, M. B. 1972. Mortality of vultures caused by electrocution. Nature 238:228.

Michell, A. R. 1974. The metabolic consequences of trauma. J. Small Anim. Pract. 15:279–291.

Modell, J. H. 1975. Pulmonary insults. Drowning-aspiration pneumonitis. Annual Refresher Course Lectures. Annu. Meet. Am. Soc. Anesthesiol., Chicago, Oct. 1975. Lecture 128:1–5.

Mole, R. H. 1960. Toxicity of radiation. In C. V. Harrison. Recent advances in pathology. 7th ed. Churchill, London.

Mortelmans, J. 1971. L'Anaesthésie des Animaux Sauvages. Ann. Méd. Vét. 115:317–332.

O'Farrell, T. P., J. D. Hedlund, R. J. Olson, and R. O. Gilbert. 1973. Radiation effects in free-ranging pocket mice, *Perognathus parvus,* during the breeding season. Science 79:289–291.

Richards, S. H. 1975a. Deer blinded by blizzard. ND Outdoors 37:2–4.

______. 1975b. Deer blinded by blizzard. Part II. ND Outdoors 38:12–13.

Rickards, D. A., P. J. Hinko, and E. M. Morse. 1972. Orthopedic procedures for laboratory animals and exotic pets. J. Am. Vet. Med. Assoc. 161:728–732.

Sargeant, A. B., and J. E. Forbes. 1973. Mortality among birds, mammals and certain snakes on 17 miles of Minnesota roads. The Loon 45:4–7.

Sevitt, S., and H. B. Stoner. 1970. The pathology of trauma. Proceedings of a symposium organized by the Royal College of Pathologists. J. Clin. Pathol. (Lond.).

Shaw, G. E., and K. A. Neiland. 1973. Electrocution of a caribou herd caused by lightning in central Alaska. J. Wildl. Dis. 9:311–313.

Siegmund, O. H. 1967. The Merck veterinary manual. 3rd ed. Merck Co., New Jersey.

Stout, I. J., and G. W. Cornwell. 1976. Non-hunting mortality of fledged North American waterfowl. J. Wildl. Manage. 40:681–693.

Sugden, J. W. 1930. White pelicans killed by lightning. Auk 47:72.

Suter, R. B., and K. S. Rawson. 1968. Circadian activity rhythm of the deer mouse, *Peromyscus:* Effect of deuterium oxide. Science 160:1011–1014.

Vaneysinga, C. R. 1969. The dietary requirements of lions, tigers and jaguars when kept outdoors during winter months. Int. Zoo Yearbook 9:164–166.

Wallach, J. D., and M. Flieg. 1969. Frostbite and its sequelae in captive exotic birds. J. Am. Vet. Med. Assoc. 155:1035–1038.

Walls, S., and M. W. Fox. 1973. Wild animals in captivity: Veterinarian's role and responsibility. J. Zoo Anim. Med. 4:7–17.

Wright, E. N. 1972. Birdstrikes and the third London airport. Animals 14:151–155.

Wynne-Edwards, V. C. 1962. Animal dispersion in relation to social behaviour. Oliver and Boyd, Edinburgh.

Young, E. 1967. Leg paralysis in the greater flamingo and lesser flamingo following capture and transportation. Int. Zoo Yearbook 7:226–227.

______, and P. J. L. Bronkhorst. 1971. Overstraining disease of game. Afr. Wildl. 25:51–52.

9 *Capture Myopathy*

GORDON A. CHALMERS
MORLEY W. BARRETT

CAPTURE MYOPATHY (CM), also known as overstraining disease, stress myopathy, polymyopathy, white muscle disease, transport myopathy, spastic paresis, muscle necrosis, and leg paralysis, is recognized primarily as a disease of recently captured wildlife. In ungulates the syndrome is characterized clinically by depression, muscular stiffness, incoordination, paralysis, metabolic acidosis, myoglobinuria, and death. Pathologically, CM resembles the myodegenerative disorders of domestic cattle, sheep, horses, and swine. Undoubtedly, this condition has existed for years as a major, but until recently unrecognized, cause of mortality in the large ungulates of Africa and North America.

Jarrett et al. (1964) observed CM and provided the first published description of the pathology of this condition in a Hunter's hartebeest, *Damaliscus hunteri.* Subsequently, numerous reports have described a similar condition in other free-ranging African ungulates (Basson et al., 1971; Ebedes, 1969; Harthoorn and Van Der Walt, 1974; Harthoorn and Young, 1974; Hofmeyr, 1974; Hofmeyr et al., 1973; Jarrett and Murray, 1967; Mugera and Wandera, 1967; Young, 1966; Young and Bronkhorst, 1971).

The occurrence of CM has been reported in the following African big game species: cape buffalo, *Syncerus caffer;* red hartebeest, *Alcelaphus buselaphus;* springbok, *Antidorcas marsupialis;* blesbok, *Damaliscus dorcas phillipsi;* bontebok, *D. d. dorcas;* tsessebe, *D. lunatus;* eland, *Taurotragus oryx;* gemsbok, *Oryx gazella gazella;* giraffe, *Giraffa camelopardalis;* roan antelope, *Hippotragus equinus;* sable antelope, *H. niger;* Burchell's zebra, *Equus burchelli;* mountain zebra, *E. zebra hartmannae;* impala, *Aepyceros melampus;* kudu, *Tragelaphus strepsiceros;* nyala, *T. angasi;* steenbok, *Raphicerus campestris;* blue wildebeest, *Connochaetes taurinus;* black rhinoceros, *Diceros bicornis;* elephant, *Loxodonta africana;* and oribi, *Ourebia ourebi* (Basson and Hofmeyr, 1973). Jarrett and Murray (1967) and Mugera and Wandera (1967) listed additional wild species affected with myopathies similar to those of CM. The condition was observed also in recently captured baboons, *Papio ursinus* (McConnell et al., 1974) and in greater flamingoes, *Phoenicopterus ruber roseus,* and lesser flamingoes, *Phoeniconaias minor* (Young, 1967).

There have been relatively infrequent reports of CM in free-ranging wildlife other than those of Africa. In Great Britain, Fairlie (1964) described myopathy suggestive of CM in a recently captured young roe deer, *Capreolus capreolus,* and Gibbs et al. (1975) suggested that mortalities that had occurred in drive-trapped roe and muntjac deer, *Muntiacus muntjac,* may have been caused by CM. In Australia, myopathy in recently captured pademelon, *Thylogale billardierii,* and Bennett's wallaby, *Protemnodon bennetti,* was described by Munday (1972).

In North America, Hebert and Cowan (1971) described white muscle disease in a herd of recently trapped mountain goat, *Oreamnos americanus,* in British Columbia. Based on the continuity of capture, clinical signs, clinicopathologic findings, and lesions, present evidence suggests that this report represents the first clear documentation of CM in free-ranging North American ungulates. Wobeser et al. (1976) reported myopathy and myoglobinuria in a live white-tailed deer, *Odocoileus virginianus,* as well as myopathy similar to that of CM in recently captured pronghorn antelope, *Antilocapra americana,* and a moose, *Alces alces.* Haigh et al. (1977) also reported CM in a moose. Capture myopathy has been observed in wild-trapped bighorn sheep, *Ovis canadensis,* in Colorado (DeMartini and Davies, 1977; Spraker, 1976) and in drive-trapped pronghorn antelope in Alberta (Chalmers and Barrett, 1977).

Myopathy of undetermined etiology was observed in a dead white-tailed deer and in a bighorn sheep that was unable to stand when captured (Hadlow, 1955, 1973). Further cases of a condition undistinguishable from CM have been observed by the authors in bighorn sheep and mountain goat, in recently captured white-tailed deer (Wobeser, 1976); mule deer, *O. hemionus* (Haigh et al., 1977); bison, *Bison bison* (Hudson, 1976); and elk, *Cervus canadensis,* (Lewis et al., 1977). A mild form of CM was suspected in a dolphin, *Tursiops gilli* (Colgrove, 1978). Paralysis of the limbs and the subsequent loss of Canada geese, *Branta canadensis,* associated with drive-trapping, handling, and translocation occur regularly, especially during hot weather (Wishart, 1977). Capture myopathy affecting the cervical, superficial, and deep pectoral gastrocnemius, lateral digital extensor, and other muscles of the hindlimb, has been confirmed in recently captured migrating snow geese, *Anser hyperborea,* and Ross's geese, *Chen rossii* (Wobeser, 1978). These observations suggest that CM-like conditions may be more common hazards for this and other recently captured avian species than has been recognized previously. Exertional myopathies of wild and domestic animals and man have been discussed (Bartsch et al., 1977).

Capture myopathy may occur irrespective of the season of the year, condition, or sex of the animals involved. Harthoorn et al. (1974c) noted that more than half of the animals captured may be lost, many of them gravid females. Occasionally, the incidence of mortality may approach 100% of captured animals (Harthoorn, 1975). With the exception of elephant and blue wildebeest, young animals appear to be less susceptible to CM than are adults (Basson and Hofmeyr, 1973). Similarly in primates, CM was found to be more prevalent in adult baboons than in juveniles (McConnell et al., 1974). This was thought to be related to the greater excitability of mature animals after capture and caging. Some species, such as blue wildebeest, cape buffalo, and impala appear to be less susceptible to CM than others, for example, roan antelope (Basson and Hofmeyer, 1973).

ETIOLOGY. The etiology of CM is not fully understood; however, there is usually a strong association between the occurrence of this condition and the concerted and vigorous use of all muscles during pursuit and capture. In most recognized cases, intense air or ground pursuit, capture with or without immobilizing drugs, and frequently, transportation precede clinical signs and death (Basson and Hofmeyer, 1973; Basson et al., 1971; Chalmers and Barrett, 1977; DeMartini and Davies, 1977; Ebedes, 1969; Harthoorn, 1975; Harthoorn and Van Der Walt, 1974; Harthoorn and Young, 1974; Hebert and Cowan, 1971; Hofmeyr, 1974; Hofmeyr et al., 1973; Jarrett et al., 1964; McConnell et al., 1974; Mugera and Wandera, 1967; Munday, 1972; Spraker, 1976; Young, 1966; Young and Bronkhorst, 1971). Immobilizing drugs that induce hyperthermia or acidosis during capture have been associated with signs and lesions of CM (Basson et al., 1971; Harthoorn and Van Der Walt, 1974; Young, 1972). This condition can occur, however, irrespective of chemical or physical methods used for capture and restraint (Basson and Hofmeyr, 1973).

Chalmers and Barrett (1977) found an increased mortality of pronghorn antelope captured during periods of warm ambient temperature and a lowered incidence in those captured during cold weather. Hofmeyr et al. (1973) emphasized the importance of capturing animals under cool conditions. Despite the absence of pursuit, CM was suspected retrospectively by the authors as the cause of the recumbency and mortality observed in bait-trapped elk and moose (Lynch, G. M., 1975). The stress of confinement and handling appeared to be the main factor associated with these mortalities. Capture myopathy was later confirmed in bait-trapped elk (Lewis et al., 1977).

Fear and Anxiety. Muscular lesions similar to those of CM have been observed in free-ranging sable antelope and zebra that were not known to have been pursued by man (Young and Bronkhorst, 1971). Harthoorn (1975) noted that incipient muscular lesions identical to those of CM have been demonstrated in animals killed by hunting. These observations suggest that CM-like lesions may be a natural result of intraspecific combat or of prolonged harassment by predators, including man (Hebert and Cowan, 1971; Young and Bronkhorst, 1971). It is conceivable that the hunting behavior of predators, particularly that of canids (Mech, 1975), may induce CM in prey species during pursuit. The role of CM, however, in improving predator success is an entirely speculative, but intriguing, possibility at present.

A related problem of some importance is the use of domestic dogs in the pursuit of big game (Young and Bronkhorst, 1971). There is speculation that the stresses of fear and anxiety are the triggering mechanisms, which may be modified by genetic or acquired predispositions to the disease. These factors in turn may be exacerbated by overexertion, exhaustion, hyperthermia, unnecessary disturbance, excessive handling, transportation, and shock (Basson and Hofmeyr, 1973; Harthoorn and Young, 1974; Hebert and Cowan, 1971; Hofmeyr, 1974; McConnell et al., 1974).

Nutritional Deficiencies. In most documented cases, the role of nutritional deficiencies as contributing causes of CM is not clear. Although it was not demonstrated, a deficiency of vitamin E may have contributed to the development of myopathy in a Hunter's antelope and perhaps in other African ungulates examined (Jarrett and Murray, 1967; Jarrett et al., 1964). Munday (1972) suggested, but did not demonstrate, that deficiencies of selenium (Se) or vitamin E, in addition to the effects of overexertion, may have been associated with myopathy observed in captured pademelon and wallaby. Analysis of 13 species of forage from the summer and winter ranges of mountain goat revealed a mean Se value of only 51 parts per billion (ppb); goats from these areas showed signs and lesions of myopathy after capture (Hebert and Cowan, 1971). These authors did not report Se values in tissues, but their account demonstrated the first apparent association between Se deficiency in forage and the development of CM-like lesions in captured wild ungulates. Basson et al. (1971) and Basson and Hofmeyr (1973) suggested that CM in African ungulates is not primarily a Se-vitamin E deficiency disease.

Harthoorn et al. (1974a), however, noted that myopathy is more likely to occur when animals from Se-deficient areas are stressed, and suggested that seasonal fluctuations of hepatic Se values might result in a temporary predisposition to CM. Barrett (1974) reported a mean Se value of 983 ppb in winter forage of pronghorn antelope; these findings suggested that CM seen in this species in Canada was unlikely to be associated with a Se deficiency. Further investigations into the importance of Se and vitamin E in the development of CM in various geographic areas of the world appear warranted.

PATHOGENESIS AND SIGNS. Clinical signs of CM may occur within hours, several days, or even weeks after capture (Basson and Hofmeyr, 1973; Chalmers and Barrett, 1977; Harthoorn and Young, 1974; Hebert and Cowan, 1971; Hofmeyr, 1974; Hofmeyr et al., 1973; Lewis et al, 1977; McConnell et al., 1974; Mugera and Wandera, 1967; Munday, 1972; Young, 1966, 1967, 1972; Young and Bronkhorst, 1971). Signs in affected wildlife are similar to those observed in acute rhabdomyolysis, or tying up, and paralytic myoglobinuria of horses and in the nutritional and transport myopathies of domestic cattle and sheep (Blood and Henderson, 1974; Hadlow, 1973; Lindholm et al., 1974). Clinically, CM resembles the porcine stress syndrome, a condition characterized by dyspnea, muscular tremors, irregular breathing, hyperthermia, collapse, and death (Topel et al., 1975). Capture myopathy bears some clinical and pathologic similarity to Type 1 idiopathic paroxysmal myoglobinuria of man, a disease in which intense muscular effort precedes signs in aproximately half of the cases (Adams, 1975).

Early clinical signs of CM include increased respiratory and cardiac rates and an elevated body temperature. Other prevalent signs are an unsteady gait, incoordination, stiffness, tremors, and torticollis. Weakness, lameness, and difficulty in swallowing may occur also. Depression and partial or total muscular paralysis are frequent findings (Fig. 9.1). In addition, labored respiration and the passage of coffee-colored urine (myoglobinuria) may be evident. Animals in the terminal stages of CM may have a thready pulse and a muffled heartbeat; collapse, prostration, and coma usually precede death. In many cases, affected animals may die suddenly without premonitory signs, either early in the course of the disease or within several days to weeks after capture.

Metabolic Acidosis. The physiologic basis of CM is incompletely understood, but recent investigations have shed light on the pathogenesis of this condition. Blesbok, subjected to forced exercise and subsequent capture, developed a metabolic acidosis that was most severe in animals pursued rapidly over a short distance and least severe in those captured after a more prolonged, less intense pursuit (Harthoorn and Van Der Walt, 1974). These observations suggested that a relatively short burst of intense activity, probably involving a high proportion of body muscle mass, has a greater effect in liberating fixed lactic acid than does prolonged exercise. Harthoorn and Van Der Walt suggested further that muscular lesions seen in CM might reflect the combined effects of increased lactic acid production and forced exercise. The resulting severe change in the hydrogen ion concentration could induce muscular spasms.

Subsequent investigations of pursued Burchell's zebra confirmed the initial observation that metabolic acidosis was a significant component of CM (Harthoorn and Young, 1974). In these animals, a mean blood pH value of 6.67 was increased, by appropriate therapy, to a mean of 7.28. The return of the blood pH to normal or nearly so was accompanied by marked clinical improvement in these zebra, findings that provided further evidence of the importance of metabolic acidosis in the genesis of CM.

Harthoorn and Young (1974) suggested that the drastic fall in the blood pH may bring about decreased cardiac output, a drop in systemic blood pressure, fibrillation and possible cardiac arrest, and death. The increased pulmonary arterial pressure that was found in chased young zebra and wildebeest was believed to be due, in part, to the action of low pH values (Harthoorn and Young, 1976). Renal failure, perhaps as the result of myoglobinuria, may account for some deaths that occur several weeks after capture. Cardiac lesions may be associated with either early or late deaths of CM-affected animals (Young, 1966).

Investigations of forced exercise in domestic

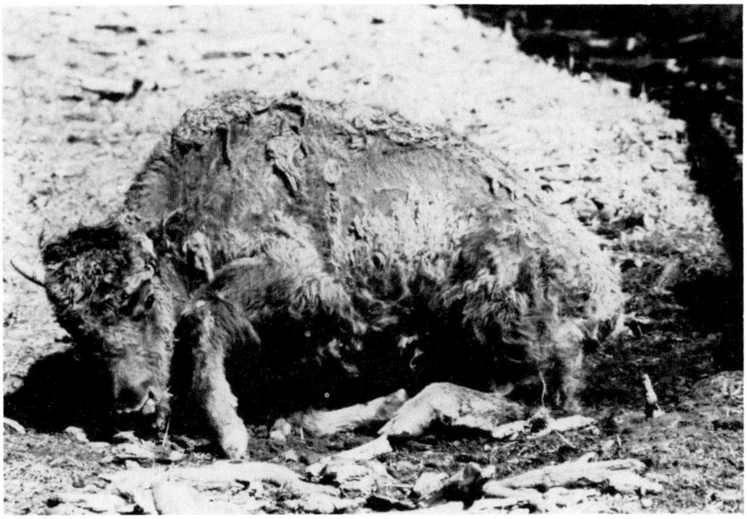

Fig. 9.1. Capture myopathy, bison, *Bison bison,* with posterior paralysis as the result of muscular lesions (Photo courtesy R. J. Hudson, University of Alberta, Edmonton).

sheep (Gericke and Belonje, 1975) and of CM in springbok (Gericke and Hofmeyr, 1976) also demonstrated that metabolic acidosis was an important sequela of strenuous exercise. Gericke and Hofmeyr (1976) concluded that CM in springbok occurred as a result of trauma, acute stress, and hyperthermia induced by forced exercise and that these factors were potentiated by an intense alarm reaction and a concurrent release of catecholamines. Under these conditions, hemoconcentration occurred, plasma glucose values increased markedly, and because of the increased workload on the muscles, the oxidative capacity of the mitochondria was exceeded. This resulted in hypoxia, increased anaerobic metabolism, metabolic acidosis, increased lactate values, and importantly, increased permeability of the cell membrane.

Elevated Serum Enzymes. Elevated values of serum enzymes, including glutamic oxaloacetic transaminase (SGOT), glutamic pyruvic transaminase, lactic dehydrogenase, and creatine phosphokinase (SCPK) have been observed in CM-affected animals (Chalmers and Barrett, 1977; Gericke and Hofmeyr, 1976; Harthoorn, 1973; Harthoorn and Young, 1976; Harthoorn et al., 1974c; Hebert and Cowan, 1971; Hofmeyr et al., 1973; Lewis et al., 1977; Wobeser et al., 1976; Young, 1966). Concurrently, elevations of serum potassium, blood urea nitrogen (BUN), creatinine, glucose, and lactate have been reported also by several of these investigators. Elevated values of serum enzymes, particularly those of SGOT and SCPK, reflect damage to skeletal and cardiac muscles; elevation of SCPK values appears to be one of the most sensitive and specific indices of muscular damage (Cardinet, 1971; Cardinet et al., 1967; Kronfeld and Medway, 1969).

Because of its important role in the cellular physiology, potassium elevations may be a further reflection of muscular or other tissue damage. Gericke and Belonje (1975) noted that in the metabolic acidosis accompanying exercise-induced stress, an exchange occurs between extracellular hydrogen and intracellular potassium ions, with resulting elevations of plasma potassium. Elevated serum creatinine values noted in some drive-trapped pronghorns probably reflected extensive muscular and renal damage (Barrett and Chalmers, 1977).

Phases of CM. Harthoorn (1973) summarized the clinical and biochemical events of CM and suggested the subdivision of the condition into four phases: hyperacute, acute, subacute, and chronic (or indefinite). In the *hyperacute* form, the profound metabolic acidosis is sufficiently severe to cause cardiac fibrillation, circulatory collapse, and sudden death; concurrently, high serum potassium values result from damage to body musculature. The *acute* form continues to be associated with severe metabolic acidosis. Affected animals show clinical signs of muscular stiffness, depression, rapid pulse, and increased respiratory rate; death from pulmonary edema occurs, often within 12 hours. The *subacute* form of CM is associated with damage to skeletal muscle and to internal organs. As a result, animals may knuckle over at the fetlocks or develop muscular paralysis. Elevated values of serum enzymes, potassium, and BUN reflect damage to various internal organs, such as muscle, liver, heart, and kidney. Affected animals may survive for several weeks, with no response to various treatments. Death appears to be related to renal failure resulting from myoglobinuric nephrosis.

The *chronic* form, which has not been demonstrated conclusively, may be characterized by the sudden death, following renewed stress, of animals that have survived the initial capture procedures for several weeks or months. Fibrotic areas in the myocardium, possibly representing previous infarcts or other areas of necrosis, may be found in these animals at necropsy.

PATHOLOGY. Grossly and histologically, muscular lesions of CM are virtually indistinguishable from those of paralytic myoglobinuria of horses and the nutritional and transport myopathies of domestic cattle and sheep (Hadlow, 1973; Jubb and Kennedy, 1970). Gross or histologic lesions of CM in ungulates, macropods, primates, and birds have been observed by several investigators (Basson and Hofmeyr, 1973; Chalmers and Barrett, 1977; Ebedes, 1969; Harthoorn and Young, 1974; Hebert and Cowan, 1971; Hofmeyr et al., 1973; Jarrett et al., 1964; Lewis et al., 1977; McConnell et al., 1974; Mugera and Wandera, 1967; Munday, 1972; Young, 1966; Young and Bronkhorst, 1971). Affected muscles may include the cardiac, pectoral, and intercostal, as well as those of the shoulder and forelimb and the large muscles of the hindlimb, including the gluteus, biceps femoris, semimembranosus, semitendinosus, and gastrocnemius. Lesions tend to be bilateral and asymmetrical in distribution and may involve the total affected muscle masses (Fig. 9.2).

In the early stages, the major gross lesions in skeletal muscle may consist of hemorrhage and edema, and a uniform pallor or blanched appearance, as well as dull white striations. Alternating light and dark areas, resulting in a banded appearance in affected muscle, may be seen (Fig. 9.3). In later stages, lesions may be more pronounced and may appear as sharply demarcated

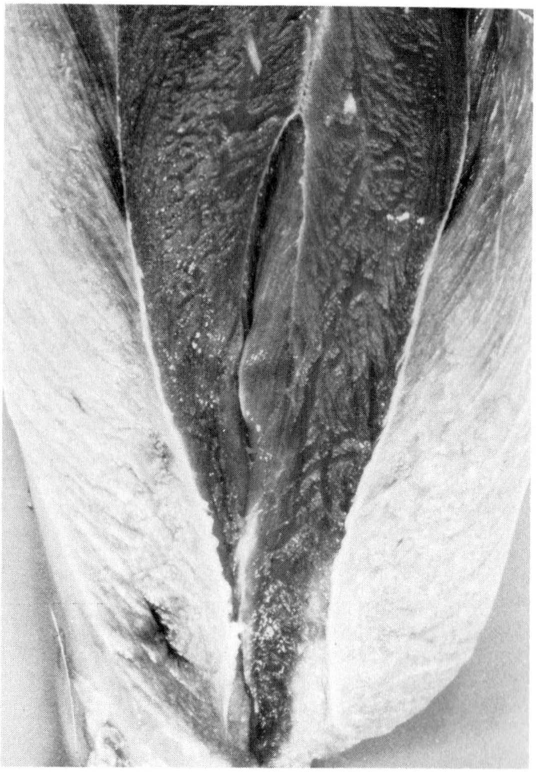

Fig. 9.2. Capture myopathy, elk, *Cervus canadensis*. Note the marked pallor of affected gastrocnemius muscle and contrasting appearance of the normal superficial digital flexor (Photo courtesy R. J. Lewis, Alberta Department of Agriculture, Edmonton).

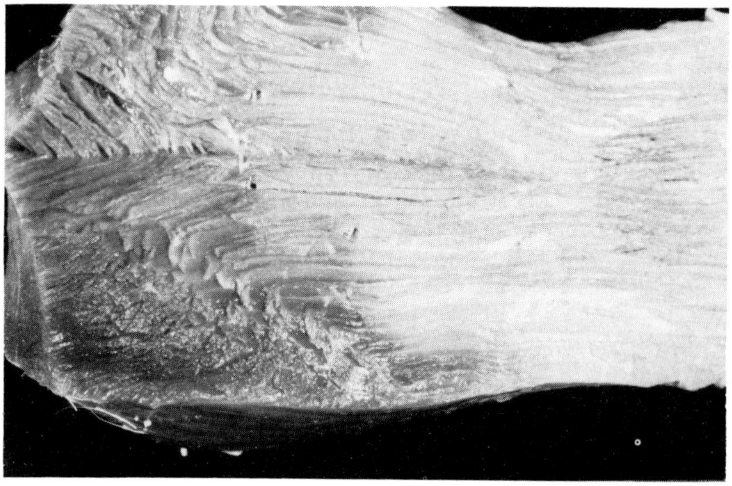

Fig. 9.3. Capture myopathy, elk, *C. canadensis*. Diffuse pallor with alternating dark and light striations (Photo courtesy R. J. Lewis, Alberta Department of Agriculture, Edmonton).

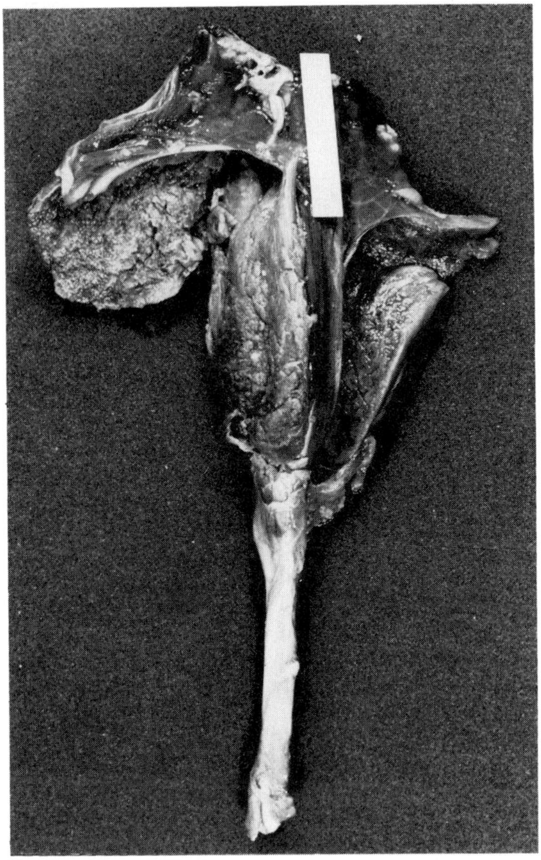

Fig. 9.4. Capture myopathy, white-tailed deer, *Odocoileus virginianus.* Note the rupture of the gastrocnemius muscle (Photo courtesy G. A. Wobeser, University of Saskatchewan, Saskatoon).

white steaks that run parallel with the plane of the muscle masses. In some cases, hemorrhage may be associated with frank rupture of affected muscles (Fig. 9.4) (Basson and Hofmeyr, 1973; Lewis et al., 1977; Wobeser, 1976).

Lesions similar to those found in skeletal muscle may be found in the heart. Pulmonary hyperemia and edema with tracheal and bronchial froth are found commonly and may be associated with some alveolar and interstitial emphysema. The liver is often swollen and pale. There may be hemorrhage or hyperemia of the adrenal cortex. The kidneys may be swollen and pale or dark, and the urinary bladder may contain red-brown or coffee-colored urine.

Histologically, lesions in skeletal muscle consist of hemorrhage and swelling of muscle fibers, loss or attenuation of cross-striations, increased eosinophilia, and a hyaline to granular degeneration (Fig. 9.5). More severe lesions are seen as transverse fragmentations and necrosis plus mild infiltrations of polymorphonuclear leukocytes. Normal muscle fibers are often interspersed with degenerating fibers. Calcification is not a consistent finding but has been reported in some cases (Chalmers and Barrett, 1977; Hofmeyr et al., 1973; Lewis et al., 1977; McConnell et al., 1974; Mugera and Wandera, 1967; Munday, 1972; Young, 1966).

More advanced changes, often associated with regeneration, are characterized by marked cellularity, including the presence of macrophages laden with yellow pigment and the proliferation of chains of swollen, vesicular sarcolemmal nuclei (Fig. 9.6). Slim, slightly basophilic new fibers are often associated with the presence of many sarcolemmal nuclei. Healed lesions may be

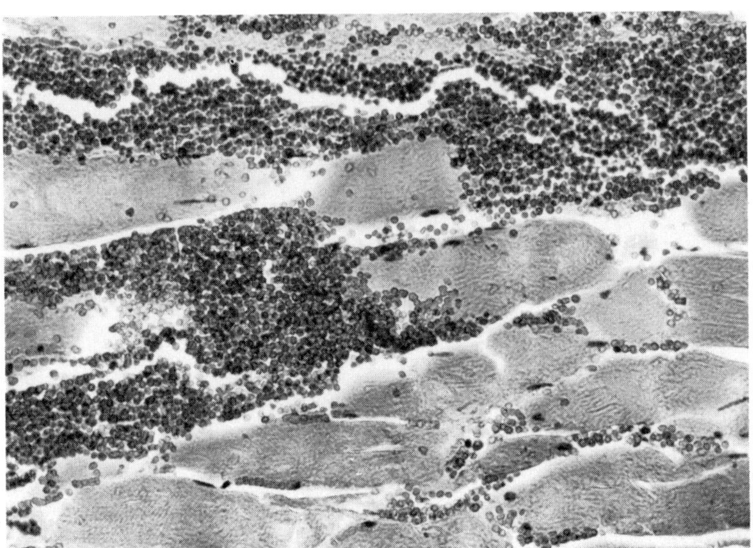

Fig. 9.5. Capture myopathy, pronghorn antelope, *Antilocapra americana.* Acute stage. Note the hemorrhage, nuclear pyknosis, loss or attenuation of cross-striations, and hyalinization of some fibers (×251).

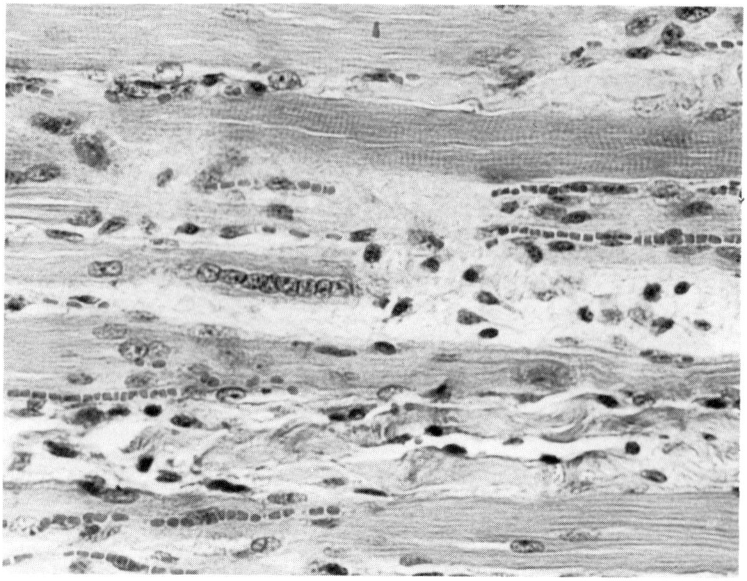

Fig. 9.6. Capture myopathy, pronghorn antelope, *A. americana*. Regenerative stage. Chains of proliferating sarcolemmal nuclei, macrophages, and degenerated sarcoplasm are evident (×251).

evident as areas of fibrosis in both skeletal and cardiac muscle. The lungs may be hyperemic, with widespread edema and occasionally, alveolar emphysema. Cloudy swelling and hyperemia may be seen in the liver. Adrenal cortices may be hyperemic or hemorrhagic. Cortical atrophy and hyaline droplets may be present in the zona glomerulosa and zona fasciculata, as well as in the outer zone of the adrenal medulla. Renal lesions may be evident as tubulonephrosis accompanied by casts and extra- and intratubular hemorrhages.

Preliminary examinations of electron micrographs of muscle from CM-affected elk (Lewis et al., 1977) revealed several lesions (Fig. 9.7A,B). Diffuse necrosis in many areas of affected muscle was indicated by lack of normal ultrastructural detail. In other affected areas, mitochondria were swollen, the Z bands were disrupted, and there was myofibrillar dissociation leading to marked alterations in sarcomeres.

DIAGNOSIS. Because of the clinical and pathologic similarity of CM to various myopathies of domestic animals, including those caused by the toxic plants, *Cassia occidentalis, C. obtusifolia,* and *Karwinskia humboldtiana* (Blood and Henderson, 1974; Hadlow, 1973; Jubb and Kennedy, 1970), the diagnosis depends, to a large degree, on a composite of history, clinical signs, clinical pathology, and gross and microscopic pathology. Therefore, in this disease, a history of pursuit, capture, physical restraint, or immobilization by drugs is important in the differentiation of CM from similar myopathies of domestic livestock.

In most reported cases, the violent and concerted use of muscles by frightened, fleeing, or restrained wild animals appears critical to the development of signs and lesions. However, chemical immobilization, with or without pursuit, may precipitate the disease; for this reason, cases of sudden death or the observation of animals showing clinical signs after chemical immobilization or physical restraint, should alert the investigator to the distinct possibility of CM.

In live animals, determinations of serum enzyme, lactate, potassium, creatinine, blood pH, and pCO_2 values may contribute additional confirmatory information to that provided by history, clinical signs, and subsequent pathologic examinations. In dead animals, a history of recent capture or immobilization, associated with gross and microscopic lesions of cardiac and skeletal muscle, provides a basis for the diagnosis of CM. The effects of low values of dietary Se may be additional complicating and possibly precipitating factors in areas in which such deficiencies are known to exist. For this reason, analysis of forage and tissues for values of Se may be useful.

TREATMENT AND PREVENTION. Early attempts at therapy for CM were often empirical and consisted of injections of preparations containing Se and vitamin E, vitamin B_{12}, calcium borogluconate, antibiotics, detoxicants, corticosteroids, and antihistamines (Hofmeyr, 1974; Hofmeyr et al., 1973). In most cases, these procedures were found to be ineffective in reversing the clinical signs (Young, 1972). Similarly, the effectiveness of injections of a vitamin B complex

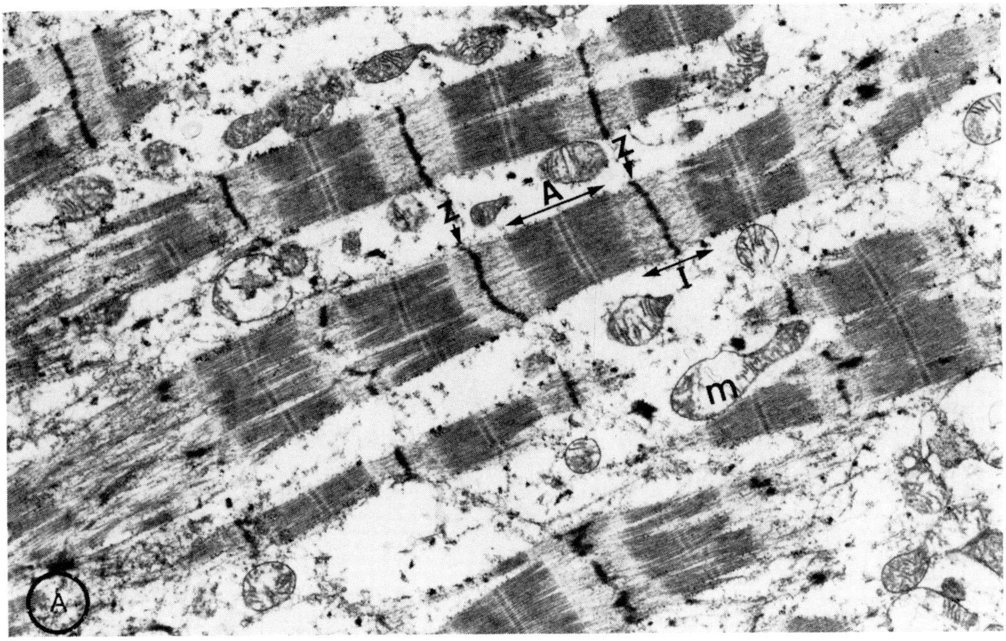

Fig. 9.7. (A) Capture myopathy, elk, *C. canadensis.* Disruption and streaming of Z bands with dissociation of myofibrils and swollen mitochondria. A = A band; I = I band; m = mitochondrion; Z = Z band (×10,000).

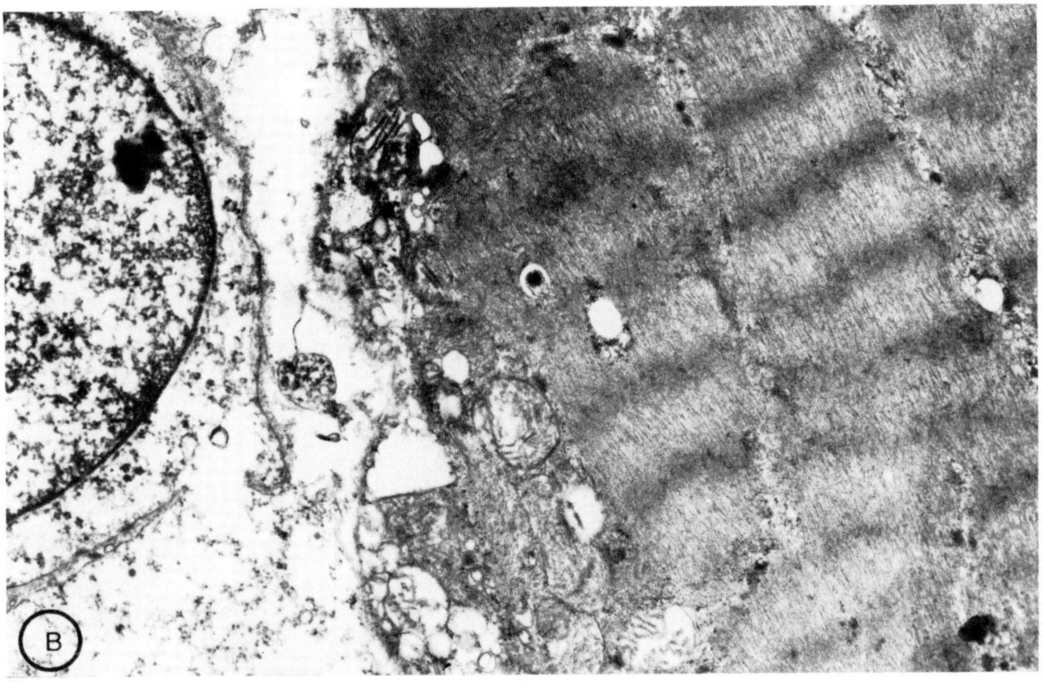

(B) Capture myopathy, elk, *C. canadensis.* Myonecrosis with swelling of mitochondria. Note the intact sarcolemmal nucleus (×32,000) (Photos courtesy R. J. Lewis, Alberta Department of Agriculture, Edmonton).

as supportive therapy in exercise-stressed tsessebe could not be established (Harthoorn and Harthoorn, 1976). However, there are indications that injections of preparations containing Se, vitamin E, and corticosteroids markedly reduced mortality rates (Basson and Hofmeyr, 1973; Hofmeyr, 1974).

Treatment consisting of the intravenous infusion of 1,000 mEq sodium bicarbonate/250 kg body weight, resulted in immediate and dramatic clinical improvement in zebra affected acutely with CM (Harthoorn, 1975; Harthoorn and Young, 1974; Harthoorn et al., 1974b). Animals treated in this manner did not exhibit further signs of illness and remained in good condition for several months. Conversely, untreated control animals died within 12 hours of pursuit and capture.

In treating exercise-stressed acidemic sheep, Gericke and Belonje (1975) used an intraperitoneal injection of sodium bicarbonate, containing a glucocorticoid and antibiotics, and an intramuscular injection of a vitamin B complex. This treatment increased values for plasma glucose and blood pH, buffer base, bicarbonate, and base excess and significantly decreased values for plasma potassium.

These observations suggest that solutions of sodium bicarbonate should provide an effective and convenient therapy for handling suspected cases of acute CM under field conditions. Based on data provided by Harthoorn and Young (1974) for zebra affected with CM, sodium bicarbonate, dissolved in sterile balanced electrolyte or physiologic saline solutions, may be given intravenously or intraperitoneally at the rate of 400 mEq (32 gm)/100 kg body weight; a suggested concentration for infusion is 1 mEq sodium bicarbonate/ml of fluid. These solutions, which are useful also in combating shock, should be administered over a period of 5 to 10 minutes.

Under field conditions, absolute prevention of CM is unrealistic, but it should be possible to limit the effects of the disease by reducing stress during capture of wildlife species (Basson et al., 1971; Young, 1972). Factors that decrease the intensity and increase the length of pursuit appear useful (Harthoorn, 1975; Harthoorn and Van Der Walt, 1974; Harthoorn and Young, 1974). Animals should not be pursued to the point of exhaustion before capture or darting (Hofmeyer et al., 1973). Procedures such as physically overpowering animals forced into water or deep snow are potentially hazardous. If indicated by clinical signs, suitable therapy as outlined previously should be instituted to reduce the risk of death.

Hofmeyr (1974) indicated that prolonged chemical immobilization and the control of heat stress were preferable to the use of crates for the capture and translocation of roan antelope by air. The use of woven plastic sheeting (Hofmeyr, 1974; Oelofse, 1970) for the walls of drive-traps and large enclosures prevents injuries and reduces psychological stress in recently captured animals; increased survival results. Similarly, the common practice of using eye shields on captured wildlife appears to be useful in reducing excitement. Young (1967) suggested that transport bags for recently captured flamingoes be replaced by supportive slings during translocation.

In areas in which there is a known or suspected Se deficiency in vegetation, injections of Se-vitamin E preparations, in addition to those of bicarbonate solutions immediately after capture or at the first signs of distress, may well be mandatory to promote survival of these animals. In CM-susceptible animals, these precautionary procedures may be necessary despite the absence of clinical signs; caution must be taken, however, to avoid unnecessary handling and agitation of the animals.

In summary, every effort should be made to select trapping and translocation procedures that 1) do not exhaust animals, 2) reduce heat stress, 3) minimize direct contact with humans, and 4) shorten the period of captivity. Trapping crews should include personnel trained in the detection and treatment of CM. The importance of CM associated with traditional capture procedures will become more apparent in future years as the condition becomes more widely recognized. The increased use of telemetry devices to monitor activities of animals following capture and release will, in all probability, provide new insights into capture-related mortalities.

REFERENCES

Adams, R. D. 1975. Diseases of muscles. A study in pathology. 3rd ed. Harper & Row, Hagerstown.

Barrett, M. W. 1974. Importance, utilization and quality of *Artemisia cana* on pronghorn winter ranges in Alberta. Proc. 6th Antelope States Workshop, Salt Lake City, 26–57.

______, and G. A. Chalmers. 1977. Clinico-chemical values for free-ranging pronghorns. Can. J. Zool. 55:1252–1260.

Bartsch, R. C., E. E. McConnell, G. D. Imes, and J. M. Schmidt. 1977. A review of exertional rhabdomyolysis in wild and domestic animals and man. Vet. Pathol. 14:314–324.

Basson, P. A., and J. M. Hofmeyr. 1973. Mortalities associated with wildlife capture operations. In E. Young. The capture and care of wild animals. Human and Rousseau, Cape Town.

______, R. M. McCully, S. P. Kruger, J. W. Van Niekerk, E. Young, V. De Vos, M. E. Keep, and H. Ebedes. 1971. Disease conditions of game in southern Africa; Recent miscellaneous findings. Vet. Med. Rev. No. 2/3: 313–340.

Blood, D. C., and J. A. Henderson. 1974. Veterinary medicine. 4th ed. Lea and Febiger, Philadelphia.

Cardinet, G. H. 1971. Skeletal muscle. In J. J. Kaneko and C. E. Cornelius. Clinical biochemistry of domestic animals. Academic Press, New York.

______, J. F. Littrell, and R. A. Freedland. 1967. Comparative investigations of serum creatine phosphokinase and glutamic oxaloacetic transaminase activities in equine paralytic myoglobinuria. Res. Vet. Sci. 8:219–226.

Chalmers, G. A., and M. W. Barrett. 1977. Capture myopathy in pronghorns in Alberta, Canada. J. Am. Vet. Med. Assoc. 171:918–923.

Colgrove, G. S. 1978. Suspected transportation-associated myopathy in a dolphin. J. Am. Vet. Med. Assoc. 173:1121–1123.

DeMartini, J. C., and R. B. Davies. 1977. An epizootic of pneumonia in captive bighorn sheep infected with *Muellerius* sp. J. Wildl. Dis. 13:117–124.

Ebedes, H. 1969. Notes on the immobilization of gemsbok, *Oryx gazella gazella,* in southwest Africa using etorphine hydrochloride (M99). Madoqua 1:35–45.

Fairlie, G. 1964. Myopathy in a roebuck. Vet. Rec. 76:1147–1148.

Gericke, M. D., and P. C. Belonje. 1975. Aspects of forced exercise and the therapy thereof in sheep. J. S. Afr. Vet. Med. Assoc. 46:353–357.

______, and J. M. Hofmeyr. 1976. Aetiology and treatment of capture stress and myopathy in springbok, *Antidorcas marsupialis.* S. Afr. J. Sci. 72: 28.

Gibbs, E. P. J., A. McDiarmid, and J. J. Rowe. 1975. Management of deer for experimental studies with foot-and-mouth disease virus. Vet. Rec. 96:503–506.

Hadlow, W. J. 1955. Degenerative myopathy in a white-tailed deer. Cornell Vet. 45:538–547.

______. 1973. Myopathies of animals. In C. M. Pearson and F. K. Mostofi. The striated muscle. Williams & Wilkins, Baltimore.

Haigh, J. C., R. R. Stewart, G. Wobeser, and P. S. MacWilliams. 1977. Capture myopathy in a moose. J. Am. Vet. Med. Assoc. 171:924–926.

Harthoorn, A. M. 1973. Physiology and therapy of capture myopathy. Second Annu. Rep., Transvaal Nature Cons. Div., Pretoria.

______. 1975. The chemical capture of animals. A guide to the chemical restraint of wild and captive animals. Ralph Curtis Books, Hollywood.

______, and L. M. Harthoorn. 1976. Parentrovite as a supportive therapy for locomotory stress in tsessebe. J. S. Afr. Vet. Assoc. 47:219–222.

______, and K. Van Der Walt. 1974. Physiological aspects of forced exercise in wild ungulates with special reference to (so-called) overstraining disease. 1. Acid-base balance and pO_2 levels in blesbok, *Damaliscus dorcas phillipsi.* J. S. Afr. Wildl. Manage. Assoc. 4:25–28.

______, and E. Young. 1974. A relationship between acid-base balance and capture myopathy in zebra, *Equus burchelli,* and an apparent therapy. Vet. Rec. 95:337–342.

______, and E. Young. 1976. Pulmonary hypertension in relation to acidaemia after maximum forced exercise. J. S. Afr. Vet. Assoc. 47:187–189.

______, W. Jenkins, J. Turkstra, and D. Mason. 1974a. Seasonal changes in liver selenium content as a possible factor in transit myopathy: a preliminary report. Proc. Am. Assoc. Zoo Vet. 1974:1–5.

______, K. Van Der Walt, and E. Young. 1974b. Possible therapy for capture myopathy in captured wild animals. Nature 247:577.

______, E. Young, and W. York. 1974c. Blood enzyme levels as indications of capture stress (capture myopathy or overstraining disease) in zebra, *Equus burchelli.* Proc. Am. Assoc. Zoo Vet. 1974:34–39.

Hebert, D. M., and I. McT. Cowan. 1971. White muscle disease in the mountain goat. J. Wildl. Manage. 35:752–756.

Hofmeyr, J. M. 1974. Developments in the capture and airlift of roan antelope, *Hippotragus equinus equinus,* under narcosis to the Etosha National Park. Madoqua 1 (8):37–48.

______, G. M. Louw, and J. S. du Preez. 1973. Incipient capture myopathy as revealed by blood chemistry of chased zebras. Madoqua 1(7):45–50.

Hudson, R. J. 1976. Personal communication. Department of Animal Science, Univ. of Alberta, Edmonton.

Jarrett, W. F. H., and M. Murray. 1967. Muscular dystrophy in antelope and gazelle in Kenya. Vet. Rec. 80:483.

______, F. W. Jennings, M. Murray, and A. M. Harthoorn. 1964. Muscular dystrophy in a wild Hunter's antelope. East Afr. Wildl. J. 2:158–159.

Jubb, K. V. F., and P. C. Kennedy. 1970. Pathology of domestic animals. Vol. 2. 2nd ed. Academic Press, New York.

Kronfeld, D. S., and W. Medway. 1969. Blood chemistry. In W. Medway, I. E. Prier, and J. S. Wilkinson. A textbook of veterinary clinical pathology. Williams & Wilkins, Baltimore.

Lewis, R. J., G. A. Chalmers, M. W. Barrett, and R. Bhatnagar. 1977. Capture myopathy in elk in Alberta, Canada: A report of three cases. J. Am. Vet. Med. Assoc. 171:927–932.

Lindholm, A., H. E. Johansson, and P. Kjaersgaard. 1974. Acute rhabdomyolysis ("tying up") in Standardbred horses. A morphological and biochemical study. Acta Vet. Scand. 15:325–339.

Lynch, G. M. 1975. Personal communication. Fish and Wildlife Div., Alberta Depart. of Recreation, Parks and Wildlife, Edmonton.

McConnell, E. E., P. A. Basson, V. de Vos, B. J. Meyers, And R. F. Kuntz. 1974. A survey of diseases among 100 free-ranging baboons, *Papio ursinus,* from the Kruger National Park. Onderstepoort. J. Vet. Res. 41:97–168.

Mech, R. D. 1975. Hunting behavior in two similar species of social canids. In M. W. Fox. The wild canids. Their systematics, behavioral ecology and evolution. Van Nostrand Reinhold, Toronto.

Mugera, G. M., and J. G. Wandera. 1967. Degenerative polymyopathies in east African domestic and wild animals. Vet. Rec. 80:410–413.

Munday, B. L. 1972. Myonecrosis in free-living and recently-captured macropods. J. Wildl. Dis. 8:191–192.

Oelofse, J. 1970. Plastic for game catching. Oryx 10:306–307.

Spraker, T. R. 1976. Personal communication. Wild Animal Disease Center, Colorado State Univ., Fort Collins.

Topel, D. G., L. L. Christian, and R. A. Ball. 1975. Porcine stress syndrome. In H. W. Dunne and A. D. Leman. Diseases of swine. 4th ed. The Iowa State Univ. Press, Ames.

Wishart, W. 1977. Personal communication. Fish and Wildlife Div., Alberta Depart. of Recreation, Parks and Wildlife, Edmonton.

Wobeser, G. 1976. Personal communication. Western College of Veterinary Medicine, Univ. of Saskatchewan, Saskatoon.

______, 1978. Personal communication. Western College of Veterinary Medicine, Univ. of Saskatchewan, Saskatoon.

______, J. E. C. Bellamy, B. G. Boysen, P. S. MacWilliams, and W. Runge. 1976. Myopathy and myoglobinuria in a wild white-tailed deer. J. Am. Vet. Med. Assoc. 169:971–974.

Young, E. 1966. Muscle necrosis in captive red hartebeest, *Alcelaphus busephalus.* J. S. Afr. Vet Med. Assoc. 37:101–103.

______. 1967. Leg paralysis in the greater flamingo and lesser flamingo, *Phoenicopterus ruber roseus* and *Phoeniconaias minor,* following capture and transportation. Int. Zoo Yearbook 7:226–227.

______. 1972. Overstraining disease (capture myopathy) in the tsessebe, *Damaliscus lunatus,* and oribi, *Ourebia ourebi.* Koedoe 15:143–144.

______, and P. J. L. Bronkhorst. 1971. Overstraining disease in game. Afr. Wild Life 25:51–52.

10 *Amyloidosis*

G. E. COSGROVE
L. C. SATTERFIELD

AMYLOIDOSIS, or amyloid degeneration, is a disease resulting from the deposition in tissues of a homogeneous, acidophilic, proteinaceous infiltrate called amyloid. It tends to occur in vertebrates in association with aging, chronic stress, or diseases associated with considerable chronic tissue destruction.

Amyloidosis has been recognized as a human disease for several hundred years. The term amyloid was apparently introduced by Virchow in 1851 to describe the waxy material seen in certain diseased organs. During the 1800s, reports of observations of amyloid in mammals and birds were fairly numerous and covered a wide range of species. During that period the terms *primary* and *secondary* amyloidosis came into use to designate cases with no accompanying disease (primary) as opposed to cases associated with other severe chronic disease processes (secondary), usually serious infections, neoplasms, or other diseases with extensive tissue breakdown.

Extensive research into the biochemical nature of amyloid and the possibilities of inducing it experimentally began in the late 1800s and has been pursued vigorously ever since (Mandema et al., 1968). With the advent of more sophisticated special staining and microscopy and from the use of electron microscopy, improved histologic demonstration of amyloid and better understanding of its morphology gradually occurred (Black, 1972; Cohen, 1965; Franklin and Zucker-Franklin, 1972; Mandema et al., 1968).

The literature on amyloidosis is voluminous, and there have been a number of recent reviews (Christensen et al., 1972; Cohen, 1965; Franklin and Zucker-Franklin, 1972; Mandema et al., 1968; Rigdon, 1974; Schwartz, 1970). When reviewing the literature on comparative species distribution of amyloidosis, one is struck by the scarcity of reports of this condition in true wildlife. There are, however, many articles reporting it in confined, controlled, or zoo mammals of wild origin or in descendants of wild ancestors (Andervont and Dunn, 1970; Gillman and Gilbert, 1955; Hjärre, 1933; Osman Hill, 1954; Ratcliffe, 1967; Rigdon, 1974; Schwartz et al., 1971; Sherwood et al., 1968; Woolf and Kradel, 1973). With the exception of the articles by Hadlow and Jellison (1962) and Helvie and Smith (1971) reporting amyloidosis in bighorn sheep, *Ovis canadensis,* the authors were unable to find reports involving mammals living in the wild. Since the authors have found amyloidosis in two road-killed wild skunks, *Mephitis mephitis* (unreported cases), it is suspected that other cases from wildlife are found and not reported but that they must be uncommon; however, amyloidosis has been reported in captive skunks (Wade-Smith and Richmond, 1975). In about one thousand autopsies of wild-derived small mammals that were kept in the laboratory for varying periods, the authors have found four cases of amyloidosis, one in *Microtus oeconomus* and three in *Peromyscus californicus insignis.*

Similarly, most of the reported cases of amyloidosis, especially those involving waterfowl, are found in confined zoo or pet bird species (Cowan, 1968a,b; Karstad, 1972; Karstad and Sileo, 1971; Keymer, 1972; Ratcliffe, 1967; Rigdon, 1974; Sauer and Zook, 1974). However, cases involving wild birds have been reported (Karstad, 1972). From personal experience with many hundreds of road- or hunter-killed wild birds, the authors have found no cases of amyloidosis.

While a few cases have been reported from reptile or amphibian autopsies, these apparently all have been captive specimens. Cowan (1968c) reviewed the Philadelphia zoo records and found only two cases, in *Constrictor constrictor* and *Boa enhydris,* out of 1,249 reptiles autopsied. Trautwein and Pruksaraj (1967) reported a case in a tortoise and the prosector's report from the National Zoo (Sauer and Zook, 1974) listed a case in the giant toad, *Bufo peltocephalus.* In personal necropsies on many hundreds of wild reptiles and amphibians, the authors have not encountered amyloidosis.

ETIOLOGY AND PATHOGENESIS. Amyloid may occur in the tissues of vertebrates with chronic infections, many other chronic diseases, neoplasms, and some hereditary diseases or spontaneously (especially in the aged) and is easily inducible experimentally (Azar, 1968; Cohen, 1965; Franklin and Zucker-Franklin, 1972; Mandema et al., 1968; Rigdon, 1974; Schwartz, 1970). Amyloidosis becomes increasingly common with age in man, animals, and birds (Schwartz, 1970). Evidence of this has been reported in farm mink, *Mustela vison* (Schwartz et al., 1971), mice (Heston and Deringer, 1948; Thung, 1957), and Pekin ducks, *Anas platyrhynchos domesticus* (Rigdon and Mack, 1969), among others. In some studies, age was seemingly less important than environmental and social stress: in mice (Hall et al., 1960; Page and Glenner, 1972); in many zoo bird species (Cowan, 1968a,b); in ducks (Cowan and Johnson, 1970); in Pekin ducks (Rigdon and Mack, 1969); and in park waterfowl (Karstad and Sileo, 1971). Species and strain differences in incidence are reportedly so marked for amyloidosis that heredity is considered extremely important. Examples are reported for man (Mahloudji et al., 1969); for laboratory mice (Heston and Deringer, 1948); for wild-derived mice (Andervont and Dunn, 1970); for domestic ducks (Rigdon, 1967; and for zoo birds (Cowan, 1968a).

There is extensive documentation on the experimental induction of amyloidosis by a wide variety of procedures in various avian and mammalian species. Techniques often involve alteration of immune mechanisms by stimulation or depression or by dietary alteration (Franklin and Zucker-Franklin, 1972; Glenner, 1972; Hass et al., 1943; Mandema et al., 1968).

The mode of deposition of amyloid is still unknown. Theories include, among others, origin from precipitation of a serum component or local secretion by a variety of cell types (Black, 1972). Considerable elucidation of the chemical nature and configuration of amyloid has occurred. It is a hydrophilic protein-mucopolysaccharide complex, not always chemically uniform and probably not an antigen-antibody precipitate in spite of the frequent association with immunologic disorders (Cohen, 1965; Franklin and Zucker-Franklin, 1972; Glenner, 1972; Glenner and Terry, 1974; Mandema et al., 1968; Schwartz, 1970). Electron microscopy has demonstrated the fibrous/fibrillar nature of the amyloid matrix, with associated pentagonal precipitates (Black, 1972). The fibrillar nature and chemical composition apparently are variable (Cohen and Calkins, 1959; Franklin and Zucker-Franklin, 1972; Hobbs, 1973; Mandema et al., 1968).

PATHOLOGY. When amyloid is present in small amounts, no gross changes are usually noted. When present in larger quantities, the involved organs are usually enlarged and heavier, firm and rubbery, with waxy, pale pink or grey smooth surfaces. Cut surfaces of involved organs have a smooth, glossy appearance in the areas of deposit and are relatively bloodless. In some areas it occurs as focal translucent patches. A wide variety of tissues and organs have been found to contain the deposits, and these may vary from case to case and from species to species (Cheville, 1976; Cowan, 1968b; Franklin and Zucker-Franklin, 1972; Karstad, 1972; Rigdon, 1967, 1974; Schwartz, 1970). Gross changes are most likely to be noted in spleen, liver, or kidney. Since amyloid is often found in individuals with large inflammatory, neoplastic, or degenerative lesions, diligent search should be made in such cases.

Microscopically, with H & E stains, amyloid appears as a lightly acidophilic, homogeneous, and amorphous extracellular material, often intimately associated with blood vessels of all sizes or found in connective or fat tissues near the basement membranes of cell layers. The principal differential diagnostic problem in microscopic examination is with hyalinized connective tissue, or fibrinoid. It has wide distribution in various organs. For example, it commonly occurs as a parafollicular band in the spleen (Figs. 10.1, 10.2), between the hepatic cell cords in liver, in glomeruli or scarred interstitial areas in the kidney, in intestinal villi, in the inner layer of the adrenal cortex, in blood vessel walls, and between heart-muscle fibers. Many other organs are less frequently involved, varying sporadically from case to case (Karstad, 1972; Rigdon, 1967; Schwartz et al., 1971).

The physical presence of amyloid in an area does not seem to invoke an inflammatory response. The surrounded and infiltrated cells seemingly survive and function until they are finally crowded out or are unable to obtain nutrition.

DIAGNOSIS AND TREATMENT. Symptomatology is of doubtful value in the antemortem diagnosis of amyloidosis because of the wide distribution and variation in extent of tissue involvement. The possibility of amyloidosis should be considered in old animals with chronic infections and other diseases historically associated with amyloidosis. It should also be more likely in situations with chronic stress, such as deer die-offs, rodent population crashes, bird migration, or breeding periods, and the like.

In advanced cases of amyloidosis, the spleen and liver may be palpable. The diagnosis may be made with the aid of the Congo red test, using dye injected intravenously. During the gross examination of tissue, iodine solution may be applied, whereupon the amyloid stains brown. With the addition of dilute sulfuric acid to the surface, the color changes to blue.

Amyloid can be identified histologically by special techniques. Although Congo red and gen-

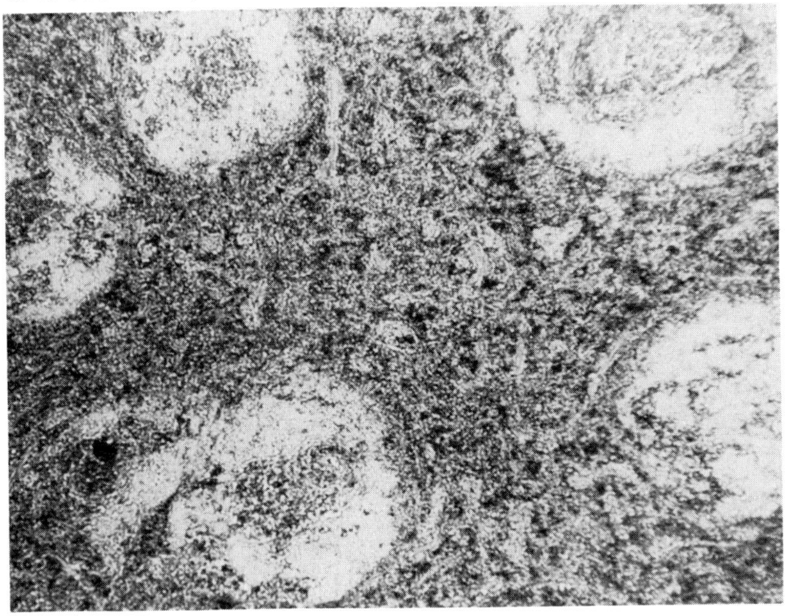

Fig. 10.1. A low-power view of several spleen follicles from a skunk, *Mephitis mephitis,* each surrounded by a wide pale zone of amyloid deposition (H & E, ×40).

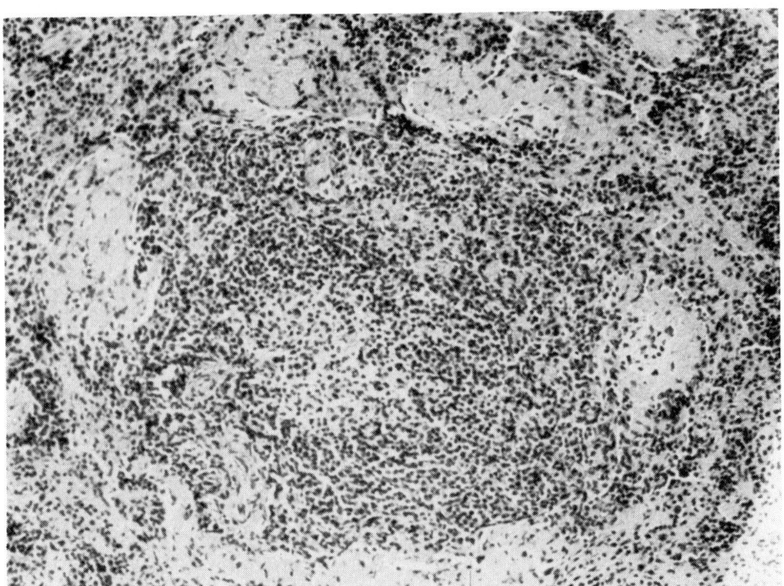

Fig. 10.2. View of a single spleen follicle from another skunk, *M. mephitis.* In this case the amyloid deposits are less severe and form a patchy ring (H & E, ×120).

tian violet stains have been used among others, thioflavin-S and -T are preferable. These fluorescent stains are excellent for the demonstration of deposits when viewed with ultraviolet light. Polarization microscopy makes possible the visualization of the earliest amyloid deposits before they can be detected by ordinary light microscopy. Schwartz (1970) has reviewed the different staining techniques for the demonstration of amyloid.

In secondary amyloidosis, partial or complete disappearance of amyloid has occurred in rare instances upon control of the underlying disease (Moschcowitz, 1936; Richter, 1954; Rosenblatt, 1936; Sagler, 1970). There is some experimental data suggesting resorption of amyloid by multinucleated giant cells (Wright et al., 1972). In two human cases treated with melphalan, amyloid deposition was thought to have been arrested (Hobbs, 1973). Apparently no therapeutic procedure has successfully eliminated amyloidosis (Parkins and Bywaters, 1959; Sagler, 1970).

SIGNIFICANCE. To date, amyloidosis does not seem to be an important disease in wildlife. With greater awareness of predisposing factors and widespread use of histopathology on diseased wildlife, an increase in reports can be expected.

REFERENCES

Andervont, H. B., and T. B. Dunn. 1970. Amyloidosis in wild house mice during inbreeding and in hybrids derived from inbred strains and wild mice. J. Natl. Cancer Inst. 44:719–727.

Azar, H. A. 1968. Amyloidosis. Pathol. Annu. 3: 105–122.

Black, M. M. 1972. The nature, pathogenesis and staining properties of amyloid. Br. J. Dermatol. 87:280–283.

Cheville, N. F. 1976. Cell pathology. Iowa State Univ. Press, Ames.

Christensen, H. E., and Editorial Committee. 1972. Dissertationes in honorem Gunnar Teilum septagenarii, 1902–1972. Acta Pathol. Microbiol. Scand. (A), Suppl. 233:1–238.

Cohen, A. S. 1965. The constitution and genesis of amyloid. Int. Rev. Exp. Pathol. 4:159–243.

______, and E. Calkins. 1959. Electron microscopic observations on a fibrous component in amyloid of diverse origins. Nature 183:1202–1203.

Cowan, D. F. 1968a. Avian amyloidosis. I. General incidence in zoo birds. Pathol. Vet. 5:51–58.

______. 1968b. Avian amyloidosis. II. Incidence and contributing factors in the family Anatidae. Pathol. Vet. 5:59–66.

______. 1968c. Diseases of captive reptiles. J. Am. Vet. Med. Assoc. 153:848–859.

______, and W. C. Johnson. 1970. Amyloidosis in the white Pekin duck. I. Relation to social environmental stress. Lab. Invest. 23:551–555.

Franklin, E. C., and D. Zucker-Franklin. 1972. Current concepts of amyloid. Adv. Immunol. 15:249–304.

Gillman, J., and C. Gilbert. 1955. Primary amyloidosis in the baboon, *Papio ursinus.* Its relationship to macromolecular syndromes and diseases of the connective tissues. Acta Med. Scand. (Suppl.) 306:155–189.

Glenner, G. G. 1972. The discovery of the immunoglobulin origin of amyloid fibrils and its pathogenetic significance. Acta Pathol. Microbiol. Scand. (A), Suppl. 233:114–121.

______, and W. D. Terry. 1974. Characterization of amyloid. Annu. Rev. Med. 25:131–135.

Hadlow, W. F., and W. L. Jellison. 1962. Amyloidosis in Rocky Mountain bighorn sheep. J. Am. Vet. Med. Assoc. 141:243–247.

Hall, C. E., E. Cross, and O. Hall. 1960. Amyloidosis and other pathologic changes in mice exposed to chronic stress. Tex. Rep. Biol. Med. 18:205–213.

Hass, G. M., R. Huntington, and N. Krumdieck. 1943. Amyloid. III. The properties of amyloid deposits occurring in several species under diverse conditions. Arch. Pathol. 35:226–241.

Helvie, J. G., and D. D. Smith. 1971. Summary of necropsy findings in desert bighorn sheep. SWRHL-62-r (microfiche), West. Environ. Res. Lab., Las Vegas.

Heston, W. E., and M. K. Deringer. 1948. Hereditary renal disease and amyloidosis in mice. Arch. Pathol. 46:49–58.

Hjärre, A. 1933. Über das Vorkommen der Amyloid-degeneration bei Tieren. Acta Pathol. Microbiol. Scand. (A), Suppl. 16:132–162.

Hobbs, J. R. 1973. An ABC of amyloid. Proc. Royal Soc. Med. 66:705–710.

Karstad, L. H. 1972. A color atlas of wildlife pathology. I. Amyloidosis in wild waterfowl. Wildl. Dis. 58: 1–52.

______, and L. Sileo. 1971. Causes of death in captive wild waterfowl in the Kortright Waterfowl Park, 1967–1970. J. Wildl. Dis. 7:236–241.

Keymer, I. F. 1972. A survey and review of the causes of mortality in British birds and the significance of wild birds as disseminators of disease. Vet. Rec. 70:713–720.

Mahloudji, M., R. D. Teasdall, J. J. Adamkiewicz, W. H. Hartmann, P. A. Lambird, and V. A. McKusick. 1969. The genetic amyloidoses with particular reference to hereditary neuropathic amyloidosis, type II (Indiana or Rukavina type). Medicine 48:1–37.

Mandema, E., L. Ruinen, J. H. Scholten, and A. S. Cohen. 1968. Amyloidosis. Proc. Symp. Amyloidosis, Univ. of Groningen, The Netherlands. Excerpta Medica Foundation, Amsterdam.

Moschcowitz, E. 1936. The clinical aspects of amyloidosis. Ann. Int. Med. 10:73–88.

Osman Hill, S. C. 1954. Report of the Society's prosector for the year 1954. Proc. Zool. Soc. Lond. 125:533–539.

Page, D., and G. G. Glenner. 1972. Social interaction and wounding in the genesis of "spontaneous" murine amyloidosis. Am. J. Pathol. 67:555–570.

Parkins, R. A., and E. G. L. Bywaters. 1959. Regression of amyloidosis secondary to rheumatoid arthritis. Br. Med. J. 1:536–540.

Ratcliffe, H. L. 1967. Report of the Penrose Research Laboratory of the Zoological Society of Philadelphia.

Richter, G. W. 1954. The resorption of amyloid under experimental conditions. Am. J. Pathol. 30:239–261.

Rigdon, R. H. 1967. Amyloid in the liver of ducks. Poult. Sci. 46:698–705.

______. 1974. Occurrence and association of amyloid with diseases in birds and mammals including man: A review. Tex. Rep. Biol. Med. 32:665–682.

______, and J. Mack. 1969. Amyloidosis: Age of occurrence and rate of progression: Experimental study in the white Pekin duck. J. Am. Geriatr. Soc. 17:514–521.

Rosenblatt, M. B. 1936. Recovery from generalized amyloidosis secondary to pulmonary tuberculosis. Report of a case. Arch. Int. Med. 57:562–565.

Sagler, F. 1970. Experimental study by skin grafting of the absorption of amyloid in local amyloidosis. Br. J. Dermatol. 83:273–276.

Sauer, R. M., and B. C. Zook. 1974. Pathology. In National Zoological Park-Smithsonian Institution. 18-Month Report (July 1, 1971–Dec. 31, 1972).

Schwartz, P. 1970. Amyloidosis. Cause and manifestation of senile deterioration. Charles C Thomas, Springfield.

______, K. B. Wolfe, and J. T. Beuttas. 1971. Spontaneous amyloidosis in mink. J. Comp. Pathol. 81:437–445.

Sherwood, B. F., D. T. Rowlands, Jr., D. B. Hackel, and J. C. LeMay. 1968. Bacterial endocarditis, glomerulonephritis, and amyloidosis in the opossum, *Didelphis virginianus*. Am. J. Pathol. 53:115–126.

Thung, P. J. 1957. The relation between amyloid and aging in comparative pathology. Gerontologia 1:234–254.

Trautwein, G., and D. Pruksaraj. 1967. Amyloid in the tortoise. DTW 74:184–186.

Wade-Smith, J., and N. E. Richmond. 1975. Care, management, and biology of captive striped skunks, *Mephitis mephitis*. Lab. Anim. Sci. 25:575–584.

Woolf, A., and D. C. Kradel. 1973. Mortality in captive bighorn sheep—clinical, hematological, and pathological observations. J. Wildl. Dis. 9:12–17.

Wright, J. R., A. Ozdemir, M. Matsuzaki, P. Binette, and E. Calkins. 1972. Amyloid resorption: Possible role of multinculeated giant cells. The apparent failure of Penicillamine treatment. Johns Hopkins Med. J. 130:278–288.

11 *Dental Anomalies in Mammals*

GERALD L. HOFF
DIANE M. HOFF

ANOMALIES of the thecodont dentition of mammals are among the most frequently encountered anomalous conditions of wildlife species. Teeth are present in almost all mammalian species but are absent in animals of the suborder *Mysticeti,* for example, whales. The normal teeth of a mammal can furnish considerable information about the life history of the individual, a property long utilized by paleontologists. Dentition can reflect food habits, genetic relationships, environmental influences, and the approximate age of the animal. Consequently, a study of dental anomalies can be revealing in terms of genetic mechanisms, nutritional and metabolic diseases, and certain types of influences.

Embryologically, teeth are derived from ectodermal and mesodermal tissues and are composed of enamel (ectodermal) and dentin, cementum, and pulp (mesodermal). Enamel covers the exposed part of the tooth, but may be partially absent from the lingual surface of the gnawing teeth of rodents and from the tusks of boars and elephants or completely absent from the teeth of edentates (Peyer, 1968). Dentin makes up the bulk of the tooth. Cementum replaces the enamel as the covering of the dentin on the roots of the teeth of all mammals. On most teeth cementum is a thin inconspicuous layer, but in advanced herbivores it becomes an important part of the tooth. In such mammals, the teeth may have deep enamel folds and the cementum may grow over the whole tooth, even filling in the depressions in the crown. Pulp is the central living portion of the tooth. In young animals, the pulp cavity is widely open at the base and is in communication with the circulatory system. In most adults the opening is reduced to a small foramen, rooted; however, in some mammals the pulp cavity does not constrict and the tooth continues to grow throughout life, rootless.

Dentition in mammals is generally heterodont, that is, the teeth are modified in shape and size to serve specialized functions in the tooth row. In most mammals four types of teeth are generally recognized: incisors, canines, premolars, and molars. The molars are further classified by their crown patterns (Cockrum, 1962). Most mammals have two sets of teeth, diphodont, with the first set of deciduous or milk teeth consisting only of incisors, canines, and premolars. The molars are never replaced and are added to the jaw from the front backward during growth. Some marsupials have no deciduous dentition and among the placental mammals, the deciduous dentition may be lost *in utero.* Since mammals suckle their young, eruption of the milk teeth can be delayed, and up to 80% of the postnatal cranial growth takes place before the first set of functional teeth is fully erupted (Crompton and Parker, 1978).

The literature concerning anomalies of mammalian teeth, exclusive of man, is extensive, but unfortunately it is widely scattered in reports, monographs, transactions, journals, and books. For the most part, these reports are of an observational nature, documenting a case or providing prevalence information for a small series of specimens. There are some excellent studies on museum collections (Archer, 1975; Choate, 1968; Colyer, 1936; Hall, 1940; Lavelle et al., 1977; McIntosh, 1929; Phillips and Jones, 1968; Swindler, 1976), but in most instances these provide little more than case or prevalence data. The reader is referred to the *Journal of Mammalogy* as a bountiful but not exclusive source of reports on dental anomalies in wildlife, excluding primates.

ETIOLOGY AND PATHOLOGY. Anomalies of the dentition may result from abnormal tissue development, dysplasia, or environmental influences. Developmental abnormalities consist of irregularities in number, size, shape, structure, singleness, position, and eruption. Nondevelopmental anomalies generally result in discoloration or damage to the integrity of the tooth structure and can affect either the primary or secondary dentition or only specific teeth.

The vast majority of reports dealing with dental anomalies in nondomestic mammals fall into the developmental category. The etiologies of these types of anomalies are varied and include genetic disorders, nutritional or metabolic disorders, inflammation, and environmental insult (Baden, 1970; Bernier, 1959; Schulze, 1970). Determination of the exact etiology is very difficult, if not impossible, in many instances. Genetic disorders, however, appear to be the most common etiology for developmental anomalies (Archer, 1975; Long and Long, 1965; McIntosh, 1929).

The complex structure of the tooth lends itself to dysplasias of the enamel. Heredity, nutritional deficiencies, endocrine imbalances, ingestion of substances that interfere with the normal maturation of ameloblasts, inflammation, and environmental insult are all possible etiologies. Dysplasia of the mesodermal tissues can cause structural abnormalities in both dentin and cementum, usually combined with a dimensional change in the tooth root. These dysplasias are generally hereditary (Bernier, 1959; Schulze, 1970).

Nondevelopmental anomalies are the result of physical injury to the tooth. The mechanisms of insult include mechanical abrasion, acid or chelate demineralization, enzymatic digestion, and cellular resorption. The etiologies are numerous and may be influenced by important secondary factors.

Injury, cysts, tumors, abnormalities of jaw structure, size and configuration, and cranial asymmetry can all contribute to dental anomalies (Colyer, 1936; Vaughn, 1961; Wagner, 1923).

DEVELOPMENTAL ANOMALIES

Anomalies of Tooth Shape and Size. Anomalies of tooth shape and size frequently coexist. Simplification of shape often goes with diminution in size. Both conditions are frequently associated with anomalies of tooth number. Anomalies of shape and size often are only micromanifestations of a genetically determined reduction in number. An increase in size may actually be a step toward hyperdontia. Recent investigations have even shown that such seemingly unrelated characteristics as time and order of eruption of certain teeth have a statistically demonstrable relationship to tooth number and size (Schulze, 1970). Individual teeth vary markedly in length, width, thickness, crown curvature, root characteristics, marginal ridge development, form and distinctness of cusps, and so on. Characteristic differences occur not only among individuals but, more important, among populations.

Accessory or abnormally formed cusps on the teeth of wild animals are not uncommon. In man, the type of anomalous cusp formation varies with the tooth involved (Schulze, 1970). With incisors and canines, the most common development is the enlargement of the lingual tubercle into a fully formed cusp. These accessory cusps occur primarily in the palatal marginal ridges and on the labial surface. Anomalies in the crown shape of the premolars can arise from alterations in the cusp-fissure relationship, and this is more variable for the mandibular teeth and the maxillary premolars. In dasyurid marsupials, abnormal premolar crown morphology is usually exhibited by fusion or division of the crowns (Archer, 1975). Fused crowns are believed to result from damage to adjacent developing teeth, while divided crowns may represent a stage in supernumerary tooth formation. Accessory labial cusps of the molars may lead to development of a supernumerary tooth called the paramolar. Other accessory cusps, such as that depicted by Nellis (1972) in a coyote, *Canis latrans,* may also develop (Fig. 11.1).

Enamel spurs or projections are found most often on the buccal side of multirooted teeth, being located at the level of root bifurcation. Only in exceptionally pronounced cases should they be

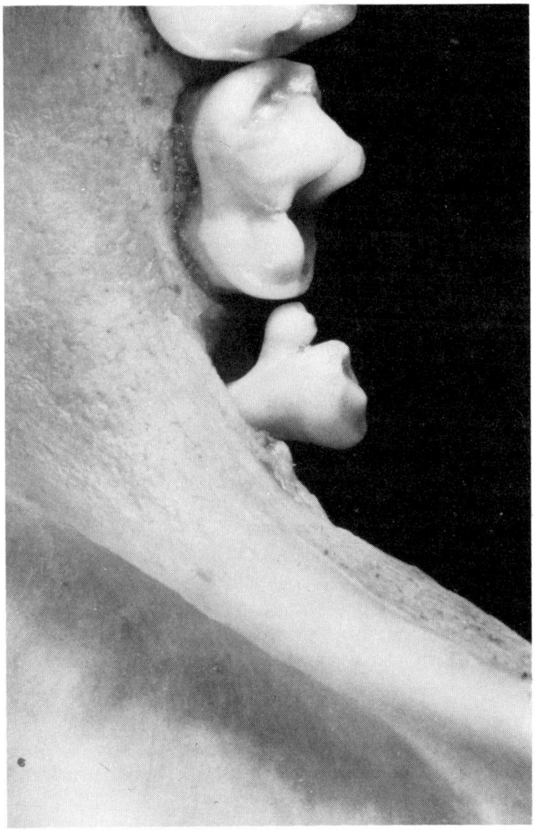

Fig. 11.1. Small bud or cusp on M_3 from a coyote, *Canis latrans* (Reprinted by permission of the National Research Council of Canada from Nellis, 1972, Figure 1-P).

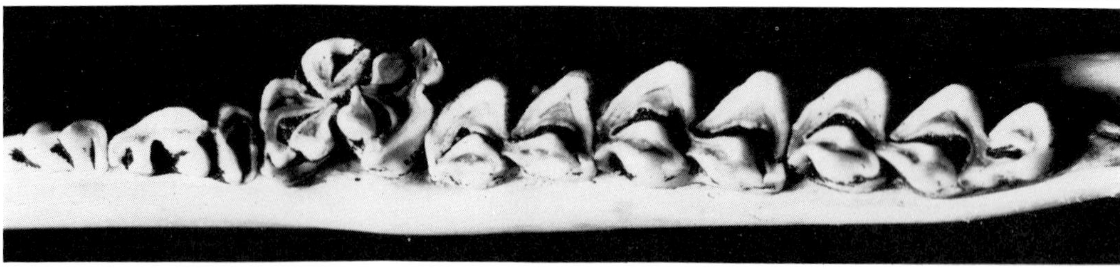

Fig. 11.2. Duplicate premolar in the mandible from a white-tailed deer, *Odocoileus virginianus* (Reprinted by permission from Wing, 1965, Figures 1, 2).

considered anomalous. On the other hand, enamel pearls, nodules, or droplets are considered anomalies. These structures are hemispheric, variable in size, and may be found at the bifurcation of multirooted teeth, at the end of a spur, or on the root surface distant from the bifurcation. They occur more frequently than one might expect from gross examination. Smaller pearls may be covered by cementum and only detected by histological examination. Structurally, pearls may consist of 1) enamel, 2) enamel with a nucleus of dentin, or 3) enamel, dentin, and pulp.

The etiology of pearls is unknown; however, because of their preferential site at the bifurcation of multirooted teeth, it is suggested that they, like enamel spurs, are caused by discrepancies during the complex transition of a single enamel organ into the several sheaths of Hertwig. It is believed that cells of the sheaths of Hertwig become differentiated into ameloblasts, which then deposit the enamel of the pearls (Schulze, 1970).

Accessory or abnormally shaped roots tend to be more common with multirooted teeth. Curved and angled roots probably are the result of disturbances in the growth of the sheath of Hertwig resulting from trauma, scar formation, or displacement of nutrient vessels. Accessory roots may be caused by branching or the attachment of a new element not preformed in the normal tooth root. Photographs of branching and root fusion in caribou, *Rangifer tarandus,* have been published by Miller and Tessier (1971).

Abnormal invaginations of the tooth crown and roots have been recorded as dens invaginatus, coronal invaginations, and radicular invaginations. Dens invaginatus and coronal invaginations are enamel lined and may alter the shape of the crown. Superficial invaginations involve only the crown while deep invaginations involve both the crown and root. These invaginations may be confused with pitting. Radicular invaginations are restricted to the roots and are lined with cementum.

Supernumerary Teeth and Twin Formation. Supernumerary teeth, by definition, are teeth in excess of normal deciduous or permanent dentition. However, the surplus may occasionally be compensated for by a deficit of other teeth. The morphology of the supernumerary teeth is variable. They may imitate the shape of normal teeth (Fig. 11.2) or they may be atypically shaped. Because of mechanical interference, supernumerary teeth seldom occupy a functional position in the dental arch. In dentistry, the terms supplementary and supernumerary are used to describe extra teeth that have eumorphic or heteromorphic shape respectively. For the purposes of this presentation, supernumerary will be used for eumorphic and dysmorphic extra teeth. Supernumerary teeth are probably the most common dental anomaly reported for wildlife species.

Supernumerary teeth may represent a phylogenetic reversion. However, according to Bernier (1959), it is more likely that they originate from local influences. Inflammation, scarring, abnormal pressure, and disturbed relationships between cells that are potentially either organizers or receptors in odontogenesis are more likely causes.

In a study of 28,890 wildlife specimens in museum collections, Colyer (1936) recorded supernumerary teeth in 1.4% of the dentitions. The percentage of specimens with supernumerary teeth varied with the order to which the specimens were assigned: carnivores 2.3%, primates 1.3%, marsupials 1.0%, artiodactyls 0.8%, conies 0.8%, and rodents 0.1%. These values compare to the 1 to 3.6% reported in humans (Schulze, 1970) and agree closely with other studies on primates (Lavelle and Moore, 1973). Colyer (1936) found the supernumeraries more often in the maxillary row, 64.4%, than in the mandibular row, 35.6%. Most frequently, they were observed in the molar region, followed by the premolars and incisors respectively.

Hall (1940) found that in insectivores and carnivores, supernumerary teeth were more common in the decreasing order of the premolar, incisor, and canine regions. The anomaly was manifested unilaterally, and this varied with the type of tooth involved. Bilateral supernumerary teeth were present in 9.1% of the specimens for incisors, 27.0% for premolars, and 50.9% for molars (Colyer, 1936). Supernumerary teeth may be present simultaneously in different regions of the dentition. This condition is regarded as uncommon, with the number of supernumerary teeth in each region seldom exceeding one.

Besides supernumerary teeth, there are double or twin teeth. These consist of two or more parts that clearly demonstrate a tendency toward independence. These double teeth may take the place of a regular tooth or of two adjacent teeth, or they may occur in addition to regular teeth. They develop either from the incomplete division of a single dental germ or from the fusion of two adjacent, regular accessory germs. No decision on the mode of development is possible from the extracted tooth alone. This type of anomaly is not as common as the supernumerary condition, but has been reported by Caldwell (1964), Colyer (1936), Fine (1964), and Neal and Kilkpatrick (1957). In a study of ferrets, *Mustela putorius,* Berkovitz and Thomson (1973) observed that supernumerary deciduous incisors were the result of a dichotomy of the medially situated deciduous first incisor tooth germ. They then suggested that the permanent supernumerary incisor teeth were lost from the functional adult dentition as a result of fusion with the medially situated permanent first incisor during development. Of the animals examined, 82% had supernumerary deciduous incisors, while only 20% had supernumerary permanent incisors.

Subnumerary Teeth. Genetically determined reductions in tooth complement are often accompanied by reduced size and peg formation of the crowns of those teeth present. Two kinds of reduction in number of teeth should be distinguished: hypodontia and oligodontia. In hypodontia, a few and more specific teeth are missing because of the absence of their anlagen, for example, third molars in man. In oligodontia, many teeth are missing, and those present are markedly reduced in size. Anomalies in other organs of ectodermal origin may be associated with oligodontia, such as decreased hair and sweat glands.

Cases of hypodontia have been recorded for a number of wildlife species; however, the condition is not as common as supernumerary teeth (Chiasson, 1955; Colyer, 1936; Hall, 1940; Knable and Werner, 1964; Mumford, 1963; Palmer, 1937; Stager, 1943; Wallace and Bader, 1966). Reports of conditions resembling oligodontia generally represent postnatal pathologic origins rather than developmental origins (Miller, 1977). A diagnosis of hypodontia in a wildlife species is difficult and at times impossible, as teeth may be absent from the dental complement through agenesis, failure to erupt, injury, or disease (Fig. 11.3). As a result, comparisons between taxonomic groups of animals are not feasible at present. Certain observations, however, can be noted. Among primates the most frequently absent teeth are the molars, the condition being most common in man and more common in anthropoid apes than

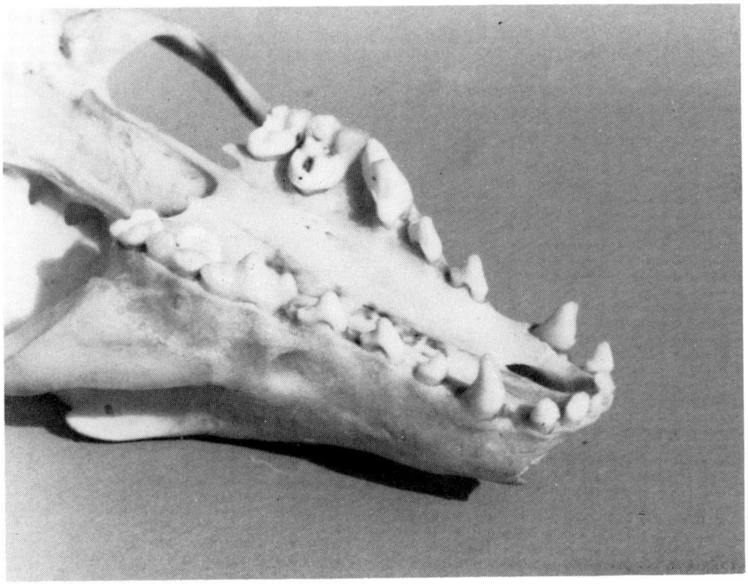

Fig. 11.3. Agenesis of PM_1 in a gray fox, *Urocyon cinereoargenteus.*

in monkeys (Lavelle and Moore, 1973). In carnivores, chiropteres, and insectivores, premolars are the teeth most commonly missing, while in pinnipeds it is the postcanines.

Studies on mice, *Mus musculus,* and moles, *Scapanus latimanus,* have revealed subspecific variations with regard to subnumerary teeth (Palmer, 1937; Wallace and Bader, 1966). With *M. musculus,* agenesis involved the third molar, usually in the mandible. Agenesis occurred in 0.63% of the mice from the western hemisphere as compared to 3.38% of the mice from Eurasia. In the mole, *S. latimanus,* agenesis involved the premolars and was more common in the *anthonyi* subspecies than in the *occultus* subspecies, in which it was more common than in the *latimanus* subspecies.

Abnormal Eruption of Teeth. Eruption of primary and permanent teeth takes place in a definite sequence and at definite time intervals. Abnormalities of tooth eruption include failure to erupt, partial eruption, eruption out of sequence, and retention of primary teeth.

Failure of teeth to erupt may only be a manifestation of another anomalous dental condition or may be mistaken as agenesis of teeth. The work of Marshall (1952) on martens, *Martes americana,* demonstrated how failure of teeth to erupt can be mistaken for agenesis. Mechanical factors, odontomas, and follicular cysts are generally responsible for the failure of the teeth to erupt. Pathological changes of the overlying bone, malposition of tooth bud, supernumerary teeth, retained teeth, and malpositioned teeth are the common mechanical factors that predispose toward failure of tooth eruption. The influence of odontomas and cysts on tooth eruption in wildlife species is well illustrated by Colyer (1936).

Partial eruption of teeth generally results from malposition of the tooth bud, injury to the jaw or developing tooth, or from impedance by other teeth. This condition is frequently seen at the end of the tooth row. In many cases, supernumerary teeth are only partially erupted. The presence of supernumerary teeth may also result in crowding of the tooth row and partial eruption of other teeth.

Abnormalities of the sequence of tooth eruption include premature and delayed eruption. Variations in the sequence are believed to be controlled genetically; however, metabolic disturbances and exogenous factors, such as untimely loss of primary teeth, also play a role. In children, premature eruption occurs 10.7% of the time as opposed to 5.7% for retarded eruption (Schulze, 1970). With the exception of primates (Colyer, 1936), little attention has been given to this condition in wildlife species, despite the fact that eruption patterns are utilized as estimates of age in many species.

The retention of primary teeth in the dentition is rarely reported for wildlife species (Conaway and Landry, 1958). Agenesis of the permanent tooth and malposition of the bud of the permanent tooth with resultant insufficient growth and eruptive force are believed to be factors in tooth retention.

Anomalies of Tooth Position and Occlusion. Malposition of individual teeth and malocclusion are not synonymous terms, although the two conditions frequently coexist. Anomalies in tooth position vary from malposition of a single tooth to involvement of all the teeth in the complement. These variations can be related to alteration in form, size, and width of jaws or they may occur independently. They may or may not interfere with occlusion. Beilly (1956) reported that 16% of the voles in a population of *Clethrionomys gapperi* had malposition of the entire dental complement but still retained perfect occlusion.

Morphologically, similar cases can be due to different etiologic factors and, conversely, similar etiologic factors can cause a variety of malpositions. Moreover, several factors may act simultaneously. Both heredity and environmental factors play important roles. The type of tooth that is commonly malpositioned differs with the various taxonomic groups of animals. In primates, carnivores, artiodactyls, and marsupials, the premolars are usually the malpositioned teeth, while in perissodactyls, proboscids, and conies it is the incisors (Colyer, 1936). Among lagomorphs, the incisors are more commonly maloccluded than the premolars and molars (Zeman and Fielder, 1969).

Abnormalies in tooth position are frequently encountered in free-ranging mammals, with the exception of rodents and lagomorphs (Colyer, 1936). The degree of malposition may vary from slight to severe. In many cases, the malposition is not noticeable unless the investigator is examining large series of specimens from the same species. The prevalence of malpositioned teeth in many groups of mammals averages between 5 and 12% of the specimens examined, and among primates, prevalences up to 40% are common. When animals raised in captivity are considered, the prevalence may double or triple (Colyer, 1936). The influence of environment upon the position of teeth remains uninvestigated.

Abnormalities in tooth position are due in a large measure to disparities between jaw and tooth size, that is, evolutionary reduction in the length of the jaw at a proportionally greater rate than the reduction in the length of the tooth series (Colyer 1936; Schulze, 1970). Both crowding and separation occur, with crowded arches being more frequently encountered. Abnormal tooth size is usually more important than a large or small jaw. Colyer (1936) felt that the rarity of positional variations in rodents and lagomorphs may be partly due to ample room in the dental arch for teeth. Tooth loss, patterns of eruption, the presence of supernumerary teeth, and injury are major influences on tooth position.

Malocclusion generally results from abnormalities in tooth position, disparities in the length of the mandible and maxillae, injury, or misshapen skulls. Protrusion of either the maxillary or manibular incisors is a common form of malocclusion for species in which the incisor teeth meet "edge-to-edge." Mandibular incisor protrusion is frequently observed in primates but not so in carnivores, whereas, the opposite is true of maxillary incisor protrusion (Colyer, 1936). It is felt that these protrusions are the result of overgrowth in the maxillae or the mandible. Malocclusion may also result from injury (Fig. 11.4).

NONDEVELOPMENTAL ANOMALIES

Anomalies of Tooth Structure and Color. All calcified components of the tooth may exhibit anomalies of the gross or fine structure or of mineralization. These abnormalities, although considered structural, may also involve tooth size, shape, or color. The etiology of structural anomalies may be either hereditary or nonhereditary and, grossly, can be classified accordingly: 1) hereditary anomalies usually involve both the primary and secondary dentitions, whereas nonhereditary anomalies affect either the primary or secondary dentition or only specific teeth; 2) as a rule, hereditary structural anomalies affect either enamel or dentin as opposed to nonhereditary anomalies, which affect both enamel and dentin; and 3) hereditary anomalies most often cause diffuse or even vertical orientation of derangements, while nonhereditary structural anomalies are primarily horizontal (Shulze, 1970).

Hereditary structural anomalies of the enamel include hypomineralization and hypoplasia or aplasia of the enamel. Hypomineralization is characterized by reduced mineralization in contrast to hypoplasia or aplasia in which mineralization is normal while there is a quantitative reduction in enamel matrix. Hypoplasia or aplasia of enamel occurs less frequently than disorders of hypomineralization.

In man, hereditary hypoplasia of the dentin occurs twice as frequently as enamel hypoplasia (Schulze, 1970), the primary disorder affecting both the dentin and pulp. In contrast to enamel hypoplasia, other components of the tooth may be secondarily involved, particularly the enamel, of which the color, contour, and functional capacity may be changed. These alterations of the enamel may be so clinically striking that they lead to confusion with enamel hypoplasia.

Nonhereditary structural anomalies may result from (1) prolonged alterations of mineral metabolism due to dietary deficiencies, vitamin disorders, and metabolic dysfunctions; (2) inclusion of chemicals or pigments into the organic ground substance or the crystals of the enamel or dentin; and (3) injury to the differentiated amelo-

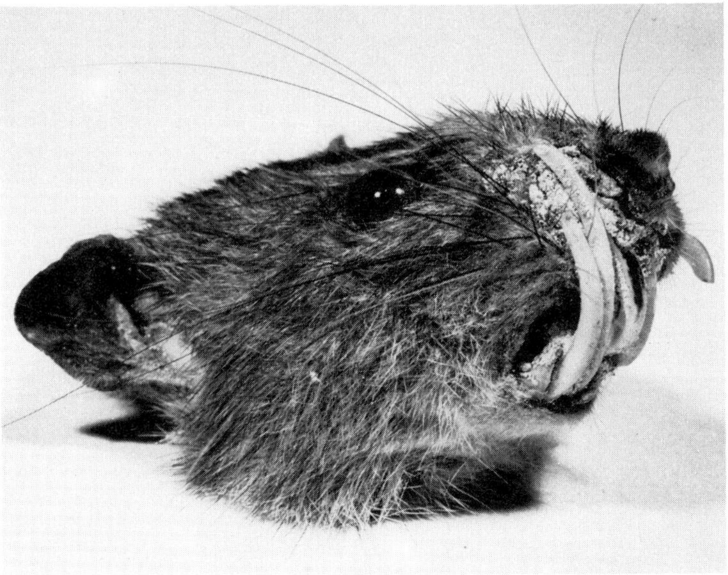

Fig. 11.4. Malocclusion and resultant overgrowth of incisors from a rat, *Rattus* sp., as the result of injury.

blasts or odontoblasts due to infection in the individual or its mother (Andersen and Holst, 1970; Cagnone, 1970; Karstad, 1967; Levy, 1970).

Structural anomalies are found frequently in the teeth of captive and free-ranging primates (Colyer, 1936). Mild cases show only a slight pitting of the enamel; in more advanced conditions the enamel becomes dark in color and studded with numerous deep pits, and in some cases there is only a slight covering of enamel. Occasionally the defect takes the form of transverse grooves, the enamel presenting a smooth glassy appearance. The dentin in these cases is seldom affected. The irregularities of the enamel surface are usually most conspicuous near the neck of the tooth, gradually lessening and disappearing as the occlusal area is approached.

These structural anomalies appear to be limited primarily to the incisors and canines, and Colyer (1936) suggested that the enamel organs of these teeth were more responsive to alterations in calcium metabolism and therefore would be the first to present defects of the enamel. In addition, Colyer (1936) noted enamel defects simulating hereditary hypoplasia in the teeth from several genera of palm civets.

It is extremely difficult to separate structural and color changes in the dentition. Hypoplasia of any of the calcified dental tissues changes the color of the teeth. Discoloration of the teeth generally refers to change in the color of the crown but may involve the root or the entire tooth as well. It may be caused by the deposition of a film, pigment, or calculus on the surface of the enamel, exposed dentin, or cementum, resulting in surface color changes or extrinsic stains that can be removed by abrasives or by chemicals. An example of this condition would be the observed staining of teeth in raccoons, *Procyon lotor,* with aluminum (Hoff, 1973). Physiologic aging also increases the surface pigmentation of the enamel. Internal changes in color affecting the calcified tissues of the teeth may be of local (dentin, cementum, and pulp) or systemic (blood-borne) origin and are called intrinsic stains. The latter are often sensitive indicators of internal homeostasis (Baden, 1970).

DIAGNOSIS. Certain types of dental anomalies are easy to recognize, whereas others require considerable knowledge of the dentition of the species. As a result, most reports deal with obvious anomalies, such as supernumerary and subnumerary teeth, deformities, gross malocclusion, malposition, and stained teeth. Large series of specimens and familiarity with the species involved may be required to achieve diagnosis of the more subtle anomalies involving tooth shape, size, structure, and eruption sequence. Histological study may be required also. All too frequently, an animal has multiple dental anomalies or a tooth has more than one anomaly.

When utilizing a large series of specimens to determine the prevalence of an anomaly, the age and sex of the individuals, the locality from which they were collected, and the manner in which the anomaly presents itself must be considered. Maxillary canines among cervid species illustrate these points.

Maxillary canines are normally present in the dentition of a few genera of cervids, such as *Rangifer, Capreolus, Elaphodus, Elaphurus, Hydropotes, Moschus,* and *Muntiacus* (Whitehead, 1972). However, for most genera maxillary canines represent a supernumerary condition. Many reports document the presence of maxillary canines in *Odocoileus,* and the subject of their occurrence, as well as in other genera of cervids, has been reviewed by Brokx (1972). These teeth usually are imbedded in alveoli and persist in museum collections. Van Gelder and Hoffmeister (1953) felt that maxillary canines occurred more frequently in *O. virginianus* from south of 24° N. latitude. This was disputed by Brokx (1972), who claimed that this was an artifact produced by the sex composition of the collections examined. In Venezuela, Brokx noted that 11% of the does examined possessed maxillary canines as opposed to 3% of the bucks. The majority of data from North America has been based upon hunter-kill collections which consisted primarily of bucks, as opposed to Central and South American collections involving both sexes.

Jackson (1976) noted that 11% of fallow deer, *Dama dama,* had maxillary canine teeth. However, none of these teeth had alveoli; they had closed roots. The teeth were found lying adjacent to the bone at or near the junction of the maxilla and premaxilla. The percentage of deer with these canines decreased with age, suggesting that teeth were lost through cuts in the gum acquired while feeding. This hypothesis is supported by Chapman and Chapman (1973) who found maxillary canines in 25% of newborn fallow deer, but in only 2% of the deer up to 18 months of age. In addition, Jackson (1976) noted that the prevalence of supernumerary canines was 18.7% in inbred herds, compared to 4.2% in "open" herds.

The most difficult aspect of dental anomalies to diagnose is etiology. While many cases are considered to be genetic in origin, this is not always easy to prove. The effects of infections, nutritional deficiencies, metabolic imbalances, and injury may or may not be obvious in the manifestation of the anomaly. Genetic mechanisms, though, are probably the etiology of the vast majority of dental anomalies reported for wildlife species.

SIGNIFICANCE. The significance of dental anomalies to the survival and health of an animal is difficult to ascertain. Oligodontia or severe malocclusion most likely would be fatal. Severe deformities of long teeth, such as rootless incisors or tusks, might lead to penetration of the cranial structure and prove fatal. Absence or malformation of specialized teeth for food procurement or defense would likewise compromise health and survival. The majority of the anomalies that have been described, however, have minimal effect upon animal survival.

Anomalies may provide information on genetic disorders or evolutionary trends among species or populations and can reflect environmental insult or serious health problems resulting from environmental sources, such as nutritional deficiencies or fluorosis. Thus as an indicator of such conditions, dental anomalies if properly utilized may serve as an important research tool for geneticists, wildlife managers, disease investigators, and the like.

REFERENCES

Andersen, J. J., and G. Holst. 1970. Endocrine disorders. In R. J. Gorlin and H. M. Goldman. Thoma's oral pathology. C. V. Mosby Company, St. Louis.

Archer, M. 1975. Abnormal dental development and its significance in dasyurids and other marsupials. Mem. Queensland Mus. 17:251–265.

Baden, E. 1970. Environmental pathology of the teeth. In R. J. Gorlin and H. M. Goldman. Thoma's oral pathology. C. V. Mosby Company, St. Louis.

Beilly, E. M. 1956. Malarrangement of teeth in *Clethrionomys gapperi.* J. Mammal. 37:298–299.

Berkovitz, B. K. B., and P. Thomson. 1973. Observations on the aetiology of supernumerary upper incisors in the albino ferret, *Mustela putorius.* Arch. Oral Biol. 18:457–463.

Bernier, J. L. 1959. The management of oral disease. C. V. Mosby Company, St. Louis.

Brokx, P. A. 1972. The superior canines of *Odocoileus* and other deer. J. Mammal. 53:359–366.

Cagone, L. D. 1970. Metabolic disorders. In R. J. Gorlin and H. M. Goldman. Thoma's oral pathology. C. V. Mosby Company, St. Louis.

Caldwell, D. K. 1964. Tusk twinning in Pacific walrus. J. Mammal. 45:490–491.

Chapman, D. I., and N. G. Chapman. 1973. Maxillary canine teeth in fallow deer, *Dama dama* L. J. Zool. 170:143–147.

Chiasson, R. B. 1955. Dental anomalies of the Alaskan fur seal. J. Mammal. 36:562–564.

Choate, J. R. 1968. Dental abnormalities in the short-tailed shrew, *Blarina brevicauda.* J. Mammal. 49:251–258.

Cockrum, E. L. 1962. Introduction to mammalogy. Ronald Press, New York.

Colyer, F. 1936. Variations and diseases of the teeth of animals. John Bale, Sons, and Danielsson, Ltd., London.

Conaway, C., and S. O. Landry. 1958. Rudimentary mandibular teeth of *Scalopus aquaticus.* J. Mammal. 39:58–64.

Crompton, A. W., and P. Parker. 1978. Evolution of the mammalian masticatory apparatus. Am. Sci. 66: 192–201.

Fine, M. D. 1964. An abnormal P_2 in *Canis latrans* from the Hagerman fauna of Idaho. J. Mammal. 45:483–485.

Hall, E. R. 1940. Supernumerary and missing teeth in wild mammals of the orders Insectivora and Carnivora with some notes on disease. J. Dent. Res. 19:103–143.

Hoff, G. L. 1973. Raccoon teeth stained with aluminum. J. Wildl. Dis. 9:323.

Jackson, J. E. 1976. Mandibular and maxillary dental abnormalities in fallow deer, *Dama dama,* from the New Forest, Hampshire. J. Zool. 180:518–523.

Karstad, L. H. 1967. Fluorosis in deer, *Odocoileus virginianus.* Bull. Wildl. Dis. Assoc. 3:42–46.

Knable, A., and W. E. Werner. 1964. Raccoon with unusual dental complement. J. Mammal. 45:493.

Lavelle, C. L. B., and W. J. Moore. 1973. The incidence of agenesis and polygenesis in the primate dentition. Am. J. Phys. Anthropol. 38:671.

______, R. P. Shellis, and D. F. G. Poole. 1977. Evolutionary changes to the primate skull and dentition. Charles C Thomas, Springfield.

Levy, B. M. 1970. Mineral metabolism. In R. J. Gorlin and H. M. Goldman. Thoma's oral pathology. C. V. Mosby Company, St. Louis.

Long, C. A., and C. F. Long. 1965. Dental abnormalities in North American badgers, genus *Taxidea.* Kansas Acad. Sci., trans. 68:145–155.

Marshall, W. H. 1952. Note on missing teeth in *Martes americana.* J. Mammal. 33:116–117.

McIntosh, W. C. 1929. On abnormal teeth in certain mammals, especially in the rabbit. Royal Soc. Edinborough, trans. 56:333–407.

Miller, F. L., and G. D. Tessier. 1971. Dental anomalies in caribou, *Rangifer tarandus.* J. Mammal. 52:164–174.

Miller, W. A. 1977. Extreme tooth loss in a specimen of *Isodon macrourus* (Peramelidae; Marsupialia). Aust. Wildl. Res. 4:229–232.

Mumford, R. E. 1963. Unusual dentition in *Myotis occultus.* J. Mammal. 44:275.

Neal, B. J., and R. D. Kilkpatrick. 1957. Anomalous canine tooth development in an Arizona peccary. J. Mammal. 38:420.

Nellis, C. H. 1972. Dental anomalies in coyotes from central Alberta. Can. J. Zool. 50:1259–1262.

Palmer, F. G. 1937. Geographic variation in the mole, *Scapanus latimanus.* J. Mammal. 18:280–314.

Peyer, B. 1968. Comparative odontology. Translated

and edited by R. Zangerl. Univ. Chicago Press, Chicago.

Phillips, C. J., and J. K. Jones, Jr. 1968. Dental abnormalities in North American bats. I. Emballonuridae, Noctilionidae, and Chilonycteridae. Kansas Acad. Sci., trans. 71:509–520.

Schulze, C. 1970. Developmental abnormalities of the teeth and jaws. In R. J. Gorlin and H. M. Goldman. Thoma's oral pathology. C. V. Mosby Company, St. Louis.

Stager, K. E. 1943. Remarks on *Myotis occultus* in California. J. Mammal. 24:197–199.

Swindler, D. R. 1976. Dentition of living primates. Academic Press, New York.

Van Gelder, R. G., and D. F. Hoffmeister. 1953. Canine teeth in white-tailed deer. J. Wildl. Manage. 17:100.

Vaughan, T. A. 1961. Cranial asymmetry in the pocket gopher. J. Mammal. 42:412–413.

Wagner, G. 1923. An odd malformation in a woodchuck. J. Mammal. 4:21.

Wallace, J. T., and R. S. Bader. 1966. Dental agenesis in wild-caught house mice. J. Mammal. 47:733–734.

Wing, E. S. 1965. Abnormal dentition in several white-tailed deer jaws. J. Mammal. 46:348–350.

Whitehead, G. K. 1972. Deer of the world. Viking Press, New York.

Zeman, W. V., and F. G. Fielder. 1969. Dental malocclusion and overgrowth in rabbits. J. Am. Vet. Med. Assoc. 155:1115–1119.

12 *Soybean Impaction of Waterfowl*

ROBERT L. JARVIS

IMPACTION of the esophagus, or crop, with soybeans, *Glycine max,* is a condition that occurs infrequently but which can cause the death of large numbers of waterfowl. Soybean impaction has also been termed "bound crop" (Hanson and Smith, 1950) and "crop impaction" (Durant, 1956). Soybeans are a widely cultivated crop frequently encountered by feeding waterfowl and other birds. Most cases of impaction can be attributed to soybeans; however, cowpeas, *Vigna sinensis,* may also cause impaction.

Although naturally occurring episodes of soybean impaction occur, only two experimental investigations of the problem have been undertaken (Durant, 1956; Jarvis, 1969). In both studies impactions were produced only when anesthetized Canada geese, *Branta canadensis,* were force-fed soybeans, and even then the procedure sometimes failed to produce an impaction. Thus, most of what is known about the initiation and progress of soybean impaction has been inferred from necropsy lesions.

EPIZOOTIOLOGY. Hanson and Smith (1950) first reported soybean impaction in Canada geese at Horsehoe Lake Refuge in Southern Illinois, but the number of geese that died was not stated. Durant (1956) estimated that about 500 Canada geese died annually from soybean impaction at Swan Lake National Wildlife Refuge in Missouri in the early 1950s. Although lesser snow geese, *Anser c. caerulescens,* were present at Swan Lake Refuge, no cases of soybean impaction were detected in this species. Mortality of Canada geese from soybean impaction occurred each year from 1963 to 1966 at Crab Orchard National Wildlife Refuge in Southern Illinois (Jarvis, 1969, 1976; Wise, 1967). The number of geese that died varied greatly, ranging from 100 in 1965 to 3,000 in 1966; the proportion of the population afflicted varied from less than 1% to nearly 20%.

Page and Lynch (1959) attributed the death of 15,000 to 20,000 mallards, *Anas platyrhynchos,* in Arkansas in January 1956 to three causes: lead poisoning, impaction of the crop with soybeans, and an unidentified microbial agent. Fourteen of the 30 birds they examined had signs typical of lead poisoning: lead shot in the gizzard and lead in the tissue of the gizzard. Lead was not found in the other 16 birds, but they had impacted and necrotic esophagi. The contribution of an unknown viral agent was inferred on the basis of low virulence in white mice and chicken eggs of tissue cultured from impacted mallards. It was postulated that the microbial agent predisposed the mallards to impaction of the esophagus with soybeans. This hypothesis has not been tested.

PATHOGENESIS. Soybean impaction is caused by the ingestion of a large number of dry soybeans that are retained in the crop. Waterfowl have a fusiform crop; the soybeans are present throughout the length of the esophagus. The dry soybeans swell rapidly upon contact with moisture, doubling in volume in approximately two hours. They produce a final volume 2.5 times the original dry volume in 17 to 24 hours (Jarvis, 1969). Although geese may frequently drink water shortly after eating soybeans, there is sufficient moisture present in the esophagus to allow the soybeans to swell fully (Jarvis, 1969). The swelling of soybeans in the filled esophagus produces pressure necrosis. The rapidity of the swelling process allows only a small portion of the soybeans to pass into the gizzard, and the pressure and ischemia produced by the swelled soybeans disrupt peristalsis of the esophagus. Even though the soybeans may eventually disintegrate, the esophagus is unable to transport the beans to the gizzard. Necrosis often extends into the proventriculus, further disrupting the digestive process.

Only dry soybeans cause impactions; ingestion of moistened or swelled soybeans is harmless (Durant, 1956; Jarvis, 1969). Death of large numbers of geese from soybean impaction usually occurs in September and October when the earliest migrating geese arrive on wintering areas and feed in harvested soybean fields before other foods are available (Durant, 1956; Jarvis, 1969, 1976). When other grains, particularly corn, become available, geese stop feeding on soybeans, and the number of impactions virtually ceases. Hanson and Smith (1950) observed mortality of geese from soybean impaction in winter during a period when foods other than soybeans had been depleted and temperatures were below normal.

Attempts to induce captive, wild geese to consume sufficient quantities of soybeans to cause impaction were unsuccessful (Jarvis, 1969). The geese were allowed only a limited amount of time to feed, after withholding food for several days. In 1964, only about 40% of the geese feeding in soybean fields at Crab Orchard National Wildlife Refuge developed impactions that proved fatal (Wise, 1967). Thus, the mechanisms involved in ingestion of a sufficient quantity of soybeans to cause impaction and the quantity of soybeans that will result in an impaction are unknown. Whatever mechanisms are involved are apparently independent of age and sex, since age and sex ratios of geese that died from impaction at Crab Orchard National Wildlife Refuge in 1966 were not significantly different from the age and sex ratios of the population (Jarvis, 1969).

Hanson and Smith (1950) suggested that lead poisoning may contribute to the formation of soybean impactions because lead poisoning occasionally results in impaction of the upper digestive tract (Jordan and Bellrose, 1951). Geese with soybean impactions at Crab Orchard National Wildlife Refuge did not contain lead shot in the gizzard, and the level of lead in tissues was minimal (Jarvis, 1969; Wise, 1967). Page and Lynch (1959) noted that about half the mallards they examined (16 of 30) had impacted, necrotic esophagi and were lead-free. Lead poisoning apparently plays no role in the formation of soybean impactions, although birds concurrently afflicted with both soybean impaction and lead poisoning may occasionally be encountered.

SIGNS AND PATHOLOGY. Soybean impaction occurs in an acute and a chronic form (Durant, 1956), and the signs of the two forms are distinct. In Canada geese with the acute form, death occurred within 24 hours after consumption of soybeans (Jarvis, 1969, 1976). Body weight and fat reserves were normal, and internal organs, except the esophagus, appeared unaffected. Usually the entire length of the esophagus was distended due to recently swollen soybeans (Fig. 12.1); occasionally the proventriculus was also distended. Obvious impressions from the swollen soybeans were evident in the lining of the esophagus, particularly at the thoracic inlet, but gross tissue damage was absent. Rupture of the esophagus of geese with acute impactions occasionally occurs: ruptured esophagi were noted in one goose in Missouri (Durant, 1956) and in three geese in Illinois (Jarvis, 1976). Page and Lynch (1959) reported ruptured crops in 9 of 30 mallards. In the geese in Illinois, ruptures were confined to the thoracic portion of the esophagus and the proventriculus. Death of geese with acute impactions is apparently due to shock (Jarvis, 1969).

In contrast to acute impaction, geese with chronic impactions have extensive esophageal necrosis (Fig. 12.2). In some cases, necrosis extends through the skin of the neck, with putrefied food items projecting from the resultant fistula. Usually necrosis is most extensive from midneck to the thoracic inlet, and the esophagus often adheres to the skin of the neck. Occasionally the thoracic portion of the esophagus is also necrotic, but only rarely does extensive necrosis extend to the proventriculus.

In chronic impactions, esophageal contents are putrefied and consist of fragments of soybeans and other seeds, but a bolus of grass is usually the most obvious content of the esophagus. Reimpaction occurs as the geese continue to feed and the soybeans that cause the initial impaction slowly disintegrate (Durant, 1956).

Starvation is the ultimate cause of death in cases of chronic impaction (Durant, 1956; Jarvis,

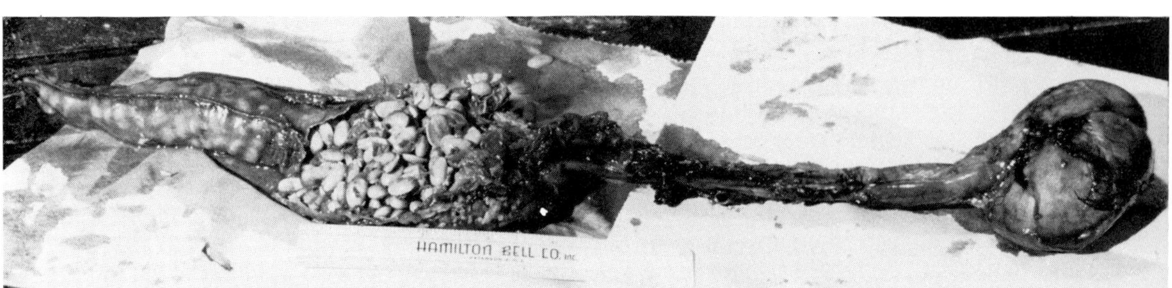

Fig. 12.1. Upper digestive tract of a Canada goose, *Branta canadensis*, from Crab Orchard National Wildlife Refuge, 1966. The impaction was restricted to the cervical portion of the esophagus. The esophagus was cut open to reveal the swollen soybeans.

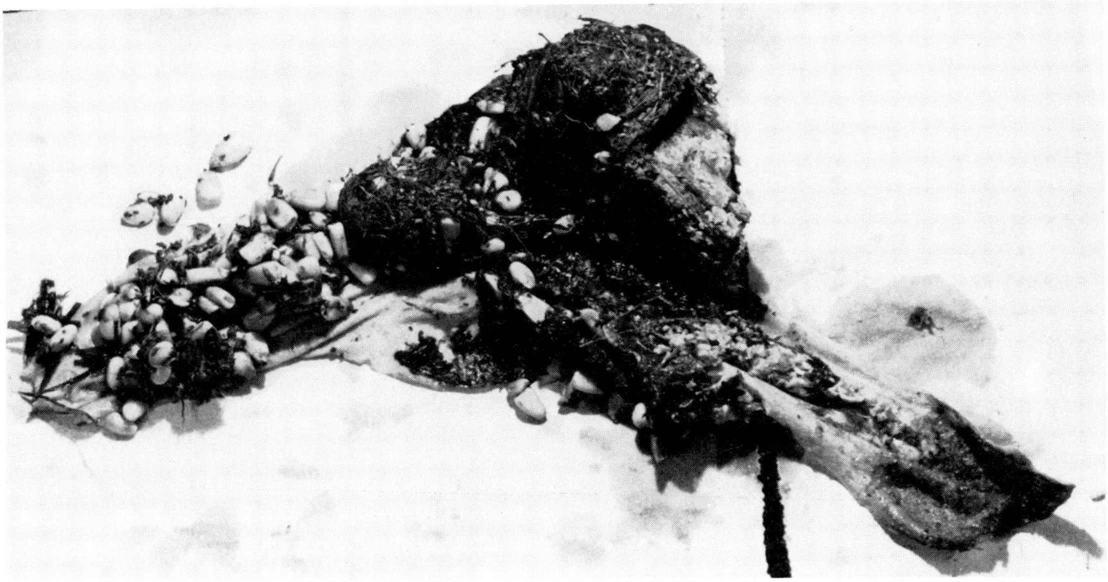

Fig. 12.2. Upper digestive tract of a Canada goose, *B. canadensis,* with a chronic impaction, from Crab Orchard National Wildlife Refuge, 1966. The dark mass in the center of the photograph is putrefied vegetative matter in the area of the thoracic inlet. The corn in the anterior portion of the esophagus was consumed from a baited trap-site. The proventriculus is in the lower right corner of the photograph.

1969, 1976). Body weight of geese with chronic impactions is about 60% of normal. The liver is also greatly reduced in size, weighing 30% of normal (Jarvis, 1969). Death from starvation occurs two to three weeks after the initial formation of impactions (Wise, 1967). This readily explains the advanced state of necrosis observed in geese that die from chronic impactions.

At Crab Orchard National Wildlife Refuge, approximately 20% of the cases of soybean impaction were acute and 80% were chronic. Durant (1956) reported that 30 to 40% of the cases in Missouri were acute.

TREATMENT AND DIAGNOSIS. Birds with impacted esophagi could be treated by lavage or surgical relief, but treatment is impractical because of the rapid death in acute cases and advanced esophageal necrosis in chronic cases. In either case, it would be very difficult to capture wild birds for treatment.

Soybean impaction is easily diagnosed, but the occurrence of two forms of the condition, which differ considerably in appearance, can be confusing. When large numbers of birds develop impactions, acute cases occur early, but chronic cases may not appear for two to three weeks. The initial stages of an outbreak may not be detected because the carcasses of the small number of birds with acute impactions are dispersed about roosting areas and consumed by scavengers. Conversely, geese with chronic impactions may be found in fields, ponds, lakes, and occasionally even in brushy and forested areas. These birds are easily recognized because of their reluctance to fly, weak flight, or inability to fly. Despite their weakened condition, geese with chronic impactions often make daily excursions between aquatic roosting areas and adjacent feeding areas. Frequently these excursions are made by walking, a highly abnormal behavior for Canada geese.

PREVENTION. Control measures are likely to be ineffective after an outbreak of soybean impaction has been detected. By the time an outbreak becomes apparent, most impactions will have already developed. However, soybean impaction occurs only when a specific set of circumstances occurs and the likelihood of the occurrence of soybean impaction can be qualitatively predicted (Jarvis, 1976). At Crab Orchard National Wildlife Refuge, below normal precipitation during the growing season (June, July, and August), lack of rain in early fall, early migration of large numbers of geese, and delayed harvest of corn were conducive to large numbers of geese dying from impaction. Since below normal precipitation is the most consistent predisposing factor to outbreaks of soybean impaction, a preventive program should be implemented in dry years before the arrival of geese in the fall.

Soybean impaction can most easily be prevented by restricting the utilization of soybeans by feeding birds. Practices such as disking of harvested fields and providing alternate foods should be effective in reducing mortality from impaction, particularly when used concurrently. Elimination of soybeans from farming programs on waterfowl refuges is another possible preventive measure but may be ineffective where soybeans are grown on private land adjacent to refuges, unless alternate preferred foods are available.

REFERENCES

Durant, A. J. 1956. Impaction and pressure necrosis in Canada geese due to eating dry hulled soybeans. J. Wildl. Manage. 20:399–404.

Hanson, H. C., and R. H. Smith. 1950. Canada geese of the Mississippi flyway, with special reference to an Illinois flock. Illinois Natur. Hist. Surv. Bull. 25 (Art. 3):67–210.

Jarvis, R. L. 1969. Ecological and physiological aspects of soybean impaction in Canada geese. Ph.D. Dissertation, Southern Illinois Univ.

______. 1976. Soybean impaction in Canada geese. Wildl. Soc. Bull. 4:175–179.

Jordan, J. S., and F. C. Bellrose. 1951. Lead poisoning in wild waterfowl. Illinois Natur. Hist. Surv. Biol. Notes 26:1–27.

Page, C. A., and J. J. Lynch. 1959. A laboratory study of an Arkansas duck die-off. Annu. Conf. Southeastern Assoc. Game Fish Comm. 13:161–164.

Wise, G. A. 1967. Canada goose mortality at Crab Orchard National Wildlife Refuge. M.S. Thesis, Southern Illinois Univ.

13 *Nutritional Diseases of Wild Birds*

JOEL D. WALLACH
JOHN E. COOPER

LIKE all forms of wildlife, wild birds depend on the availability of adequate food supplies for survival and propagation. When the food supply is suboptimal during the breeding and rearing season, a great number of hatchling birds fail to reach maturity. Unlike neonatal mammals that suckle, young birds depend on residual yolk material for an initial energy source. After a few days, the young bird either becomes self-sufficient, as with precocious species, such as game birds and waterfowl, or they depend on the parent bird for a source of food, for example, raptors, which makes them more acutely dependent on environmental sources of food.

It is very difficult to determine the exact numbers of wild birds that succumb during lean food seasons to the specific forms of malnutrition encountered in the free-ranging state because the weak birds are lost to predators or aggressive members of their own species. Probably the birds for which the most data are available are the raptors, and 60 to 80% of these birds in North America and Great Britain die in their first year of life (Snow, 1968). Such individuals often succumb to territorial aggression; however, death is almost invariably due to starvation. Since damage to the carcass of dead individuals in the field makes it impossible to perform an accurate differential diagnosis of nutritional diseases, it is useful to study the scope of nutritional diseases to which wild birds are susceptible as captive individuals.

The advances in research and management of commercial poultry and zoo animal nutrition have been a boon to game bird and waterfowl hobbyists and falconers. The nutritional requirements of captive raptors and fancy birds are now more easily met by standard pelleted or mixed rations. Nutritional disease is, therefore, now most often observed in birds that have some other management problems, for example, insufficient feeder space for the number of birds being fed or the feeding of unbalanced home-mixed rations.

ETIOLOGY, PATHOLOGY, DIAGNOSIS, TREATMENT

Carbohydrates. Carbohydrates are an important source of calories to game birds and waterfowl, especially young growing birds, laying females, and birds housed outdoors during inclement weather (Wallach, 1969, 1971a). A common error made by the owner of the Easter duck and beginning hobbyist in keeping wild species is that they feed too much succulent green material to growing birds. The palatable greens are often consumed to excess and less of the pelleted ration may be consumed, thereby resulting in caloric exhaustion.

An experiment was set up by Wallach (1969, 1970, 1971a) to illustrate this phenomenon of caloric exhaustion with four groups of day-old mallard ducklings, *Anas platyrhynchos* (Fig. 13.1). Each group consisted of 25 birds. Group 1 was fed lettuce only, Group 2 was fed hydroponic grass only, Group 3 was fed a commercial waterfowl ration, and Group 4 was fed a mixture of waterfowl ration and hydroponic grass. Nearly all of the birds in Groups 1 and 2 died of caloric exhaustion by 11 days of age while the birds in Groups 3 and 4 nearly doubled their hatching weight.

Grit of appropriate size must be provided for the gallinaceous birds if they are to obtain the maximum amount of calories from any ration (Wallach, 1969, 1970, 1971a). Undigested grain will appear in the feces if a grit deficiency exists.

Carbohydrates make up a minimal part of the diet of a normal free-ranging raptor; however, commercial diets can employ a reasonable percentage of carbohydrates for captive birds. A range of 1,760 to 2,200 total calories/kg of diet should be provided for raptors, the major portion being derived from deamination of protein sources. Commercial rations contain a calorie range of 2,450 to 2,850 kilocalories (kcal) of metabolizable energy/kg (Norris and Scott, 1965).

Excessive intake of calories produces obese

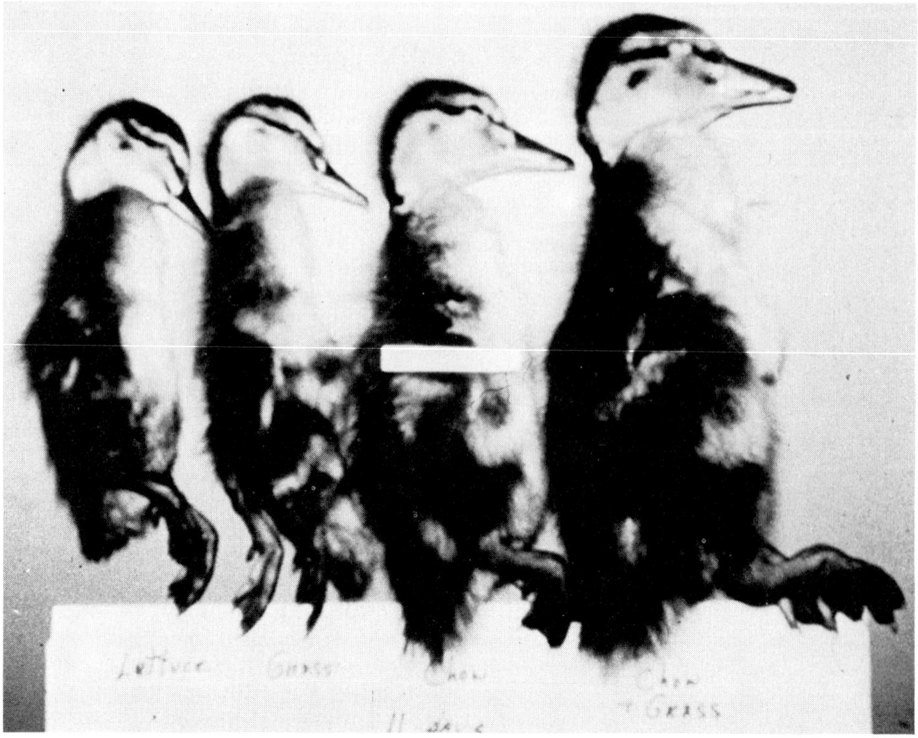

Fig. 13.1. Eleven-day-old mallard ducklings, *Anas platyrhynchos*, showing disparity in growth rate when fed on four different rations.

birds, which can result in infertility, more susceptibility to heat stress, and in hens, more liability to the "egg-bound" syndrome. Thin birds that have exhausted fat depots will have a prominent keel and a small liver, which is due to the depletion of glycogen and protein stores.

Fats. Lipids act as a source of energy, a carrier for fat-soluble vitamins, and a source of the essential fatty acids, linoleic, linolenic, and arachidonic (Norris and Scott, 1965; Renner, 1971; Wallach, 1970). Dietary fat levels of 2 to 3% are recommended. A linoleic acid deficiency in Japanese quail, *Coturnix coturnix japonica*, produces a 50% decrease in egg production. Lipids can play a major role as a calorie source for raptors; 5 to 6% of the total diet is recommended. Excessive dietary fat will produce obese birds, malabsorption, and possibly diarrhea (Wallach, 1970).

It is of interest to note that for many centuries, falconers have recognized excessive "fatness" in their birds as being undesirable. This was evidenced by poor flying shown by the birds and was also seen as a possible predisposing cause of disease. Methods of reducing the fatness of a trained hawk were discussed as early as the 15th century (Bernes, 1486).

Protein. Protein provides amino acids and acts as a major energy source for young growing birds (Norris and Scott, 1965). As a rule of thumb, the younger growing birds require a higher percentage of protein for the first six to eight weeks; also, the smaller the species, the higher the percent of protein required in the diet. Protein requirements of game birds, raptors, and waterfowl for the first six to eight weeks are as follows: chickens 20%; turkeys 28%; ducks and geese 17%; raptors 18%; pheasants 30%; quail 28%; and Japanese quail 23% (Anon., 1966; Norris and Scott, 1965).

Protein deficiencies result in poor feathering, stunted growth, high mortality rate of hatchlings, emaciation of adult birds, and infertility (Giroud, 1968; Wallach, 1969). Deficiencies of crude protein rarely occur; however, inadequate levels of specific amino acids have been recognized. Deficiencies of methionine result in "shock marks" or notched feathers or in patchy feather loss. This is especially common in birds on an all-fruit diet. Deficiencies of lysine result in the periodic loss of feather coloration (Fig. 13.2). There is a theory among falconers that "shock marks" may also be associated with periods of stress, for example, a drop in temperature or traumatic injury. In an effort to provide high-quality meat protein, the

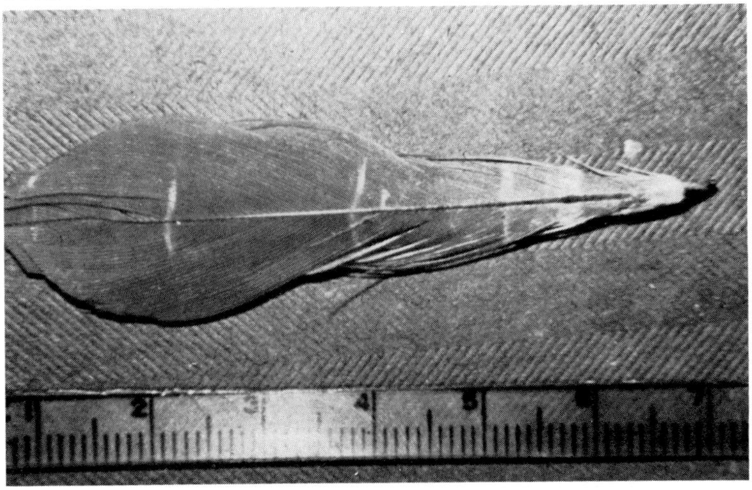

Fig. 13.2. Tail feathers from an African gray parrot, *Psittacus erithacus*. The colorless bands have resulted from periodic lysine deficiency.

falconer often restricts the diet to beef steak, pigeon muscle meat, liver, or horse meat. It is recommended that diets fed to captive raptors consist of whole rodents or a commercially prepared diet for birds of prey.

Excesses of dietary protein have produced visceral and arthritic gout (Wallach, 1969). Diets containing high levels of DNA, for example, fish, heart, liver, kidney, brain, shrimp, or meat meal, as well as dehydration predispose birds to gout. A diagnosis of gout may be made in the live bird by finding elevated levels of blood uric acid.

Birds are uricotelic and they normally excrete the majority of their nitrogenous wastes as uric acid (Austic and Cole, 1971). The total quantity of uric acid excreted increases in direct proportion to the level of excess dietary nitrogen. Renal pathology and/or extreme excesses of dietary nitrogen produce hyperuricemia and visceral gout (Austic and Cole, 1971; Wallach, 1970; Ward and Slaughter, 1968). Renal pathology may also result from hypovitaminosis A or dehydration. There is a practice among falconers and aviculturists to give little or no water to captive birds of prey (Brown and Amadon, 1968). Fresh water should always be available, even if overt consumption is rare. In the tropics, birds drink frequently, and it is particularly important that water is available for well-fed captive specimens.

Articular gout (Fig. 13.3) occurs less frequently than the visceral form. Articular gout has been reproduced experimentally in domestic birds by feeding all-meat or 80% protein diets. Clinical signs include sudden death in the visceral form and chronic lameness in the arthritic form.

In visceral gout (Fig. 13.4), pearl-colored,

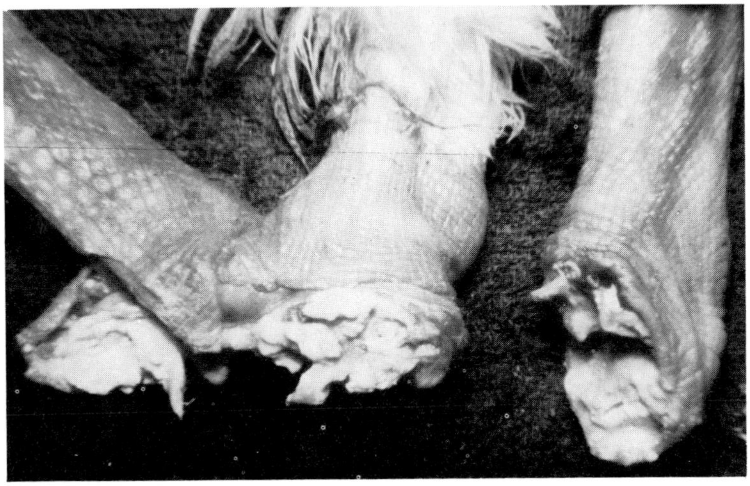

Fig. 13.3. Advanced articular gout in the hock joint of a goose.

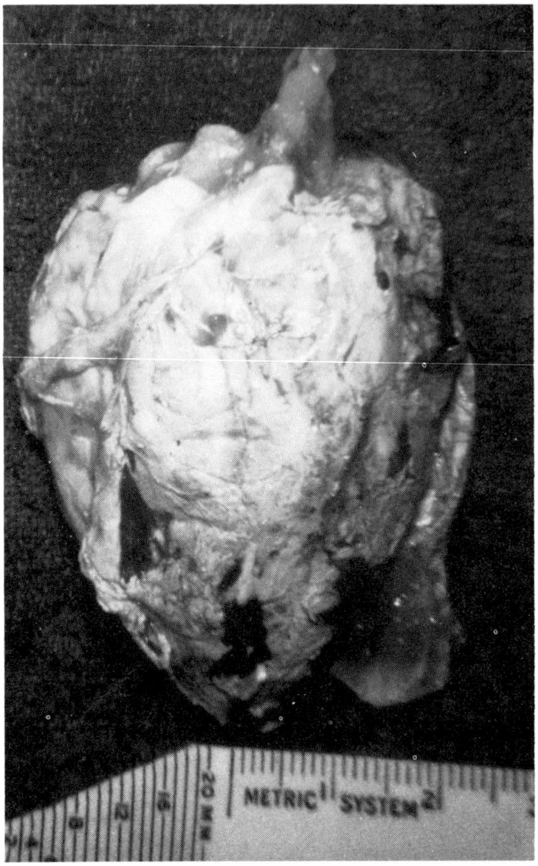

Fig. 13.4. Visceral gout in a goose as evidenced by a large collection of uric acid crystals in the pericardial sac.

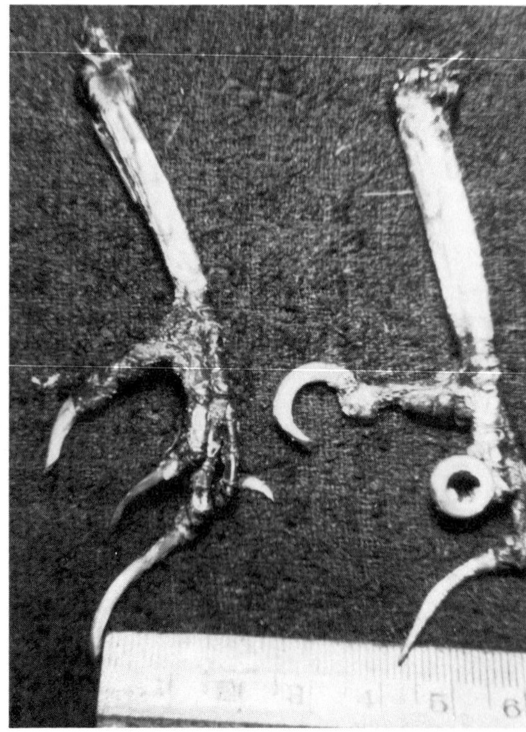

Fig. 13.5. Overgrown claws in a perching bird have resulted from continuous feeding of a high-protein diet. This problem occurs more frequently in males.

chalky crystals are found adhering to the serosal surfaces of the thoracic and abdominal viscera (Wallach, 1969, 1970). The arthritic form is characterized by uric acid granulomas, tophi, in the periarticular tissue and in the synovial sac (Wallach, 1969, 1970). The incidence of gout in captive wild birds is usually low, but heavy losses may occur in flocks of laying females that become dehydrated, a condition which causes renal shutdown. The losses may be arrested by reducing the protein level of the diets and providing surplus drinking water (Wallach, 1970).

Beak and claw overgrowth syndrome (Fig. 13.5) may be associated with excess feeding of high-quality protein (Wallach, 1970). This syndrome occurs more frequently in male specimens. Cosmetic intervention and correction of the diet will normally correct or arrest the overgrowth.

Vitamins. Deficiencies of vitamin A produce clinical signs in growing chicks within two to three weeks and at a somewhat slower rate for mature birds (Scott and Norris, 1965; Wallach, 1969, 1970). Growth is generally retarded. There is general weakness, emaciation, ataxia, ruffled plumage, sinusitis (Fig. 13.6), keratinization of the third eyelid, conjunctivitis, pustular pharyngitis (Fig. 13.7), and esophagitis (Scott and Norris, 1965; Wallach, 1969, 1970, 1971a). The pustular pharyngitis and esophagitis are produced by a squamous metaplasia of the mucous gland ducts, which results in keratinous plugs (Scott and Norris, 1965; Wallach, 1970). Keratinization and desquamation of the tracheal epithelium often occur to such a degree that a pseudomembrane is produced. Deficiencies of vitamin A predispose birds to air sacculitis and esophagitis that may be mistaken for trichomonad infestation. More recently, bumble foot is thought to be associated with chronic vitamin A deficiency (Cooper, 1978). Egg production and the hatchability rate are also much reduced (Giroud, 1968). Specific diagnosis depends on clinical and postmortem lesions and an accurate dietary history.

Treatment of vitamin A deficiencies for most species of birds should include the use of 11,000

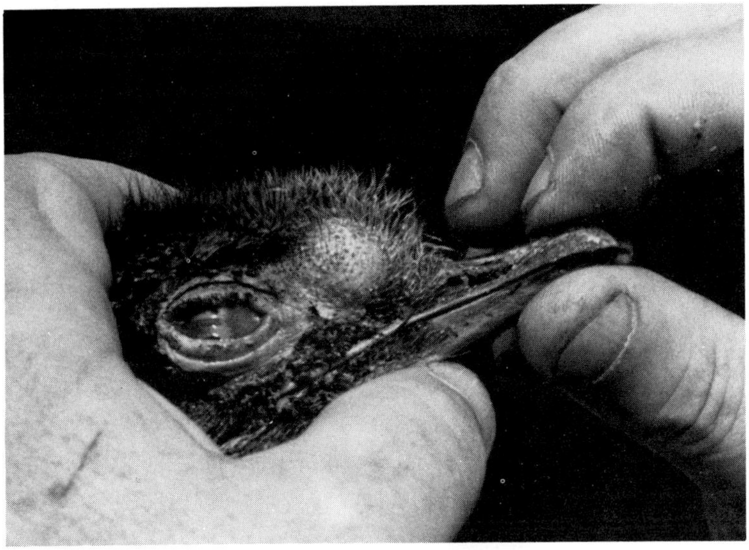

Fig. 13.6. Sinusitis in an immature rhea, *Rhea americana*, resulting from a vitamin A deficiency.

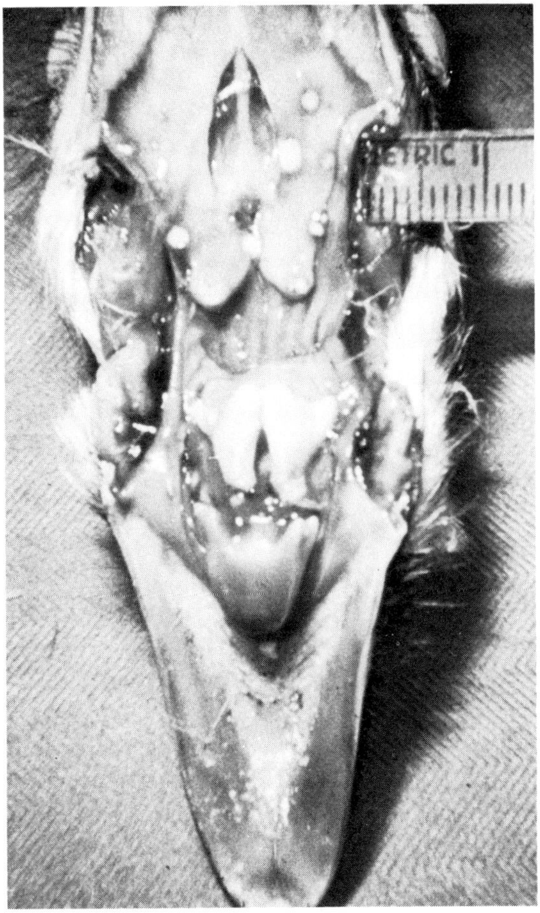

Fig. 13.7. Pustular pharyngitis in a rhea, *R. americana*, with advanced avitaminosis A.

IU vitamin A/kg of ration. After the clinical signs disappear the diet should be returned to the recommended levels of vitamin A. Vitamin A requirements (USP units)/kg of feed may vary with the species, for example, chicks 2,000; laying hens 4,000; turkey poults 4,000; and quail 13,000 (Anon, 1966; Scott and Norris, 1965).

Some typical cases of vitamin A deficiency fail to respond adequately to oral vitamin A therapy, and it is possible that in such cases either absorption of the vitamin from the digestive tract or its metabolism is impaired. In such cases, vitamin A should be administered parenterally (Cooper, 1978).

Deficiencies of vitamin B_1, have been reported in a peregrine falcon, *Falco peregrinus*, fed primarily on young chicks (Ward, 1971) and in gulls, *Larus* sp., fed smelt, *Osmerus* sp. (Wallach, 1970). The syndrome has been recognized by the senior author in storks, penguins, herons, and egrets fed smelt. Food fishes used for birds often contain dangerously high levels of thiaminase (Green et al., 1942; Wallach, 1970, 1971a).

Clinical signs include progressive weight loss, head swinging, rearing backward, opisthotonus, and clonic-tonic seizures (Scott and Norris, 1965; Wallach, 1970). The bird's appetite will usually remain normal. Deficiencies of vitamin B_1 produce polyneuritis in chicks within 9 to 12 days of hatching. Clinical signs include emaciation, digestive upsets, star gazing, ataxia, and convulsions. Aspergillosis and aspergillosis air sacculitis are common sequelae to chronic vitamin B_1 deficiency (Friend and Trainer, 1969; Wallach, 1970). Shore birds and waterfowl fed fish diets are particularly susceptible because of the thiaminase activity of fish tissue. Fish most incriminated include the smelt and the goldfish, *Carassius auratus*. Smelt thiaminase will inactivate 26 mg vitamin B_1/kg of smelt fed. To compensate for this factor one should use 33 mg vitamin B_1/kg of fish.

Treatment should include parenteral administration of 100 to 200 mg vitamin B_1/day along with a correction of the diet. A minimum of 5 mg of usable vitamin B_1 should be available daily in the diet following recovery from clinical signs.

Deficiencies of riboflavin produce diarrhea, retarded growth, leg paralysis, and a characteristic deformity known as curled toe paralysis (Scott and Norris, 1965; Wallach, 1969, 1970, 1971a). The affected birds walk on their hocks with the toes of one or both feet curled medially (Fig. 13.8). The birds appear otherwise alert and maintain their appetite. Minimal dietary levels of riboflavin for game birds and waterfowl range from 3.6 to 4.0 mg/kg of feed, the higher range being required by ducks (Austic and Cole, 1971; Scott and Norris, 1965). Treatment of the clinical disease should include parenteral administration of a total dose of 4 mg of riboflavin in addition to correction of the diet.

Deficiencies of pantothenic acid produce retarded feather growth, generalized epidermal desquamation (Fig. 13.9), crusty exfoliations of the eyelids, and commissures of the beak (Scott and Norris, 1965). Minimal dietary requirements of pantothenic acid range from 4.6 to 35.2 mg/kg of feed; the higher values are required by ducks and turkeys (Anon., 1966; Scott and Norris, 1965). Treatment should include parenteral administration of pantothenic acid at the total daily rate of 20 mg in addition to correction of the diet.

Deficiencies of niacin produce a black discoloration of the tongue and oral mucosa, retarded growth, anorexia, poor feather development, and scaly dermatitis of the feet and skin (Scott and Norris, 1965). Hock disorders similar to perosis occur in the larger species fed niacin-deficient diets. Minimal dietary requirements of niacin range from 55 to 70 mg/kg of diet (Austic and Cole, 1971; Scott and Norris, 1965). Treatment of niacin deficiency in game birds and waterfowl should include parenteral administration at the total daily rate of 100 mg of niacin.

Deficiencies of pyridoxine produce retarded growth, excitability, convulsions, aimless running, paddling of the legs in the air, twisted neck, polyneuritis, and complete exhaustion following convulsions (Scott and Norris, 1965). Minimal daily requirements of pyridoxine range from 2.6 to 3.0 mg/kg of diet (Anon., 1966; Scott and Norris, 1965). Treatment of pyridoxine deficiency should include parenteral administration of a total daily dose of 5 mg of pyridoxine in addition to correction of the diet.

Deficiencies of choline produce retarded growth, disrupted fat metabolism, and perosis (Scott and Norris, 1965; Wallach, 1970). Postmortem lesions include a pale, swollen, fatty liver. Minimal dietary requirements for choline range from 1,300 to 1,900 mg/kg of diet (Anon., 1966; Scott and Norris, 1965).

Deficiencies of biotin produce exfoliative dermatitis similar to that found in pantothenic acid deficiency (Scott and Norris, 1965). Lesions are particularly obvious on the plantar surface of the feet (Fig. 13.10). The toes may become gangrenous and slough off; the dorsal surfaces of the feet

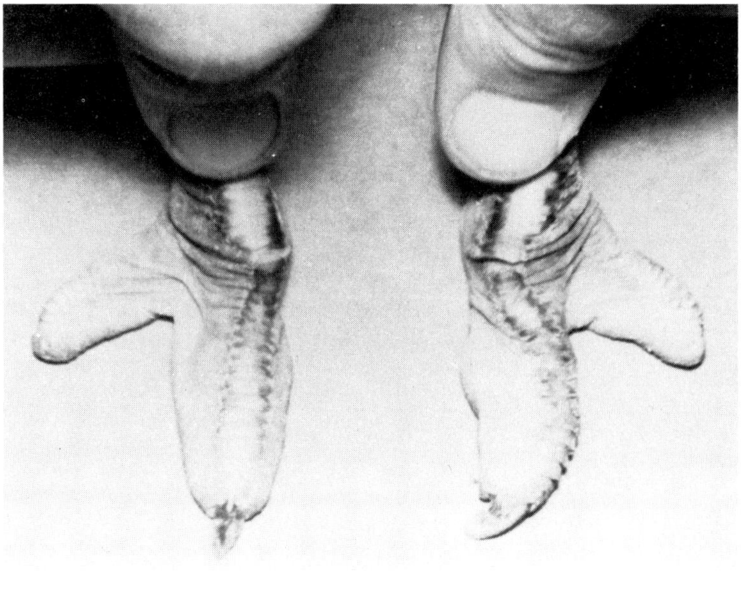

Fig. 13.8. Riboflavin deficiency in an immature ostrich, *Stuthio camelus*. Note medial curling of the anterior toe.

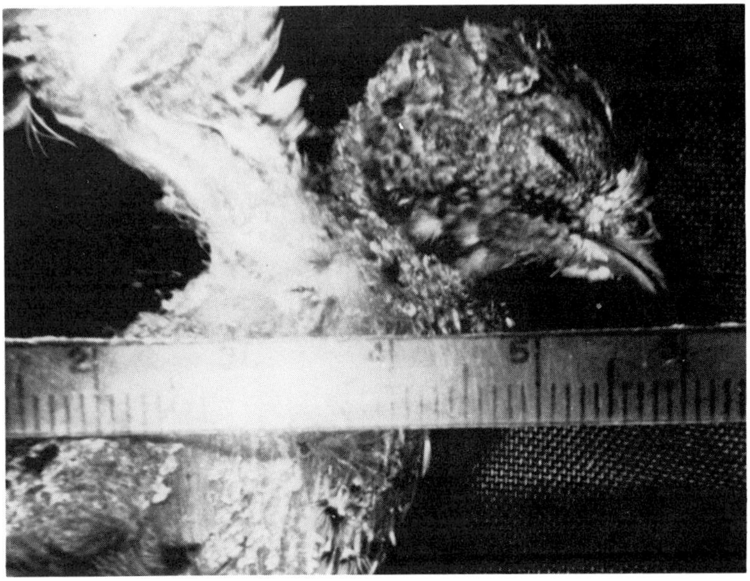

Fig. 13.9. Generalized epidermal desquamation characteristic of pantothenic acid deficiency in a quail.

and the legs show a scaly dermatitis. Minimal dietary requirements range from 0.09 to 0.15 mg/kg of diet (Anon., 1966; Scott and Norris, 1965). Treatment of biotin deficiency should include oral administration of a total daily dose of 3 to 5 mg of biotin in addition to correction of the diet.

Deficiencies of folic acid produce retarded growth, poor feather development, loss of feather pigment, achromocytic anemia, fragile red blood cells, and hock disorders (Renner, 1971). Minimal dietary requirements of folic acid range from 0.8 to 1.25 mg/kg of ration (Anon., 1966; Scott and Norris, 1965).

Deficiencies of vitamin B_{12} produce slow

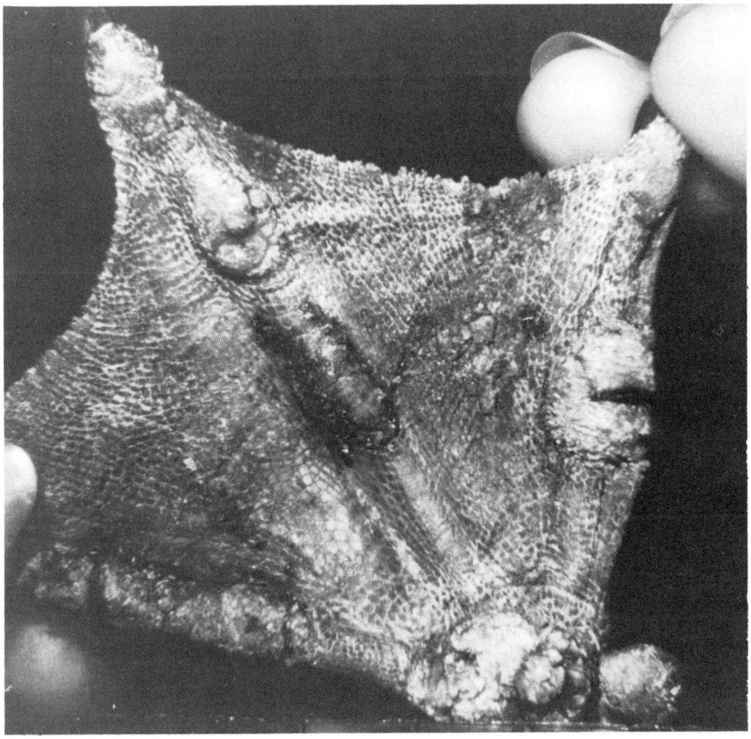

Fig. 13.10. Exfoliative dermatitis characteristic of a biotin deficiency on the plantar surface of the foot of a wood duck, *Axi sponsa.*

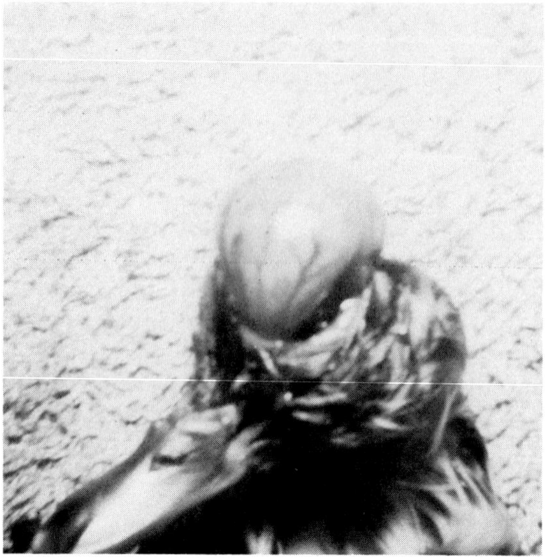

Fig. 13.11. Hydroencephalocele in a mallard hatchling, *A. platyrhynchos,* characterizes a vitamin B_{12} deficiency in the hen's diet.

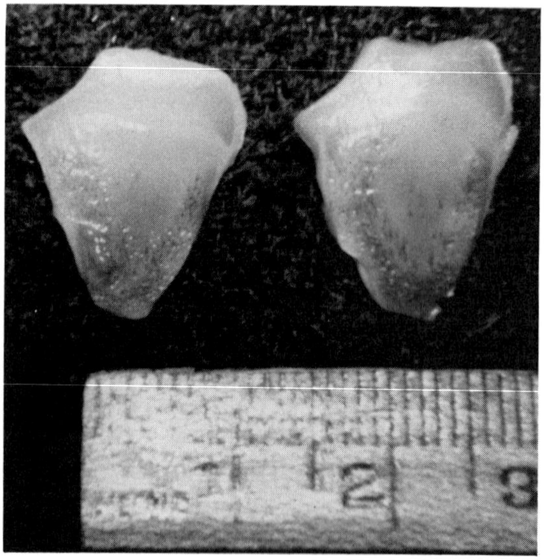

Fig. 13.12. Articular ends of the tarsometatarsal bones of a two-week-old ostrich, *S. camelus,* with the typically enlarged epiphyseal plates characteristic of rickets.

growth, myodystrophy of the legs, poor hatchability, high mortality of young birds, and hatching defects, including hydroencephalocele (Fig. 13.11), in hatchlings (Giroud, 1968; Scott and Norris, 1965). Minimum dietary requirements range from 0.009 to 0.25 mg/kg of ration (Anon., 1966; Scott and Norris, 1965).

Deficiencies of vitamin D_3 produce rickets in all birds. Young birds show retarded growth, lameness, immobilization, unthriftiness, spinal column deformities, leg deformities, breastbone deformities, enlargement of the hock joints, and "beading" of the costochondral junctions. The beak or bill becomes dystrophic and bends with only slight digital pressure (Scott and Norris, 1965; Wallach, 1969, 1970, 1971a). Birds efficiently use vitamin D_3 from fish oils and irradiated animal sterols, but do not effectively use the vitamin D_2 from irradiated ergosterol (Scott and Norris, 1965; Wallach, 1969, 1970).

Rickets are observed frequently in ratites and raptors, as young birds are normally taken while still rapidly growing and are often placed in a shed or basement without direct exposure to sunlight. Affected birds are often fed unsupplemented diets or diets supplemented with vitamin D_2. The classical signs of rickets are easily recognized on radiographs of the skeletal system: enlarged painful epiphyses (Fig. 13.12), bowed long bones, spontaneous fractures, and fibrous osteodystrophy or nutritional secondary hyperparathyroidism (NSH).

Diagnosis of rickets is easily made through radiographic examination. Rachitic epiphyseal plates are classically wider than normal (up to five times normal) producing an enlarged or "beaded" appearance of the articulation (Wallach, 1970).

Treatment of rickets can be successful in individual birds if the condition is recognized early. A single daily parenteral dose of 1,000 to 15,000 IU of vitamin D_3 associated with a correction of the diet normally effects a cure if the problem is diagnosed early enough (Scott and Norris, 1965). Dietary requirements for vitamin D_3/kg of feed include 200 IU for chicks, 500 for laying hens, 900 for turkey poults, 900 for laying turkeys, 220 for ducks, and 1,200 for pheasants (Anon., 1966; Scott and Norris, 1965).

Deficiencies of vitamin E in young birds produce a variety of clinical syndromes, including nutritional encephalomalacia (Scott and Norris, 1965; Wallach, 1969, 1970, 1971a). Clinical signs of this syndrome include prostration, opisthotonus, twisted neck, and ataxia. Postmortem lesions are characterized in the cerebellum and cerebrum as reddish to brown necrotic areas. Subcutaneous edema, edema, exudative diathesis, and myocardial and pericardial edema may also occur. Vitamin E deficiency in older or mature birds produces infertility, sterility in the male, a lowered hatchability rate, nutritional myopathy of the gizzard, muscular dystrophy of the large muscle masses of the breast and legs, spraddle legs, and steatitis (Scott and Norris,

1965; Wagner and Dietlein, 1970; Wallach, 1969, 1970, 1971a).

Clinical signs of white muscle disease include elevated serum creatine phosphokinase levels and daily exhaustion following minimal exercise. Vitamin E requirements are increased as the fat level of the diet increases. A minimum of 50 IU should be present in each kg of diet. Diagnosis in the living bird may be made from elevated serum creatine phosphokinase levels. Values above 40 units are considered a signal of advanced muscular dystrophy. Postmortem lesions include the classical pale muscle often called "fish flesh" in birds. Treatment of vitamin E deficiency should include oral administration of 300 IU vitamin E/day. This should be immediately followed by a correction of the diet.

Deficiencies of vitamin K produce delayed clotting with resultant hemorrhages from minor trauma (Scott and Norris, 1965; Wallach, 1969). Common sites of hemorrhage include subcutaneous or intramuscular tissues and the peritoneal cavity. Vitamin K deficiencies will occur in raptors routinely fed rodents poisoned with dicumarol rodenticides or in grain-eating birds that eat dicumarol-treated grain. Clinical signs include diffuse subcutaneous hemorrhages, bloody droppings, pale mucous membranes, and ataxia. Rations should include 0.4 to 1.8 mg of vitamin K/kg of diet (Anon., 1966; Scott and Norris, 1965). Sulfaquinoxaline in the drinking water or feed will aggravate the signs of vitamin K deficiency (Scott and Norris, 1965; Wallach, 1969). Treatment of dicumarol poisoning should include parenteral administration of vitamin K at the total daily rate of 1 mg. Recommended dietary levels are 1.8 to 3.3 mg/kg of diet.

Minerals. Deficiencies and imbalances in the ratio of calcium and phosphorus (Ca:P) produce NSH (Miller, 1969; Norris and Scott 1965; Wallach, 1969, 1970, 1971a, 1971b; Wallach and Fleig, 1967, 1969, 1970). This nutritional disease occurs with great frequency in captive raptors (Miller, 1969; Wallach and Fleig, 1970) and fairly often in game bird and waterfowl collections of aviculturists. In many cases, this occurs because the home-mixed rations offered are formulated primarily to ensure palatability and high levels of "proteins" and energy. Most noncommercial avian diets provide inadequate total levels of calcium or an imbalanced Ca:P ratio (Table 13.1). Adequate Ca:P ratios in avian diets are listed as 1.5:1.0 (Anon., 1966; Miller, 1969; Wallach, 1970, 1971a, 1971b; Wallach and Fleig, 1967, 1969, 1970). Avian diets that result in NSH when consumed, often contain a high proportion of red meat, oil-bearing seeds, fish, or insects. Many professional aviculturists and hobbyists incorrectly believe that an unsupplemented diet of insects provides sufficient calcium to insect-eating birds. This could not be further from the truth, since the exoskeletons of insects do not contain calcium.

Table 13.1. Calcium and Phosphorus Content of Common Bird Feeds

Feed	Calcium (%)	Phosphorus (%)	Ca:P Ratio
Alfalfa meal	2.11	0.26	8:1
Animal carcass	11.56	5.37	2:1
Apple	0.13	0.12	1:1
Grape	0.016	0.012	1:1
Sardines	0.150	0.975	1:6
Mackerel	0.008	0.274	1:34
Millet	0.050	0.280	1:6
Milo	0.020	0.380	1:14
Oats (rolled)	0.053	0.405	1:8
Corn (yellow)	0.003	0.111	1:37
Sunflower seeds	0.120	0.837	1:7

The Ca:P ratios of seeds commonly included in bird feed range from 1.0:6.0 to 1.0:37.0 (Table 13.1) (Wallach, 1970, 1971a, 1971b). A frequent problem occurs in psittacines fed a high percentage of sunflower seeds in their diet. The Ca:P ratios of meat and fish commonly offered as bird feed for raptors and shore birds range from 1.0:17.0 to 1.0:44.0, respectively (Wallach, 1970, 1971a, 1971b; Wallach and Fleig, 1967, 1969, 1970). High-fat diets considerably reduce the availability of dietary calcium because of the formation of calcium soaps in the gut. Lack of dietary vitamin D_3 and excessive dietary phosphorus and manganese prevent normal intestinal absorption of available calcium.

Normally, blood calcium originates from dietary calcium and from mineral reserves of the skeletal system, being maintained at physiologic concentrations by the parathyroid hormone. In the early stages of NSH, blood calcium concentrations may be within the normal range of 8 to 12 mg/100 ml of serum, or even elevated because of increased parathyroid activity (Wallach and Fleig, 1967, 1969, 1970). This rise may be as high as 46.0 mg/100 ml of serum (Hurwitz and Griminger, 1961). However, serum alkaline phosphatase is also elevated at this time and may be used as a diagnostic aid. A sample of 0.1 to 0.5 ml of blood can be withdrawn from the radial vein into a heparinized syringe or capillary tube, and the activity of serum alkaline phosphatase determined in a blood analyzer.

Female birds in egg production may show an increase in the alkaline phosphatase activity from the normal range of 11 to 21 Bessey-Lowry (BL) units in as little time as seven days on a high-phosphorus, low-calcium diet (Hurwitz and Griminger, 1961). The high alkaline phosphatase values indicate demineralizing activity in the skeletal system and, thus, indirectly reflect the degree of dietary calcium absorption and parathyroid activity (Hurwitz and Griminger, 1961). A physiological hypercalcemia occurs in egg-laying females and must be considered along with other clinical information.

Parenteral vitamin D therapy is contraindicated at the time NSH is diagnosed, as it does not promote intestinal absorption of calcium, but increases the blood calcium concentration by drawing upon the skeletal system (Wallach, 1971b). Prolonged vitamin D therapy at this time would completely demineralize the bird's skeletal system unless appropriate adjustments were made in the diet. It has been well documented that laying females offered diets adequate in vitamin D_3, but deficient in calcium, can lose up to 38% of their skeletal calcium after laying only six eggs. An egg of the domestic chicken, *Gallus domesticus,* may contain as much as 2.2 gm of calcium. While the shell is being formed, 100.0 to 150.0 mg of calcium is removed from the blood per hour. The ribs and sternum lose up to 50% of their mineral.

It has been demonstrated experimentally that pullets fed 3.0 gm calcium/day retain 1.83 gm and excrete 0.33 gm via the urine, resulting in net intestinal absorption of 2.16 gm/day. Grain-eating birds can have their diets supplemented with commercially prepared pellets meant for egg-laying pigeons. Care should be taken to ensure that birds have continuous access to appropriate-sized oyster shell grit. Carnivorous birds should be fed the commercially prepared bird-of-prey diet or whole laboratory rodents.

The more advanced clinical stages of NSH appear as "cramps" of the large muscle groups (Wallach and Fleig, 1970). The owner may describe this as an involuntary flapping of the wings (Miller, 1969; Wallach and Fleig, 1970). At this point, the serum calcium concentrations have reached the individual bird's critical low value but may appear as values at or near the lower limit of the normal range. The local muscle spasms progress to tetanic grand mal seizures, and this condition is usually described by the client as "fits" (Wallach and Fleig, 1970). This episode is usually stimulated by a stress, such as the sudden appearance of the owner, a large meal high in phosphorus (for example, fish, liver, heart muscle, or sunflower seeds), a loud noise, or the turning on of lights at night. The episode will begin with the flapping of wings, progressing to a grand mal seizure; the helpless bird may pitch forward or backward. In many instances, gallinaceous birds and birds of prey remain affixed to the perch hanging upside down (Wallach and Fleig, 1970). At that moment, the serum calcium concentration drops below the critical physiologic value and hypocalcemic tetany results.

Experimentally, serum calcium concentration drops precipitously to 5 mg/100 ml in parathyroidectomized birds. Mortality is high at this time, with most birds dying in hypocalcemic tetany. Many clinicians presented with birds in hypocalcemic tetany have achieved apparent "clinical success" by administering barbiturates to produce anesthesia, but when seizures are allowed to proceed unabated, a percentage of birds often recover spontaneously. This occurs at least for the first few episodes. Apparently, the parathyroids are able to draw on the nearly depleted reserves to cope with the precipitous drop in serum calcium concentration. If NSH is allowed to progress to the chronic state, the parathyroids eventually have difficulty in mobilizing calcium from depleted skeletal stores. Radiographs of such birds reveal advanced NSH and folding fractures. In advanced cases of NSH uncomplicated by a concurrent vitamin D deficiency, the width of epiphyseal plates and articular cartilages will appear relatively normal with some peripheral lipping (Wallach, 1971; Wallach and Fleig, 1967, 1969, 1970). Conversely, true rickets, vitamin D deficiency, is manifested radiographically by a widening of epiphyseal plates and a significant enlargement of the articular ends of long bones (Wallach, 1969, 1970, 1971a, 1971b; Wallach and Fleig, 1967, 1969, 1970).

Treatment of acute episodes of hypocalcemic tetany is quite specific: slow intravenous administration of calcium gluconate fortified with 5% dextrose to effect will provide immediate relief (Wallach, 1971b). A stock solution is made by adding 1 ml of 17% calcium borogluconate to 10 ml of 5% dextrose in saline. The solution is administered intravenously at the rate of 0.2 ml/30 gm of body weight to effect (Wallach, 1971b). It is essential at this time to recommend dietary alterations necessary to prevent a clinical relapse. Growing birds and laying females require greater percentages of calcium in the diet than do males and nonlaying females.

The clinical progress of the bird may be measured after seven days on a calcium-supplemented diet by analyzing serum alkaline phosphatase activity (Hurwitz and Griminger, 1961). It has been reported that serum alkaline phosphatase activity will drop from 41 to 18 BL units within seven days after the beginning of proper calcium or phosphorus supplementation. This indicates an increase in the rate of skeletal mineralization (Hurwitz and Griminger, 1961). It has also been reported that birds found to have 11.0 BL units of alkaline phosphatase activity when on a diet of 2.5% calcium, will experience

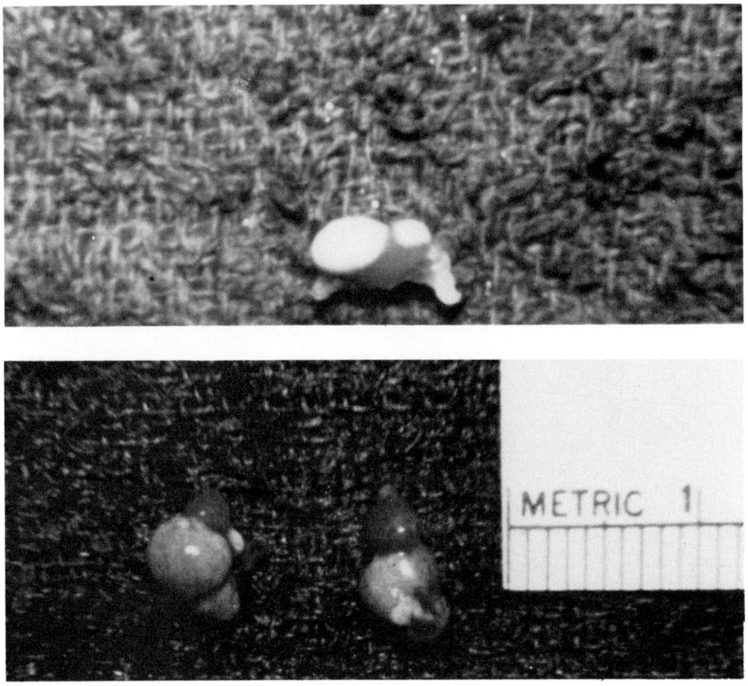

Fig. 13.13. Hypertrophic parathyroids of a parrot (above) and a heron (below) with chronic nutritional secondary hyperparathyroidism (NSH).

an increase in activity to 45 BL units if the dietary calcium is dropped to 1.0% (Hurwitz and Griminger, 1961).

Birds chronically affected with NSH usually have a markedly enlarged parathyroid (Fig. 13.13) at postmortem (Wallach, 1970, 1971a, 1971b; Wallach and Fleig, 1967, 1969, 1970). The normal avian parathyroid weighs approximately 10.0 mg/kg body weight (Wallach and Fleig, 1967, 1969, 1970). Hypertrophic parathyroids may weigh up to ten times the normal values. Physiologic hypertrophy exists in egg-laying females, but not to such a degree, nor do the bone lesions of NSH exist.

The skeletal system of the bird affected with NSH is always found to have some degree of fibrous dysplasia (Miller, 1969; Wallach, 1970, 1971a, 1971b; Wallach and Fleig, 1967, 1969, 1970). The ribs, sternum, ilium, ischium, and pubis are affected to a greater degree than the skull, metatarsus, and phalanges. The cortex of affected bones can be compressed with digital pressure and cut easily with a knife. In advanced NSH, large amounts of mineral are depleted from the long bones. Folding fractures and reduction of the caliber of the medullary cavities may be almost obliterated, with the exception of cyst formation, which can often be visualized radiographically.

Kidneys of birds with NSH may display calcified microliths. These lesions appear to be the result of prolonged hypercalcemia initiated by the release of parathyroid hormone. In the absence of calcification of elastic arteries and of other viscera, these intratubular calculi cannot be attributed to excessive vitamin D.

Deficiencies of manganese produce perosis (Fig. 13.14) (Norris and Scott, 1965; Wallach, 1969, 1970, 1971a). The syndrome has been reported in free-ranging Canada geese, *B. canadensis* (Jensen, 1968), and this disease has been observed in a great variety of captive wild birds. It is characterized by a swelling and a flattening of the lateral condyles of the hock joint, allowing the gastrocnemius tendon to slip laterally out of the articulation. The tibia and the tarsometatarsus often exhibit a lateral rotation that may affect both legs. Egg production is lowered and deformities of the embryos are produced, for example, chondrodystrophy, "parrot-beak," wiry down, and extreme shortening of the long bones. High dietary levels of calcium aggravate the deficiency by producing calcium-manganese complexes that reduce the efficiency of absorption of manganese. Minimum dietary requirements range from 55 to 60 mg/kg of ration (Anon., 1966).

Deficiencies of magnesium result in retarded growth and lethargy. Convulsions follow excitement and this results in a coma. Minimum dietary levels for birds range from 475 to 550 mg/kg of the ration (Anon., 1966; Norris and Scott, 1965).

Deficiencies of salt produce dehydration and diarrhea. Minimum dietary requirements range from 5 to 10 gm/kg of ration (Anon., 1966; Norris

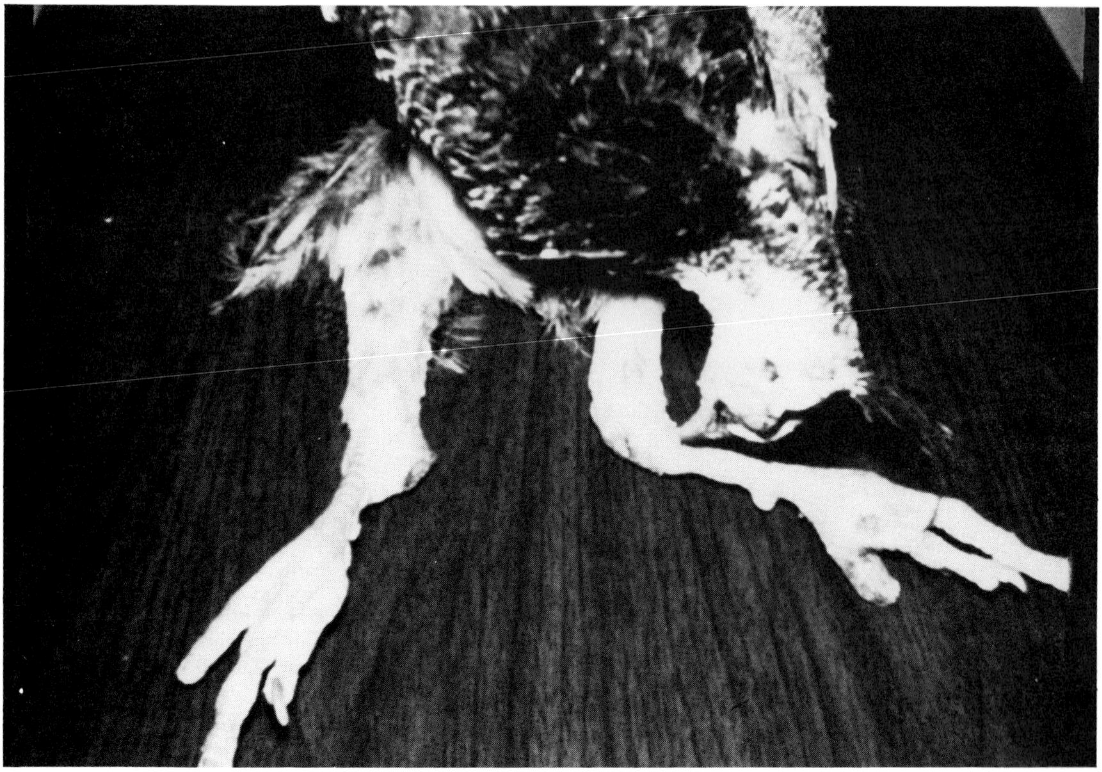

Fig. 13.14. Peacock, *Pavo* sp., with a rotated tarsometatarsus characteristic of a manganese deficiency.

and Scott, 1965; Wallach, 1969, 1970). Salt poisoning may occur during the winter when road salt is put out to melt ice or when brine is allowed to puddle up. Affected birds will show depression, ataxia, thirst, convulsive seizures, and prostration (Trainer and Karstad, 1960).

Deficiencies of potassium produce an unusually high mortality rate in growing birds with no specific clinical signs. Minimum dietary requirements range from 1.7 to 4.0 gm/kg of the ration (Anon., 1966; Norris and Scott, 1965).

Deficiencies of iodine result in enlargement of the thyroid (Wallach, 1969, 1970). The enlarged thyroids often cause pressure upon the esophagus, resulting in dysphagia in the smaller birds. The displaced trachea may produce a characteristic whistle on expiration. Minimum dietary levels range from 0.4 to 1.1 mg/kg of ration (Anon., 1966; Norris and Scott, 1965; Wallach, 1970).

Deficiencies of iron and copper produce anemia that is characterized by lower hemoglobin levels (Wallach, 1969, 1970). Birds reared and maintained on wire or concrete are particularly subject to iron and copper deficiency. Loss of or a decrease in degree of feather or skin pigment may occur in adult birds fed a diet chronically deficient in copper and iron. The minimum dietary requirement of the total ration for iron is 40 ppm and for copper 4 ppm (Austic and Cole, 1971; Norris and Scott, 1965).

Deficiencies of zinc produce retarded growth, poor feathering, enlarged hocks, slipped tendon, and scaling of the skin and feet. The minimum dietary requirement for zinc ranges from 45 to 55 ppm of the total ration (Anon., 1966; Norris and Scott, 1965).

Deficiencies of selenium produce subcutaneous edema of the embryos, or exudative diathesis (Fig. 13.15) (Gries and Scott, 1971). Hatchlings fed diets containing selenium at less than 0.005 ppm grow slowly and have a poor feather covering. At two weeks of age, 50% of the birds will develop exudative diathesis. By three weeks of age, most of the birds will die. Extra dietary levels of vitamin E and bile salts will delay death of the birds until six weeks of age.

Microscopically, selenium-deficient birds show cytoplasmic vacuoles in the acinar cells of the pancreas (Gries and Scott, 1971). Interacinar fibrosis develops even when plasma vitamin E is maintained at normal levels. The minimum die-

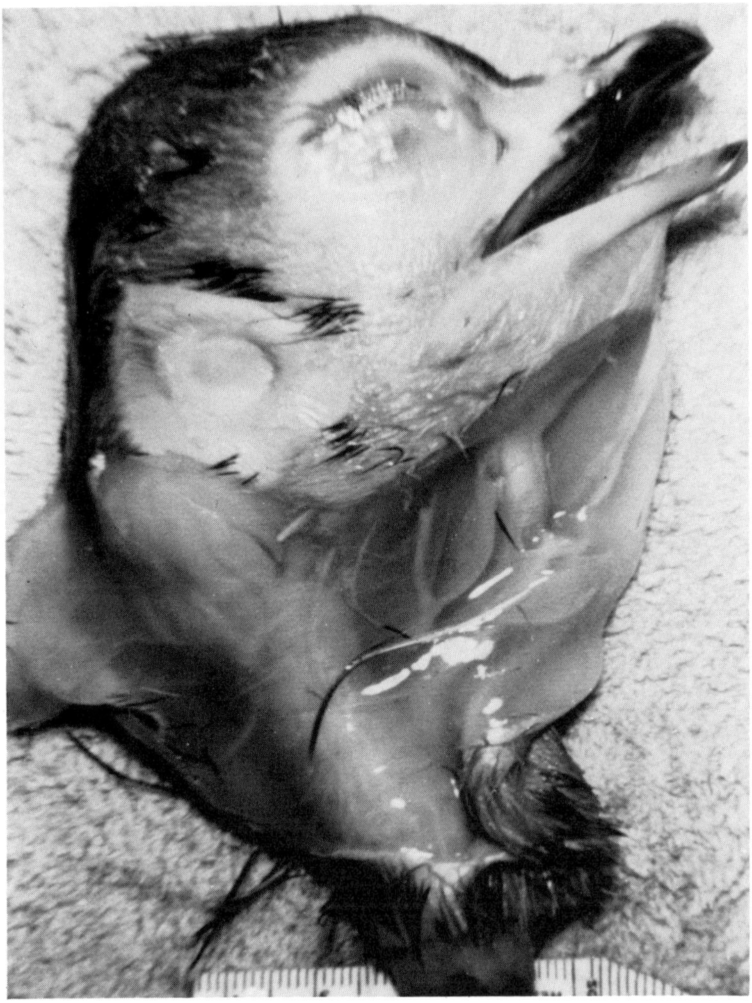

Fig. 13.15. Subcutaneous edema in an ostrich chick, *S. camelus,* characteristic of a selenium deficiency.

tary requirement for selenium is 0.05 to 0.3 ppm of the total diet. Selenium levels of 10.0 ppm or more produce toxicity, which is manifested as dead embryos, short-beaked embryos, edema of head and neck, and aplasia of the toes and eyes. Chicks on selenium-deficient experimental diets showed a remarkable recovery when the diet was supplemented with 0.1 ppm of selenium (Gries and Scott, 1971).

CONTROL. In actual practice, nutritional disease in captive wild birds is quite common. However, most nutritional deficiencies appear as a specific clinical sign of a more general condition of malnutrition. Multiple deficiencies of specific nutrients are indicative of a need to correct the entire diet, as well as to supplement for the individual nutrient deficiencies that can be recognized.

Aviculturists have historically attributed many of the nutritional problems discussed to "inbreeding"; however a hard look at statistics and real data will in most cases show such suggestions to be incorrect. A detailed investigation of the dietary history is essential to the proper diagnosis of a nutritional disease and for the correction of the problem.

REFERENCES

Anon. 1966. Nutrient requirements of poultry. Natl. Acad. Sci. Natur. Res. Coun. 5th ed. Publ. 1345.

Austic, R. E., and R. K. Cole. 1971. Impaired uric acid excretion in chickens selected for uricemia and articular gout. Proc. 1971 Cornell Nutr. Conf. Nov. 2–3, Buffalo.

Bernes, J. 1486. The Boke of St. Albans. Printed at St. Albans by the Schoolmaster Printer. Reprinted, Elliott Stock, London 1881.

Brown L. H., and D. Amadon. 1968. Eagles, hawks and falcons of the world. Country Life Books, Hamlyn House, Middlesex.

Cooper, J. E. 1978. Veterinary aspects of captive birds of prey. Standfast Press, Saul, Gloucestershire.

Friend, M., and D. O. Trainer. 1969. Aspergillosis in captive herring gulls. Bull. Wildl. Dis. Assoc. 5:271–275.

Giroud, A. 1968. Nutrition of the embryo. Fed. Proc. 27:163–184.

Green, R. G., W. E. Carlson, and C. A. Evans. 1942. The inactivation of vitamin B_1 in diets containing whole fish. J. Nutr. 23:165–174.

Gries, C., and M.L. Scott. 1971. Pathology of selenium deficiency in the chick. Proc. 1971 Cornell Nutr. Conf., Nov. 2–4, Buffalo.

Hurwitz, S., and P. Griminger. 1961. The response of plasma alkaline phosphatases, parathyroids and blood and bone minerals to calcium intake in the fowl. J. Nutr. 73:179–190.

Jensen, W. I. 1968. Perosis in Canada geese, *Branta canadensis.* Bull. Wildl. Dis. Assoc. 4:95–99.

Miller, R. M. 1969. Nutritional secondary hyperparathyroidism. Vet Med. Small Anim. Clin. 64:400–408.

Norris, L. C., and M. L. Scott. 1965. Proteins, carbohydrates, fats, fiber, minerals and water in poultry feeding. In H. E. Biester and L. H. Schwarte. Diseases of poultry. 5th ed. Iowa State Univ. Press, Ames.

Renner, R. 1971. Carbohydrate requirements and availability for chickens. Proc. 1971 Cornell Nutr. Conf. Nov. 2–4, Buffalo.

Scott, M. L., and L. C. Norris. 1965. Vitamins and vitamin deficiencies. In H. E. Biester and L. H. Schwarte. Diseases of poultry. 5th ed. Iowa State Univ. Press, Ames.

Snow, D. W. 1968. Movements and mortality of British kestrels, *Falco tinnunculus.* Bird Study 15:65–83.

Trainer, D. O., and L. H. Karstad. 1960. Salt poisoning in Wisconsin wildlife. J. Am. Vet. Med. Assoc. 136:14–17.

Wagner, J. G., and D. R. Dietlein. 1970. Steatitis in an American white pelican. Int. Zoo Yearbook 10:174.

Wallach, J. D. 1969. Common diseases and recommended treatments for waterfowl and game birds. Mod. Game Breed. 5:18–25.

________. 1970. Nutri[illegible] of exotic animals. J. Am. Vet. Med. A[illegible]599.

______. 1971a. Nutriti[illegible] in zoos. Proc. 1971 Cornell Nutr. Conf. Nov. 2–4, Buffalo.

______. 1971b. Nutritional secondary hyperparathyroidism in caged birds. In R. F. Kirk, Current veterinary therapy. Vol. IV. Small animal practice. W. B. Saunders, Philadelphia.

______, and G. M. Fleig. 1967. Nutritional secondary hyperparathyroidism in captive psittacine birds. J. Am. Vet. Med. Assoc. 151:880–883.

______, and ______. 1969. Nutritional secondary hyperparathyroidism in captive birds. J. Am. Vet Med. Assoc. 155:1046–1051.

______, and ______. 1970. Cramps and fits in carnivorous birds. Int. Zoo Yearbook 10:3–4.

Ward, F. P, 1971. Thiamine deficiency in a peregrine falcon. J. Am. Vet. Med. Assoc. 159:599–601.

______, and L. J. Slaughter. 1968. Visceral gout in a captive Cooper's hawk. Bull. Wildl. Dis. Assoc. 4:91–93.

14 *Nutritional Diseases of Mammals*

JOEL D. WALLACH
GERALD L. HOFF

THE NUTRITIONAL STATUS of free-ranging and captive wild mam[illegible]sic and primary importance to in[illegible] and group management programs. [illegible]sistance to environmental changes, infectious and parasitic diseases, and maximal reproduction and infant survival rates can only be expected from animals having optimal levels of nutrition. The qualitative value of feed must be considered as important to long-term health as is its total availability. The successful completion of the entire food chain cycle depends on the availability of nutrients in the soil for the food plants.

The dynamic effect of severe environmental disasters upon the short-term nutritional health of free-ranging wildlife has been recognized for centuries. The individual and herd health effects of differences in regional soil compositions, forage quality, and pollution of feed by agents that interfere with the normal nutritional processes are of more recent interest.

Cellular and subcellular biochemical requirements for metabolic activities are similar for all mammalian species; only the raw material form eaten by various species differs. The digestive tracts of the different mammalian species differ sufficiently in anatomy and physiology to reduce the widely divergent proteins into the amino acids necessary for life. General body condition, nearness to the taxonomic norm, rate of reproduction, and the microscopic examination of tissues may be used to evaluate the nutritional status of wild mammals (Wallach, 1970, 1971a; Wallach et al., 1978).

ETIOLOGY, PATHOLOGY, DIAGNOSIS, AND TREATMENT

Ruminants. Ruminants are very adaptable animals, being found on five of the seven continental land masses. Their ability to flourish under widely different and severe environmental conditions is due in part to their efficiency in converting a wide variety of coarse roughage into usable nutrients. The vast majority of species that are most actively engaged in grazing or browsing do this during a four-hour period in the early morning and another four-hour period in the late afternoon. During extreme deprivation, additional feeding periods may be necessary.

Feeding habits of exotic ruminants vary considerably. The wildebeest, *Connochaetes taurinus,* a grazing species, prefers vegetation 2.5 to 10.0 cm high, while the giraffe, *Giraffa camelopardalis,* and greater kudu, *Tragelaphus strepsiceros,* both browsing species, prefer their roughage at eye level. All of these ruminants are physically able to eat feed placed at a level of 1 meter, but each would consume less than an optimal amount if the only available feed was placed at that level. It is true that fully adapted captive animals can be conditioned to accept feed at any reasonable level; however, such alterations should be made gradually and only after the individual has fully adjusted to a captive diet. Delicate feeders such as duiker, *Cephalophus* sp.; dik-dik, *Rhynchotragus* sp.; chevrotain, *Hyemschus aquaticus;* and suni, *Nesotragus moschatus,* require the leafiest legume hay available because of their highly selective browsing habits. In the native state they feed on leaves, buds, and blossoms and will lose condition rapidly if only stemmy mature roughage is fed.

These differential feeding habits have resulted in specialized anatomical adaptations of the rumen and omasum to increase digestive efficiency. For example, the giraffe gazelle, *Litocranius walleri,* and the giraffe belong to different taxonomic families but have similar feeding patterns when browsing. Both have a voluminous rumen, the lining of which is densely covered with papillae, reticular cellulae that are low, and in the giraffe gazelle, an omasum that is relatively larger than that found in other species of gazelle.

Classical roughage eaters consume great quantities of high-fiber plant material. They have a relatively large rumen that displays well-developed pillars. The rumen is heavily cornified and devoid of papillae in its dorsum. The reticulum is relatively small with high thick-walled crests and deep cellulae. There are distinct subdivisions of the reticulum by secondary and tertiary crests. The omasum is spherical, large, and possesses numerous thin laminae; the abomasum is very large and spacious.

Selective browsers have a relatively small

rumen with poorly developed pillars. These ruminants have a relatively large reticulum with low crests and shallow cellulae; the walls are studded with long, pointed, cornified papillae. Secondary crests are frequently absent, and tertiary ones are nearly always missing. The omasum is a flat kidney-shaped organ of extremely small size. The omasum contains only a few thick laminae that are covered with long "bird claw" papillae. The abomasum is relatively small but has a very thick glandular mucosa. Selective browsers are thought to have a higher rumenal fermentation rate than larger ruminants.

Transitional forms of digestive tracts are found in marshland antelope, such as reedbuck, *Redunca* sp.; waterbuck, *Kobus* sp.; and kob, *K. kob* (Abrams, 1968). These species have reduced ruminal and omasal size. However, the latter organ possesses numerous thin leaves that are highly cornified.

WATER. Free-ranging ruminants may drink only in the late afternoon or early evening after the last feed. However, many species drink infrequently, often with many days separating visits to a water source. Ruminants' water consumption is directly affected by environmental temperatures, water content of forage, and levels of dietary protein and salts. Dehydration in ruminants commonly occurs in the winter when drinking water freezes or when there is some pathological condition of the upper digestive tract that interferes with normal water consumption. The classical postmortem signs of desiccation are well-demarcated collections of peach-colored urates in the corticomedullary junction of the kidney and dehydration of the carcass.

Wild ruminants that are intermittent drinkers use a variety of methods to conserve body water. The camel's, *Camelus* sp., body temperature can rise considerably during the day without ill effect. The excess body heat is tolerated until late in the day when the environmental temperature drops, at which time the camel cools by radiation. The camel absorbs minimal environmental heat during the heat of the day because of its elevated body temperature and the insulating qualities of the wool. The camel does not pant or sweat excessively, thereby conserving a great deal of body water. Water turnover in the camel is 61 ml/kg/24 hours compared with 110 and 148 ml for sheep and cattle respectively. Lastly, the camel can concentrate urine twice as efficiently as cattle.

Oryx, *Oryx* sp.; Grant's gazelle, *Gazella grantii;* Thomson's gazelle, *G. thomsoni*; and zebu, *Bos indicus*, also have impressive water-conserving capabilities that permit them to maintain a constant body weight with a total water intake of 2% body weight/day in an environmental temperature of 22° C. Hereford cattle require more than twice that amount when fed identical rations.

The buffalo, *Syncerus caffer,* and eland, *Taurotragus* sp., have similar water requirements; however, eland can live in the desert scrub independent of surface water, but buffalo only enter such areas during or right after the rainy season (Treus and Lobanov, 1971). Eland are able to more efficiently conserve water by selectively browsing on succulent plants, avoiding the midday sun, and forming dry pelletized feces. They also possess a narrow thermal neutral zone for this purpose.

Reindeer, *Rangifer tarandus*, lose 11 to 18% of body weight after only three days of water deprivation (Steen, 1968). In contrast, domestic sheep can lose 25% of their body weight following five days of water deprivation and 31% after ten days.

CARBOHYDRATES. A convenient rule of thumb for calculating minimum energy requirements for all ruminants is a function of the basal metabolic rate. The formula, $70.5W^{0.73}$ kcal/day is considered to be 95% accurate, so one must add a safety margin of 10 to 20% to ensure an adequate supply of calories (Rogerson, 1968). Energy for adult ruminants is normally derived from carbohydrates, while the major calorie source for the immature ruminant is protein and butterfat. When a very coarse mature roughage is consumed by adult ruminants, a supplemental source in the form of high-energy grain must be available to prevent a negative energy imbalance. There is normally a 10% increase in energy requirement during the last trimester of pregnancy and an increase by a factor of 1.5 to 2.5 times the maintenance level for lactation, growth, and stability of body heat during severe weather conditions. The basic metabolic rate increases 13% with each degree of increased body temperature because of increased water required to keep cool.

Experiments with domestic cattle, wildebeest, and eland indicate that all three species derive similar quantities of metabolizable energy from a constant amount of the same forage. The efficiency of use is also similar, being 82% for wildebeest, 80% for eland, and 80 to 85% for cattle and sheep (Rogerson, 1968). However, further evidence indicates that the eland and wildebeest require 20% more total metabolic energy than cattle, and since the efficiency is the same, an increased food intake or more concentrated energy source is required.

Deer fed alfalfa or poor grass hay alone show a relatively constant level of digestibility (Nordan et al., 1968). A digestibility level of 52 to 56% for roughage can be improved considerably by the consumption of high-energy grain, fruit, or seeds.

Ketosis occurs in exotic ruminants fed roughages that are too coarse (Church, 1971). Roughage such as very dry grass, hay, and straw contain most of the carbohydrate as usable cellulose. Even though the animal may consume considerable quantities of this material, a state of negative energy imbalance will occur and the animal will be forced to draw on its fat store. Ketosis also may occur in ruminants that have not eaten for several days or in animals with rumen atony associated with some other primary illness. Pregnancy ketosis occurs in wild sheep that have been fed poor-quality grasses, and twinning increases the rate of occurrence. Signs of ketosis include anorexia, central depression, acidosis, and unconsciousness. Ketosis may be diagnosed by testing for and finding ketone bodies in the urine or milk and/or finding reduced blood pH. Treatment includes administration of intravenous glucose, corticosteroids, and an increased dietary carbohydrate level that should initially include some molasses. Postmortem lesions of ketosis include severe fatty degeneration of the liver and kidneys and hemorrhages of the epicardium and icterus.

PROTEIN. Free-ranging ruminants are forced to suffer an annual protein cycle. Grass protein levels of 12 to 25% may be available for only two or three months of the year if the population does not migrate (Abrams, 1968; Crawford et al., 1968). Rapidly growing browse has protein levels of 15 to 40% and tends to maintain higher protein levels for longer periods than grass, which drops precipitously to protein levels of 5 to 9%. In general, grazers tend to suffer a greater reduction in nitrogen intake during the dry season since high-protein levels only occur during the rapid growth stages of grass. Migrating grazers follow the seasonal rains for great distances, thereby extending the periods during which they have access to high-protein forage.

Many wild ruminants possess the ability to conserve nitrogen during protein deprivation (Crawford et al., 1968). Urea excretion in the camel falls from 13.0 to 0.2 gm/day when protein intake is severely reduced (Church, 1971). Under adequate nutritional conditions, 40% of the urea filtered by the glomerulus is excreted; when protein intake is reduced, the urea excretion drops to 2%.

Optimal forage protein levels for white-tailed deer, *Odocoileus virginianus,* and aoudads, *Ammotragus lervia*, range between 13 and 16% (Brady and Ulrey, 1975; Church, 1971). Levels of 10 to 12% are adequate for large-bodied ruminants such as bison, *Bison* sp.; buffalo; banteng, *Bos banteng;* and yak, *B. grunniens*, but should be raised to a minimum of 18 to 20% for growing and lactating individuals. Small ruminants and delicate feeders should have forage protein levels of 13 to 20%.

Protein deprivation during pregnancy results in small, weak, or aborted calves, kids, and lambs. Acute excesses of protein have resulted in laminitis and enterotoxemia. Chronic excesses of protein at levels higher than 20% have resulted in overgrown hooves in captive ruminants, despite abrasive substrates. The latter problem appears to be sex related, with a predominance of hoof overgrowth in the males of the herd (Wallach, 1971a). This is thought to be the result of excessive intake by the dominant male in combination with the anabolic effect of testosterone.

FATS. Dietary fat is not required by wild ruminants. Volatile fatty acids are among the major by-products of rumen fermentation. The volatile fatty acids, that is, propionic acid and acetate, are sources of immediate energy and also the raw material required to produce essential fatty acids and fat.

Ingested fats undergo hydrolysis in the rumen and are converted into volatile fatty acids. Dietary fat levels of 2 to 5% increase the efficiency of energy conversions, while levels above 5% interfere with cellulose digestion, change the character of body fat, and interfere with assimilation of other nutrients.

VITAMINS. In the natural state, the ruminant obtains most of the fat-soluble vitamins, A, D, E, K, or their precursors, from growing plants (Church, 1971). The excesses are stored in times of plenty following the rainy season and drawn upon during the dry season. The B-complex vitamins are normally synthesized by the rumen bacterial flora.

Dietary vitamin A, or carotene, is required by the ruminant for metabolism, growth, the maintenance of epithelial surface, proper embryonal growth, and fertility (Church, 1971; Mitchell, 1967; Wallach, 1971a). Recommended levels are 22 to 44,200 IU/kg of feed, with higher levels being fed to smaller ruminants (Mitchell, 1967). Deficiencies are often seen in ruminants in semiarid or arid environments because they will readily consume poor-quality mature roughage that other ruminants will not eat. Continuous nitrate levels in the diet will interfere with the conversion of β-carotene into vitamin A.

Excesses of dietary vitamin A have not been reported in free-ranging or captive ruminants. Deficiencies lead to emaciation, poor growth, anasarca, dull hair, opacities of the cornea, excessive lacrimation, infertility, and weak or deformed offspring. Birth defects associated with vitamin A deficiencies in wild ruminants include diaphragmatic hernias, cleft palates, cardiovascular defects, microphthalmia and metaplasia, and keratinization of cuboidal and columnar epithelium to squamous epithelium.

Dietary sources of B-complex vitamins are of great importance to immature and nonruminating adult ruminants. They are required cofactors for the metabolism of carbohydrates, lipids, and proteins. Vitamin B_1 is essential for intracellular carbohydrate metabolism. Vitamin B_1 deficiencies occur in immature, nonruminating, free-ranging ruminants feeding on unsupplemented forage and in adults that have a disruption of rumen function. Feeding on toxic plants that contain thiaminase, for example, *Pteris aquilina, Equisetum polustre,* and *E. arvense,* will produce signs of overt vitamin B_1 deficiency (Church, 1971).

Clinical signs of vitamin B_1 deficiency include anorexia, dehydration, weight loss, diarrhea, blinking, head twitching, convulsions, opisthotonus, and bradycardia. Postmortem lesions are characterized by hydrothorax, hydroperitoneum, polioencephalomalacia, emaciation, flaccid skeletal muscle, and right ventricular dilatation. At least two episodes have been reported in white-tailed deer (Kurtz and Karns, 1969; Reed et al., 1976).

Diagnosis of vitamin B_1 deficiency in exotic ruminants requires recognition of the clinical signs, the collection of a history of unsupplemented diet, or diet that includes toxic thiaminase-containing plants. Low blood vitamin B_1 levels and an elevated pyruvate level will confirm the diagnosis. Treatment with parenteral vitamin B_1 at the rate of 250 to 500 mg is specific and dramatic (Church, 1971). Seemingly moribund animals will rise to their feet within hours and begin feeding.

Vitamin B_2 deficiency in immature exotic ruminants produces anorexia, anemia, lacrimation, and excessive salivation, diarrhea, erosions in the commissures of the mouth, alopecia, and death. This clinical problem appears when artificial diets are improperly supplemented. Recommended levels of dietary vitamin B_2 are 20 to 30 mg/kg body weight/day.

Vitamin D is essential to the absorption of calcium from the intestine and mineralization of the skeleton by calcium. Recommended levels are 5.5 to 6.6 IU/kg body weight for small ruminant species and 4.0 to 5.0 IU/kg body weight in larger species (Wallach, 1970, 1971a). Because wild ruminants are not under stresses of heavy milk production, vitamin D deficiency is not seen in adult ruminants. Severe excesses from overzealous use of vitamin-mineral mixes or vitamin D_3 in rations for captive wild ruminants result in excess absorption of calcium. This can result in interference with phosphorus, copper, and zinc utilization and in the development of fibrous osteodystrophy and fibrous interstitial nephritis of adults and newborn. Calcium deposits can often be found in connective tissue and the elastic vascular tree when excesses of vitamin D are fed.

Vitamin E functions as a biological antioxidant and is interrelated physiologically with selenium (Basson and Hofmeyr, 1973; Basson et al., 1971). Recommended levels are 55 to 176 IU/kg of diet, with the higher level being used for smaller species. Deficiency of this vitamin produces anemia, weak and spraddle-legged newborn, axonal dystrophy, and muscular dystrophy. Addition of cod liver oil or other polyunsaturated oils as a source of vitamins A and D to the diet of captive ruminants will interfere with vitamin E utilization and precipitate a clinical deficiency. Newborn and suckling ruminants are most often affected with higher rates of disease appearing in the smaller species (Decker and McDermid, 1977).

Immature or adult animals will exhibit exhaustion or hemoglobinuria following exercise. Blood samples taken at this time will show an elevated creatine phosphokinase (CPK). Normal CPK levels in ruminants are below 150 IU. Individuals having CPK levels of 160 to 400 IU are considered to have muscular dystrophy. Parenteral vitamin E-selenium complexes and increased dietary levels of vitamin E may arrest the condition. Despite treatment, animals showing CPK levels greater than 400 units will normally die following severe physical exercise or stress. Postmortem lesions include hyaline degeneration of skeletal (Fig. 14.1) and cardiac muscle, calcification, and chronic fibrous muscular dystrophy (Bartsch et al., 1977).

Vitamin K is required for liver synthesis of prothrombin. This is the only fat-soluble vitamin normally produced in the rumen. Ingestion of dicumarol produced in moldy hay, from rodenticides, or extended treatments with sulfonamides will interfere with vitamin K utilization. Early stages of deficiency are mainly associated with spontaneous nasal or rectal hemorrhaging.

MINERALS. Free-ranging ruminants obtain minerals from the roughage they consume and from mineral-bearing soils and water. In warm climates, ant heaps and termite mounds are often used as mineral licks. Streambeds cut through limestone deposits and expose mineral-rich surfaces as sources for ruminants to use. Limestone roadbeds in game parks often contain depressions in areas where wildlife have used them as a source of minerals. From the data available, it appears that the basic principles of mineral metabolism and daily requirements that apply to domestic ru-

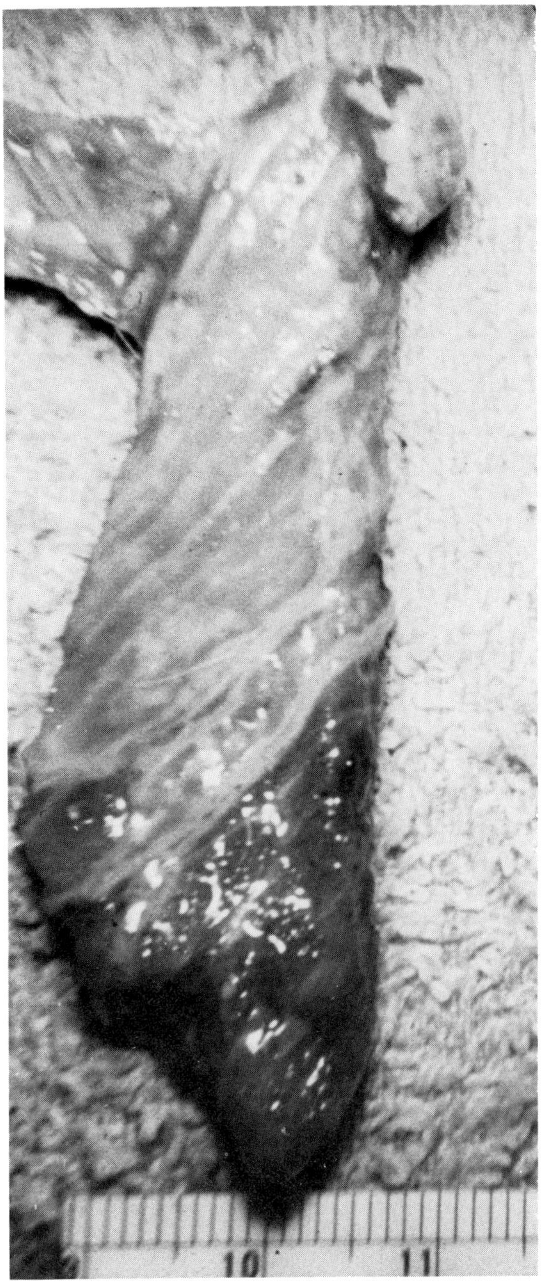

Fig. 14.1. Zenker's necrosis in iliopsoas muscle of aoudad, *Ammatragus lervia,* with vitamin E-selenium deficiency (left). Normal muscle is at the right.

minants apply to free-ranging and captive exotic ruminants (Ulrey, 1974; Wackernagel, 1966; Wallach, 1971a).

Calcium and phosphorus are required for mineralization of the skeleton, antlers, rumen nutrition, and cellular metabolism. A calcium:phosphorus ratio (Ca:P) of 1.1 to 2.0:1.0 is required for proper utilization. Minimum dietary levels of calcium and phosphorus are 0.29% and 0.21% of the ration respectively (Church, 1971). In general, the calcium requirement is satisfied when a good quality legume is consumed. Excessive supplementation of calcium will interfere with the utilization of zinc, copper, and manganese. Phosphorus usually needs to be supplemented for many wild species, including wild ruminants. Body size and antler size of a single widely ranging species such as the white-tailed deer vary considerably, depending on the availability of phosphorus. Excessive levels of dietary phosphorus can result in NSH with the associated skeletal fibrous osteodystrophy and the formation of urinary calculi (Wallach et al., 1978; Woolf et al., 1976).

Inadequate dietary levels of phosphorus result in weight loss and osteoporosis (Wobeser and Runge, 1975). Phosphorus is required for the nutrition of the rumen flora, as well as of the animal itself. Excessive levels of zinc or copper in the ration will reduce the efficiency of phosphorus utilization. Overt deficiency produces rather classical signs that include a peculiar gait described as "walking on egg shells," spontaneous lameness, spontaneous fractures, erosion of the articular cartilages, anorexia, loss of body weight, pica, reduced fertility, toe dragging of the hindlimbs, hyperirritability, and dyspnea.

High levels of dietary fat interfere with the absorption of both calcium and phosphorus. Proper levels of vitamin D are essential for proper intestinal absorption and skeletal mineralization of these minerals. Major vitamin D problems are most often reported in rapidly growing bottle-reared wild ruminants of considerable body size.

Magnesium is required as an essential catalyst of cellular metabolism. Deficiencies have been observed in bottle-reared ruminants and appear as ataxia, depression, or hypersensitivity to tactile or auditory stimuli. Associated muscle tremors and convulsions are often mistaken for enterotoxemia or tetanus. Recommended minimum levels are 0.6 gm/45.4 kg body weight (Church, 1971).

The standard level of 0.5% sodium chloride in domestic animal rations is sufficient for exotic ruminants. Trace mineral blocks with a minimum of 95% salt should be available at all times, in the absence of naturally occurring salt licks. Levels lower than 95% render the blocks unpalatable and they are rarely used. Excesses occur in the winter when drinking water freezes and salt is used to melt road ice. The clinical and postmortem signs of salt poisoning are enteritis, neurological disorder, and dehydration. Deficiencies of salt occur often in collections of captive wild ruminants where bran and oat concentrate mixes are used as the total energy and protein source without salt supplementation. Early signs of salt deficiency are constant licking of the stall walls and drinking of urine.

Iron is required for the production of hemoglobin with dietary levels usually adequate for adult wild ruminants. Deficiencies have been observed in bottle-reared ruminants. Supplementation of milk formulas with iron is essential. Dietary levels of 78 mg/day for the smaller species and 94 mg/100 kg for the larger species are recommended. Deficiency results in classical hypochromic anemia characterized by pale mucous membranes, weakness, dyspnea, and increased susceptibility to infection.

Copper is required as a catalyst of cellular metabolism and for proper hair, hoof, elastic connective tissue, and bone growth. The liver levels of copper in wild ruminants vary considerably, depending upon the species (Howard, 1964). Low levels of 29.3 ppm in liver have been reported without any clinical symptoms being recognized. Minimum levels of 17 mg/day are recommended. Complete absence of copper from the ration may result in molybdenum intoxication. Excesses of copper result in reduced liver function, hemolysis, and jaundice. Deficiencies produce hypochromic anemia, diarrhea, poorly keratinized wool and hair, achromotrichia, ataxia, lameness, and acute cardiac failure following a stressful event (Fig. 14.2). Free-ranging moose, *Alces alces,* feeding on browse with copper content of 5.72 ppm developed deficiencies (Flynn et al., 1977). Winter levels of copper in many food plants are less than 1.0 ppm, while late autumn levels range from 5 to 17 ppm. Pacing, a symptom of copper deficiency, is often noted in captive wild ruminants and a differential diagnosis must be made between a stereotyped behavior pattern and a copper deficiency. Diagnosis may be made by examining the serum copper levels. Normal levels of copper in serum are between 0.5 and 1.5 ppm. Ceruloplasmin levels have been used as an indicator of copper deficiency in free-ranging moose, an annual mean of 5.83 mg/100 ml was considered low.

Iodine is required for the production of thyroxin by the thyroid gland. Requirements are met by the use of salt with 0.01% stabilized potassium iodide. Deficiencies have been observed in captive wild ruminants. In most cases, plain salt blocks are offered to the ruminants "because the animals use them more." Congenital goiter and dead fetuses at birth are signs of iodine deficiency. Goitrogens, such as nitrate fertilizers, may occur in forages in sufficient levels to produce goiter in a ruminant having an otherwise adequate iodine intake. Effects of goitrogens will first appear in the smaller ruminants (Wallach, 1970).

Cobalt is essential for the rumen synthesis of vitamin B_{12}. Recommended levels for small and large captive wild ruminants are 0.08 to 0.2 mg/45 kg body weight and 1 mg/45kg body weight respectively. Deficiency results in lacrimation, anemia, emaciation, and death by apparent starvation.

Selenium has a physiological relationship to vitamin E and is thought to act as a biological antioxidant and cell membrane protector. Most commercial ruminant rations contain sufficient amounts. Deficiencies of selenium produce liver necrosis and nutritional muscular dystrophy, which is, perhaps, the most frequently reported nutritional disease in free-ranging, feral, and captive ruminants. It is one of the more easily recognized nutritional diseases, which may partially explain its high reporting frequency in relation to other nutritional diseases. Muscle stiffness and hyaline degeneration of striated muscle (Fig. 14.1) with some calcification occur. Elevated CPK levels are diagnostic for nutritional muscular dystrophy. Excesses of dietary selenium, such as 8.4 to 495 mg/kg of food, produce ataxia, alopecia of the tail switch, sloughing of the hooves, and malformed young (Church, 1971). Environmental pollution with sulfur dioxide has interfered with utilization of forage selenium.

Zinc acts as an enzyme activator and is an essential component of insulin. Excess dietary calcium interferes with its utilization and increases the dietary requirement. Clinical signs of zinc deficiency include salivation; pruritis; rumen parakeratosis; alopecia of the muzzle, flank, and neck; and birth defects involving the neural tube (Wallach et al., 1978). One should look for deficiencies in captive animals fed top-quality legume hay and in free-ranging animals on soils deficient in zinc.

Rodents and Lagomorphs. Rodents and lagomorphs are found on all land masses and are capable of utilizing a large variety of plant materials as a primary food source. Rodents and lagomorphs themselves are important prey for small and medium-sized carnivores in the food cycle. A great volume of nutritional data is available for the rodent and lagomorph as a result of basic nutritional studies in the laboratory species (Adams et al., 1967; Porter, 1967; Yerganian, 1967).

CARBOHYDRATES. A wide variety of carbohydrate forms, such as grain, seeds, hay, and vegetables,

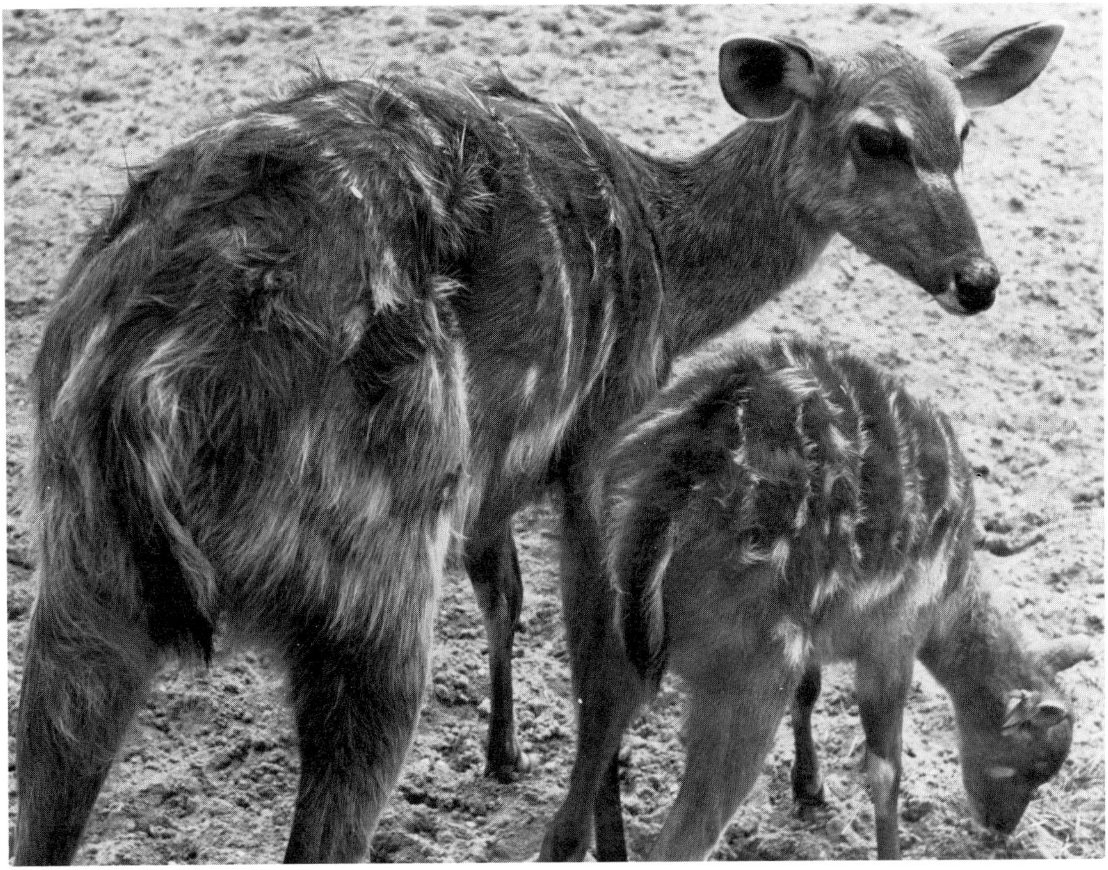

Fig. 14.2. Achromotrichia in sitatunga, *Tragelaphus spekei,* with a copper deficiency (left). Normal color pattern is seen in the animal on the right.

may be used by wild rodents and lagomorphs as energy sources. There should be a minimum of 2,500 and 2,700 cal/kg of diet for rabbits and rodents, respectively. An insufficient intake of calories will result in a loss of body weight, reduced growth rate, low reproduction rate, and starvation. Starvation is particularly common when captive specimens are fed unsupplemented vegetable diets of lettuce and carrots.

PROTEIN. Plant protein is the primary source of nitrogen for rodents and lagomorphs; however, these mammals will feed on animal carcasses. Crude protein levels of 15% are required. All of the known essential amino acids are required in the diet of rodents and lagomorphs. Deficiencies of methionine and lysine in the diet will result in alopecia and achromotrichia (Sheldon, 1971). Soybean protein is particularly rich in arginine and lysine, whereas egg protein and casein have limited amounts of these amino acids. Therefore, if casein or eggs are consumed as the sole source of protein by growing rabbits, they will be stunted in the rate of growth and total body size (Fisher, 1976).

FATS. Rodent and lagomorph diets should contain a minimum of 1% fat and may contain up to 8% without producing diarrhea. Deficiencies of linolenic, linoleic, or arachidonic acids will produce infertility, reduced hair growth, alopecia, scaly skin, caudal necrosis of the tail, renal disease, hematuria, anemia, and cutaneous ulceration.

VITAMINS. Deficiencies of vitamin A in rodents and lagomorphs produce squamous metaplasia of epithelial tissue, retarded bone development, retarded growth, xerophthalmia, corneal opacity, infertility, renal and genital deformity, diaphragmatic hernia, cleft palate, and ataxia (Giroud, 1968). A minimum of 55,000 IU/kg of diet should be available. Also, excesses of vitamin A are known to be teratogenic. Experimental doses of 1,000 IU/rat proved to be teratogenic.

Vitamin B_1 deficiencies result in anorexia, weight loss, circling, convulsions, and diarrhea. A minimum of 6.6 mg/kg of diet should be available. Bilateral polioencephalomalacia, loss of the myelin sheath in myelinated nerves, emaciation, and cardiac dilatations are common postmortem lesions.

Deficiencies of vitamin B_2 produce retarded growth; rough hair; pale feet, nose, and ears; anemia; scaley dermatitis; alopecia; depression; and cataracts (Giroud, 1968). A minimum of 8.8 to 13.0 mg/kg of diet should be available.

Pyridoxine deficiencies produce anorexia, retarded growth, ataxia, thinning of hair, convulsions, rapid whirling in a cage, hyperirritability, and paraplegia. A minimum of 6 to 14.15 ppm in the diet should be available.

Deficiencies of pantothenic acid result in weight loss, fatty liver, diarrhea, porphorin incrustations around the mouth, achromotrichia, exfoliative dermatitis, ataxia, alopecia and teratogenesis (Giroud, 1968; Sheldon, 1971). Diets should contain a minimum of 15 to 22 mg/kg.

Niacin deficiences produce retarded growth, anorexia, drooling, diarrhea, pale extremities, lowered packed cell volume, and porphorin-encrusted nose. Diets should contain a minimum of 37 to 53 mg/kg.

Choline deficiencies result in weight loss and lowered hematological values. Diets should contain 880 to 1,540 mg/kg.

Folic acid deficiencies produce megaloblastic bone marrow anemia and diarrhea. The role of folic acid in DNA metabolism, RNA metabolism, and protein synthesis in the embryo is of great importance. Deficiency of folic acid in early pregnancy produces embryo toxicity and a variety of birth defects, including hydrocephalus (Giroud, 1968). Diets should contain a minimum of 1.0 to 4.4 mg/kg. Feeding sulfonamides at the rate of 1% of the total ration produced folic acid deficiency anemia in hamsters, *Mesocricetus auratus.*

Vitamin B_{12} interacts with folic acid in its metabolic function (Woodward and Newberne, 1966). Deficiencies result in retarded growth, renal atrophy, anemia, teratogenesis, and anorexia. Diets should contain a minimum of 11 to 66 mg/kg.

Deficiencies of biotin are produced by consumption of the antivitamins in raw egg whites, amphibian egg jelly, or sulfonamides over extended periods. Deficiencies produce dermatitis, alopecia, ataxia, and achromotrichia. Diets should contain 0.12 to 0.34 ppm.

Vitamin C deficiencies have been reported in guinea pigs, *Cavia porcellus.* This species lacks the enzyme required for the conversion of L-gulonolactone to L-ascorbic acid. Diets for guinea pigs should contain vitamin C at the rate of 11 to 55 mg/kg. Deficiencies result in hemorrhage of the epiphyseal plate, painful articulations, subcutaneous hemorrhages, and death. Guinea pigs fed unsupplemented mixed seed diets are particularly prone to scurvy.

Deficiencies of vitamin D in the growing rodent and lagomorph produce classical rickets, characterized by imperfect calcification of the epiphyseal plates, stiffness, bone and joint enlargements, and hypocalcemic tetany. Hypervitaminosis D characterized by medial calcification of the major elastic arteries and metastatic calcification of soft tissues has been reported (Dieterich, 1969; Sargent, 1974). Hypervitaminosis D has been produced in captive beaver, *Castor canadensis,* and woodchucks, *Marmota monax,* by feeding commercial monkey pellets containing vitamin D_3 as a major portion of the diet (Wallach et al., 1978). Diets for rodents and lagomorphs should contain a minimum vitamin D level of 3.5 to 9.0 IU/gm of feed as activated plant sterol.

Vitamin E deficiencies have been reported in free-ranging woodchucks (Fleming et al., 1977). Deficiencies in laboratory rodents and lagomorphs produce muscular dystrophy, steatitis, anemia, hemoglobinemia, elevated CPK levels, elevated urinary creatine, and electrocardiographic changes. Diets should contain a minimum vitamin E level of 40 to 89 IU/kg of feed, the higher levels being required by the rabbit (Church, 1971). Selenium protects rodents and lagomorphs from liver necrosis.

Deficiencies of vitamin K result in a decrease in prothrombin levels producing increased clotting time and persistent hemorrhages. Vitamin K is synthesized by rodents and lagomorphs; therefore, deficiencies are rare. The synthetization process is interfered with by extended sulfonamide therapy. Vitamin K is not normally added to commercial diets for rodents and lagomorphs. Ingestion of dicumarol pesticides will produce clinical vitamin K deficiency and death.

MINERALS. Calcium and phosphorus deficiencies in growing animals produce fibrous osteodystrophy, tooth loss, malocclusion, increases of serum alkaline phosphatase, and tetany (Wallach et al., 1978). Deficiencies in the adult rodent or lagomorph produce osteomalacia, ataxia, and infertility. Diets rich in sunflower seeds are especially poor in available calcium and have produced fibrous osteodystrophy in captive gray squirrels, *Sciurus carolinensis,* and flying squirrels, *Glaucomys volans,* kept as pets and laboratory animals. Diets should contain a minimum of 0.94 to 1.30% calcium and 0.53 to 0.94% phosphorus. In addition to the correct absolute amount of calcium, a Ca:P ratio of 1.5:1.0 should be maintained.

Sodium deficiencies produce retarded growth, dehydration, corneal lesions, and urine drinking. Diets should contain a minimum sodium level of 0.20 to 0.49%.

Deficiencies of chlorine result in retarded growth, reduced serum chloride, and renal disease. Diets should contain a minimum chlorine level of 0.40 to 0.52%.

Deficiencies of potassium result in reduced appetite, stunted growth, abnormally short hair, diarrhea, lethargy, ascites, hydrothorax, coma, and death. Diets should contain a minimum potassium level of 0.80 to 1.19%.

Magnesium deficiencies produce vasodilatation, hyperirritability, seizures, cardiac arrhythmia, and mineral deposits in soft tissue, especially renal tissue (Woodward and Reed, 1969). Diets should contain a minimum of 0.19 to 0.27%.

Manganese deficiencies result in poor growth and considerably shortened long bones. Diets should contain a minimum manganese level of 40.0 to 120.7 ppm, the higher values being required by guinea pigs.

Deficiencies of iron and copper produce anemia, depression, and death. Extended copper deficiencies also result in achromotrichia. Diets should contain a minimum iron level of 200 to 350 ppm and a minimum copper level of 13 to 20 ppm.

Deficiencies of zinc result in teratogenesis, retarded growth, hyperirritability, alopecia, and parakeratosis (Smith et al., 1977). Zinc deficiency alopecia is especially noticeable in female guinea pigs and chinchillas, *Chinchilla laniger,* at about the 50th day of gestation. The hair will usually regrow in two to three weeks following parturition if the animals are on an adequate zinc diet. Diets should contain a minimum zinc level of 20 to 122 ppm.

Iodine deficiencies result in goiter, stunted growth, and stillbirths. Diets should contain a minimum iodine level of 0.6 to 2.2 ppm.

Selenium deficiencies produce varying degrees of liver necrosis. No minimum dietary levels have been established for rodents and lagomorphs.

Canines. The nutritional requirements of free-ranging and captive canids parallel those of the domestic dog. Taxonomically canids are considered carnivores; in fact, they are omnivorous and use a high percentage of plant material in their diet. Free-ranging canids meet their nutritional needs by consuming a variety of small mammals, birds, reptiles, amphibians and arthropods, fruits, and seeds. A wide variety of commercial dog foods have been used successfully to maintain captive specimens.

CARBOHYDRATES. No specific requirement for carbohydrates has been demonstrated for the canid. However, they have an important role in canid nutrition because of their availability in nature and low cost in the formulation of commercial diets. To allow for adequate protein, fat, and trace element levels in the canid, a maximum of 65% carbohydrate in the total diet has been established on a dry basis (Anon., 1965). Excessive carbohydrate levels can produce diarrhea. During gestation the caloric requirements of canids are 84 to 101 cal/kg body weight as compared to 79 to 92 cal/kg body weight for maintenance. Lactation will raise the requirement to 136 cal/kg body weight for the first week; then it will jump to 275 cal/kg body weight/day for the eight weeks of lactation. The large volume of feed required to meet this demand can be offset by frequent daily feedings. As the pups are weaned, the food intake of the bitch should be reduced to the original level. The young canid has a much higher energy requirement than the adult. Doubling the quantity of standard commercial food fed in four to five daily meals may be necessary for captive pups. It is recommended that the high-energy, high-protein commercial puppy formulations be utilized.

PROTEIN. The canid is capable of using vegetable forms of protein almost as well as animal sources, with percentages of digestibility as follows: horse meat, 91%; meat scraps, 86%; fishmeal, 88%; liver meal, 88%; blood meal, 78%; soybean meal, 86%; and linseed meal, 81%. In the formulation of commercial canid diets a minimum of 12% of the calorie source comes from the protein content; however, sufficient protein is usually supplied to provide 20 to 25% of the calories. As a rule of thumb, the authors consider that if the fat content of a diet does not constitute more than 5% by weight of the dry matter of the feed, protein levels of 22 to 25% of the dry matter will provide 25% of the calories.

When any of the essential amino acids are omitted from the diet or consumed in inadequate amounts by the wild canid, growth will be retarded and infertility and poor skin and hair coat quality will result. Total protein deficiencies can result in negative nitrogen balance and loss of condition will result. If not corrected, this condition may eventually lead to death.

FATS. Lipids provide a good concentrated energy source, 9.3 cal/gm compared with 4.1 cal/gm for carbohydrates, and a transport media for fat-soluble vitamins. The essential fatty acids, linoleic and arachidonic, are important for the health of skin and hair. On a dry matter basis, commercial canned rations have an average fat content of 10% and dry rations have 5 to 8%.

VITAMINS. Micronutrients play an important part in the enzyme reactions and metabolic pathways of the embryo, growing young, and the adult canid. Acquired congenital defects, deformities during growth, and impairment of body functions will occur in the absence of sufficient levels of vitamins.

Either carotenes or pure vitamin A can be used efficiently by the canid. However, the ability to store excess carotene that is not converted to vitamin A is limited. Carotene is more susceptible to oxidative reduction in the intestinal tract. Avitaminosis A in the fetus during the first trimester can result in abortion, cleft palate, diaphragmatic hernia, ophthalmic deformities, and other anomalies (Fig. 14.3) (Giroud, 1968; Wallach, 1970). Deficiency of vitamin A in the neonatal canid can result in retarded growth and predisposition to upper respiratory, intestinal, ocular and cutaneous disease. Vitamin A at 198 IU/kg/day is recommended for the growing canid, while 99 IU/kg/day appears adequate for adult maintenance. Hypervitaminosis A during pregnancy can produce early abortion, term stillbirth, or malformations (Giroud, 1968).

Vitamin B_1 plays a fundamental role in carbohydrate metabolism. The need for this vitamin increases in proportion to the amount of carbohydrate burned in the body; therefore, the active canid requires more than a sedentary individual. Ordinarily, 0.013 to 0.017 mg/kg of body weight will be adequate for maintenance and twice as much is required for growth.

Chastek paralysis from vitamin B_1 deficiency was first described in ranch-reared foxes fed fish

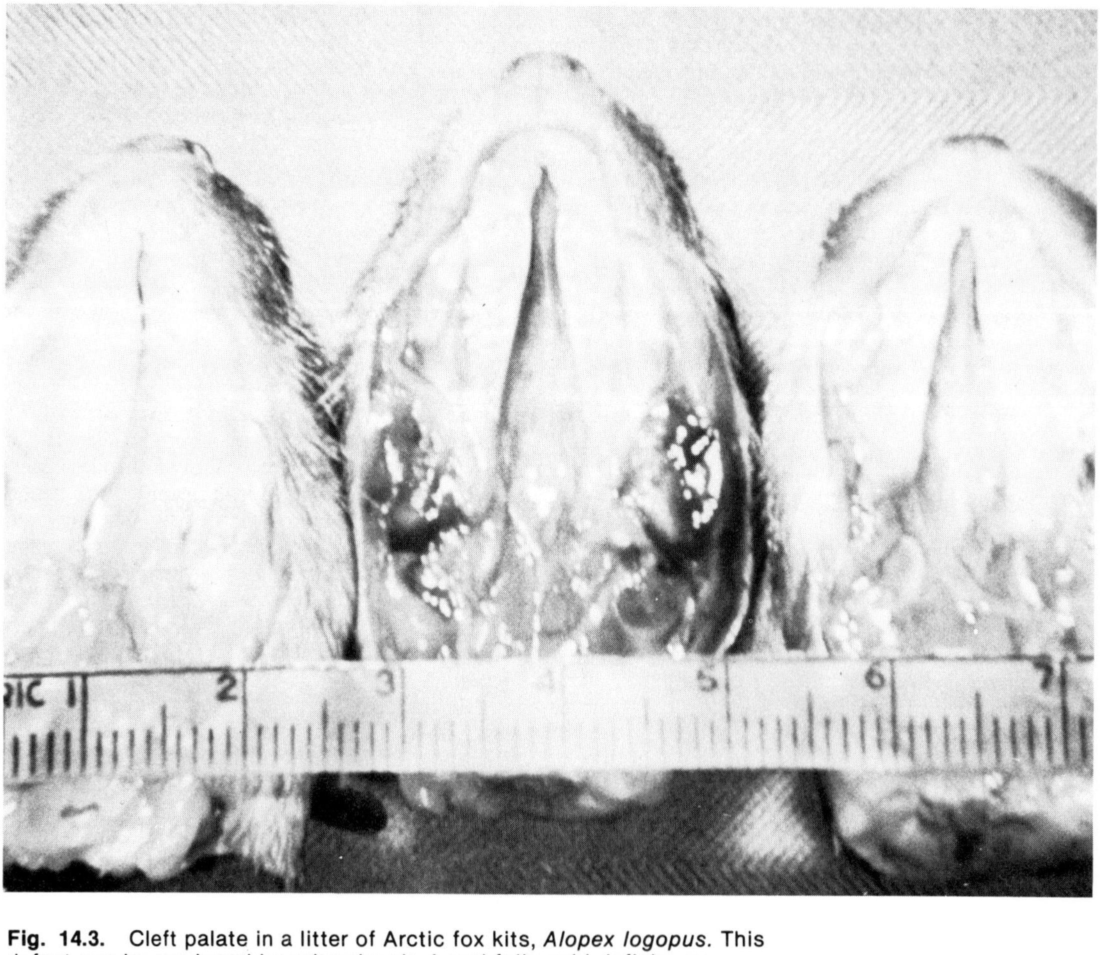

Fig. 14.3. Cleft palate in a litter of Arctic fox kits, *Alopex logopus*. This defect can be produced by avitaminosis A and folic acid deficiency.

that had high levels of thiaminase in their tissues (Jubb and Kennedy, 1970). The syndrome may develop after two to four weeks of deficiency. Anorexia, salivation, ataxia, incoordination, pupillary dilatation, loss of body weight, and convulsions that are easily induced have been observed in animals with Chastek paralysis. Administration of 25 to 100 mg of vitamin B_1 parenterally will cause a dramatic response even in individuals with advanced paralysis. Unrecognized or untreated, Chastek paralysis will progress until death occurs. Histological lesions in the central nervous system are characterized by edema, vascular dilatation, hemorrhage, and necrosis, especially in the periventricular gray matter (Yoshimura et al., 1976).

Vitamin B_2 deficiency in early pregnancy may produce syndactyly, shortened limbs, and cleft palate. The vitamin B_2 requirement of the canid seems to vary with the environmental temperature, for example, at 29° C the requirement is 1.4 mg/45 kg of body weight, while at 6°C the requirement is 4.2 mg/45 kg. Chronic deficiency may result in dry scaly dermatitis of the hindlimbs, thorax, and abdomen; anemia; muscular weakness; purulent ocular discharge; and sudden collapse. Conspicuous recovery occurs in a few days following parenteral administration of vitamin B_2 at the rate of 0.0099 mg/kg/day.

Severe niacin deficiency will produce pellagra in canids. This syndrome occurs most often when unsupplemented corn forms a large part of the diet of free-ranging or captive animals. Clinical signs of niacin deficiency include distortion of conditional reflexes, anorexia, weight loss, reddening of the oral mucosa, and persistent diarrhea. In the absence of dietary niacin, high-quality protein rich in tryptophane, which converts to niacin in the intestine, may be substituted. Parenteral injections of niacin at 0.66 mg/kg/day will relieve signs of pellagra very quickly (Anon., 1965).

Pyridoxine is important in the metabolism of amino acids and its presence is extremely vital in diets containing high levels of methionine. A general retardation of growth and skin disorders are observed in young canids on pyridoxine-deficient diets. Deficiency of pyridoxine results in a microcytic and hypochromic anemia. This anemia is accompanied by a two- to four-fold increase in plasma iron level and hemosiderosis of the liver, spleen, and bone marrow. The condition is refractory to supplementation with iron and copper but responds quickly to pyridoxine administered parenterally at the rate of 0.005 mg/kg/day.

Pantothenic acid is present in all canid cells and is essential in the diet as it cannot be manufactured in the body, although the intestinal bacterial flora produce a significant amount. Deficiency in the growing canid is characterized by a decrease in the blood levels of raw protein nitrogen, glucose, and chlorides. Skin and hair coat problems, gastroenteritis, and terminal collapse and coma occur in severe and prolonged deficiency. Parenteral administration of 0.1 mg/kg/day of pantothenic acid will alleviate the deficiency.

Biotin is a dietary essential in the canid although its exact requirement level is unknown because the intestinal flora produce significant amounts. Intestinal antibiotics and avidin in raw egg white or amphibian egg jelly will produce biotin deficiency manifested as a scaly dermatitis. Parenteral administration of biotin at the rate of 0.5 to 1.0 mg/day will alleviate the deficiency.

Folic acid deficiency produces anemia, leukopenia and thrombocytopenia, weight loss, and occasional oral ulcerations. Oral or parenteral administration of folic acid will produce reversal of signs.

Choline deficiency produces "fatty liver" and cessation of growth in young canids. When choline is added to the diet, the hepatic fat accumulation disappears. Dietary supplementation with 55 mg/kg/day of choline is recommended.

There is a metabolic relationship between folic acid and vitamin B_{12}, both being required for erythropoiesis. Vitamin B_{12} is synthesized by intestinal organisms and is dependent upon sufficient animal protein in the diet. Deficiencies in a pregnant bitch can result in fetal hydroencephalocoele. Parenteral injection of 1,000 μg of vitamin B_{12} and supplementation of the diet with 0.022 mg vitamin B_{12}/kg of dry ration will reverse the deficiency.

Vitamin C is not present in the average commercial diet for canids. Adequate amounts appear to be produced by the intestinal flora, and in free-ranging canids, vitamin C is obtained by ingestion of fresh plant materials. In cases of chronic illness or stress, the vitamin C requirement is greater than normal flora production. This situation may result in a relative deficiency manifested by slow healing, capillary fragility, dermatitis, and neonatal mortality. Supplementation of the diet of the pregnant bitch and chronically deficient canids with 50 mg/day of vitamin C is recommended.

Rickets may occur in the canid with a vitamin D deficiency, as the substance is essential for the utilization of calcium and phosphorus (Farrell, 1974). Rickets is most often seen in larger species that grow rapidly in the first 9 to 12 months of life, such as *Canis lupus* and *C. latrans.* If the Ca:P ratio is correct, supplementation of the diet with vitamin D at the rate of 13.2 IU/kg of body weight/day is sufficient for the correction of rickets. Excessive calcium increases the vitamin D requirement. Hypervitaminosis D can cause poor growth, dry hair coat, anorexia, polyuria, bloody diarrhea, polydipsea, and metastatic calcifications.

Deficiency of vitamin E or the vitamin E-selenium complex during pregnancy will result in stillbirths or weak pups with muscular dystrophy. The affected muscle has an abnormally elevated oxygen requirement that can be reduced by tocopherol supplementation. Creatine phosphokinase (CPK) levels in the plasma are indicators for the vitamin E status of skeletal and cardiac muscle. Normal CPK levels for the canid range from 19 to 31 Sigma units. Levels of up to 40 to more than 160 Sigma units/ml indicate vitamin E deficiency (Van Fleet, 1975). Elevated CPK levels occur 10 days prior to the appearance of clinical signs in experimental cases. Clinical signs include muscular weakness, myoglobinuria, and subcutaneous edema. Myocarditis and endocarditis in canids have been reported to respond to supplementation of the diet with vitamin E at the rate of 3 mg/kg/day. For growth, 44 mg/kg/day of vitamin E is required on a dry diet.

Vitamin K in the liver is required for prothrombin production. Normally sufficient levels of the vitamin are synthesized by the canid's intestinal flora. Accidental poisoning with dicumarol rodenticides or bile duct blockage will result in a secondary vitamin K deficiency. Parenteral administration of vitamin K will produce clinical improvement and correct the clotting deficiency.

MINERALS. When commercial diets are fed, few if any mineral deficiencies occur, except when dealing with weanling wolves that require a slight supplementation of calcium. Despite this fact, many canids are fed diets of improperly supplemented raw meat, which can result in recognizable nutritional disease (Fig. 14.4).

The improper balance or outright deficiency of calcium and phosphorus in the meat diet continues to be one of the greatest problems. The Ca:P ratio imbalance or deficiency produces retarded growth, lordosis, bowed leg bones, and pathological fractures. The epiphyseal plate retains its normal width in an uncomplicated calcium deficiency as opposed to a widening of this structure in true rickets caused by vitamin D deficiency. "Lipping" of the edges of the epiphyseal plate is characteristic of calcium deficiency. When the Ca:P imbalance or deficiency continues, NSH results.

For proper utilization of dietary calcium and phosphorus by the exotic canid, these minerals should occur at the rate of 264 mg of calcium and 211 mg of phosphorus/kg of body weight/day or as 1.0% and 0.8% of the diet respectively. These levels provide the recommended CA:P ratio of 1.2:1.0.

Diagnosis of calcium deficiency can be made through history and physical examination, radiography, and clinical pathology. The blood levels of calcium and phosphorus will usually remain in the lower range of the normal values; the alkaline phosphatase levels will rise way above the normal 3 to 6 Bodansky units. Pathological levels of alkaline phosphatase range from 40 to 400.

Iron deficiency occurs in young bottle-reared

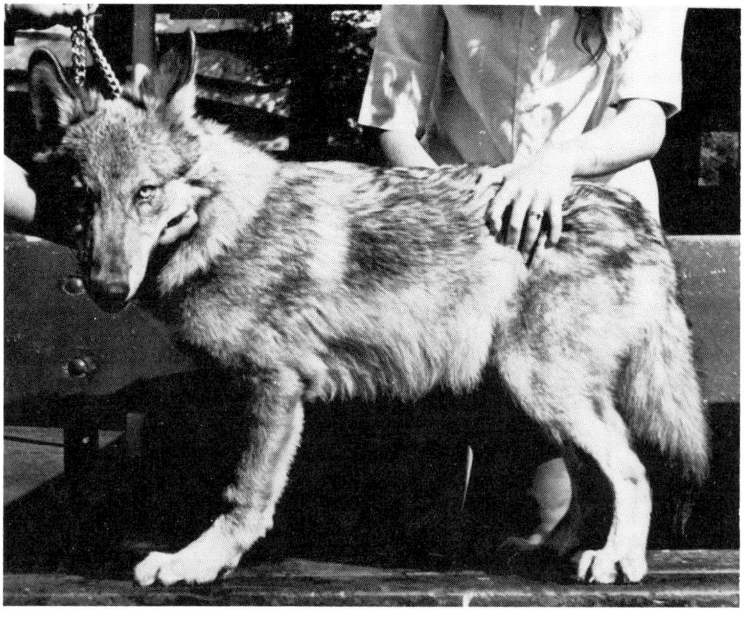

Fig. 14.4. Stunted wolf cub, *Canis lupus,* fed a ground meat diet.

canids fed improperly supplemented formula. Usually the deficient animal is housed in a scrupulously clean incubator or enclosure with a concrete or wooden floor. Iron is found in myoglobin in sufficient amounts so weanlings fed meat protein usually procure sufficient iron. Iron absorption in the canid is determined by need and is very efficiently conserved. In canids with normal iron levels the daily requirement is very small. When the canid is anemic for any reason, absorption of iron from the intestinal tract occurs. Diagnosis of iron deficiency anemia is easily made from the history of milk diet and a lowered PCV and hemoglobin level. Treatment should include parenteral administration of iron dextrose and the supplementation of the diet with iron at the rate of 1.3 mg/kg of body weight/day. Excesses are eliminated in the feces unabsorbed; therefore, slight overdoses of dietary iron are tolerated.

Copper deficiencies produce anemia, enlarged joints, osteoporosis, and achromotrichia. Treatment should include dietary supplementation with copper at the rate of 0.165 mg/kg of body weight/day.

Cobalt deficiency or a heavy infestation with *Diphyllobothrium latum*, which competes with the host for vitamin B_{12}, produces pernicious anemia. A level of 0.055 mg/kg of body weight/day is recommended.

Potassium is present in plant materials; therefore, most commercial rations have more than adequate amounts. Much of the ingested potassium is absorbed in the intestine and promptly excreted in the urine. Potassium deficiency in canids produces a paralytic syndrome that is quickly reversed with potassium supplementation. Chronic potassium deficiency produces interstitial fibrosis in the kidney and susceptibility to renal infections. Potassium should be supplemented at the rate of 440 mg/kg of body weight/day and returned to 220 mg/kg/day after symptoms abate.

Magnesium deficiency produces neuromuscular instability similar to hypercalcemia. The metabolism of magnesium in the canid is closely associated with calcium and phosphorus. Supplementation of magnesium should be made at the rate of 22 mg/kg of body weight/day.

Sodium chloride deficiency in canids produces weight loss, alopecia, dryness of skin, and death within eight weeks. Conservation and balance of the sodium is regulated by the adrenal hormone, desoxycorticosterone. Sodium chloride should be consumed at the rate of 1.5% of the dry diet or 0.33 gm/kg of body weight/day.

The use of iodized salt will provide 4.4 mg of iodine/kg of diet, which is sufficient to reverse early signs of goiter produced by iodine deficiency. Goiter, alopecia, weakness, and stillbirths are all characteristic of iodine deficiency in the canid. Enlarged thymus and spleen may occur in puppies born to an iodine-deficient bitch. Thyroid adenocarcinomas are common in canids with iodine-deficient diets (Wallach et al., 1978).

Zinc deficiency produces retarded growth, emaciation, decreased amylase activity, emesis, conjunctivitis, and keratitis and dermatitis localized on the abdomen and extremities. Excessive calcium supplementation will interfere with zinc absorption. Treatment of zinc deficiency should include supplementation at the rate of 0.22 mg/kg of body weight/day.

Felines. Felines are true carnivores; therefore, the nutritional status of the prey animal and the food carcass tissue preference of the feeding feline directly affect the cat's nutritional status. Environmental stresses increase total food consumption and caloric requirements.

WATER. A 3.2 kg cat requires 200 ml of water/day, of which 25% is normally obtained from food. The same-sized animal fed a dry commercial diet must necessarily receive a minimum of 200 ml or more of water/day.

Newly acquired exotic cats should be offered high-moisture diets as these tend to be more palatable than dry diets. If a newly acquired animal initially refuses to eat the commercial diets offered, a previously quarantined laboratory mouse, cat, rabbit, or chicken may be eviscerated and the body cavity filled with commercial diet. Usually after four to five such feedings the cat will accept the frozen or canned commercial diet alone. Dry feeds for the small species may initially require soaking in milk or beef blood. Water should be available at all times. The young weanlings are the easiest to introduce to commercial diets.

CARBOHYDRATES. Domestic cats can utilize dextrine and cooked starch. However, uncooked starch or cellulose is poorly digested. Sugars such as lactose may cause violent fermentation in the intestinal tract that results in diarrhea. Sucrose is tolerated to a greater degree than other sugars, but dextrin is the most efficiently used carbohydrate. The vitamin B complex requirement of the cat is increased approximately three times when carbohydrates are fed, as opposed to calories derived from meat.

PROTEIN. The cat has an animal protein requirement nearly twice that of the canid; therefore, commercial dog foods containing grain or cereal are unsuitable for cats. The normal animal can effectively utilize a diet containing 30% or more protein calories, especially for growth and reproduction. When the protein source is lowered so that it provides less than 18% of the caloric source, food intake is lowered and a weight loss results. The absolute minimum protein required in a cat diet is 20% of the calories or 8% protein in a canned food or 23% in a dry diet.

FATS. The cat is capable of utilizing large quantities of animal and vegetable lipids, up to two-thirds of the dry weight of the diet. Despite large quantities of dietary fat, the fat content of the feces remains constant in normal cats. One percent of linolenic acid in the diet is enough to prevent dermatitis.

VITAMINS. Felids are not able to synthesize vitamin A from β-carotene; therefore, they must obtain it from the diet. Acute and chronic vitamin A deficiencies are common (Scott, 1968). Reserves are reduced by 50% in pregnancy and lactation, and may drop to one-sixth in a normal kitten with pneumonia. Blood plasma levels of vitamin A are maintained at 200 IU/100 ml of serum until the liver stores become depleted. Plasma levels below 100 IU/100 ml indicate severe deficiency.

Clinical signs of avitaminosis A include anorexia, loss of body weight, poor hair coat, and follicular hyperkeratosis with alopecia. Conjunctivitis is accompanied by an ocular discharge stained red with porphyrins due to abnormal functioning of the lacrimal glands. The surface of the cornea becomes dry because of squamous metaplasia of the epithelium and corneal vascularization occurs. Ophthalmoscopic examination will show swelling of the optic disc and reduction in caliber of the retinal blood vessels. Retinal changes are characterized by a gradual change in distribution of rod and cone cells. Photophobia and a slowing of the irritable pupillary response from the normal one to two seconds to ten seconds occurs in severely deficient animals. Pupils may be dilated in normal light and cats may behaviorally exhibit loss of vision in strange surroundings.

The reproductive activity of the free-ranging and captive cat is severely affected by avitaminosis A. Testicular atrophy occurs with loss of production of spermatozoa. Reduction in size of seminiferous tubules and reduction in cell division and Leydig tissue are typical. Estrus may cease. Mild deficiencies allow conception but absorptions may occur at implantation or at the 30th to 50th day of gestation when the placenta normally has taken over the function of the corpus luteum. Kittens born to a vitamin A-deficient female are weak. There is a high incidence of stillbirths, neonatal deaths, and birth defects (Fig. 14.5). Avitaminosis-A-produced defects are often attributed to "in-breeding."

Abnormal bone modeling may occur. High rates of flattened thoracic rib cages occur, and if the kitten survives to the 5th week it may develop fibrous changes in the skull and the vertebrae. Pathologically thickened areas of bone press directly on the brain and spinal cord, especially in the region of the cerebellum and foramen magnum. Clinical signs associated with these changes include ataxia, tremors, spasticity, or paralysis. The degree of effect varies in different newborn of the litter; this condition was thought to be genetic in origin but is now known to be nutritionally based.

Demonstration of squamous metaplasia of the parotid duct and respiratory tract and low plasma levels of vitamin A confirm the existence of vitamin A deficiency. Parenteral administration of 5,000 to 10,000 IU of vitamin A and correction of the diet will cause recovery.

Vitamin B_1 is destroyed by overheating of the commercial preservative, sulfur dioxide, and the enzyme thiaminase that is present in fish. The onset of signs of vitamin B_1 deficiency takes about six weeks in adult cats and considerably less in kittens. Anorexia, emesis, weight loss, dehydration, polyneuritis, disordered cardiac function, convulsions, ataxia, paralysis, and prostration characterize the deficiency. A parenteral dose of vitamin B_1 brings rapid recovery in 45 minutes to 12 hours if the disease is caught in the early stages. If the condition is chronic, the response to therapy will be considerably slower and may be incomplete as the result of permanent damage to the central nervous system. A good rule of thumb for calculating the vitamin B_1 requirement for an exotic cat is to allow 0.1 mg/50 calories of food.

Deficiency of vitamin B_2 produces anorexia, weight loss, loss of hair around the head, occasional cataracts, and birth defects. Prompt recovery occurs following parenteral treatment. Cats require 0.2 mg/day, especially when on a high-fat diet (Scott, 1968).

Pyridoxine deficiency results in an accumulation of oxalic acid as the cat attempts to rid its system of oxalate in the form of calcium oxalate. High circulating levels of oxalate result in severe urolithiasis. Anemia in the free-ranging felid is more likely to be due to a pyridoxine deficiency than to an iron deficiency. Raw meat diets usually provide sufficient amounts of iron but tend to be low in vitamin B complex. Overt signs of deficiency are anemia, weight loss, and in the latter stages, convulsions. Levels of 0.2 to 0.3 mg/day are sufficient to prevent the oxalate form of urolithiasis and anemia in a 3.2 to 4.5 kg cat.

Niacin deficiency probably does not exist as a spontaneous clinical problem in the cat and has been recognized only with purified experimental diets. Reported signs include diarrhea, weight loss, neonatal death, oral ulceration, production

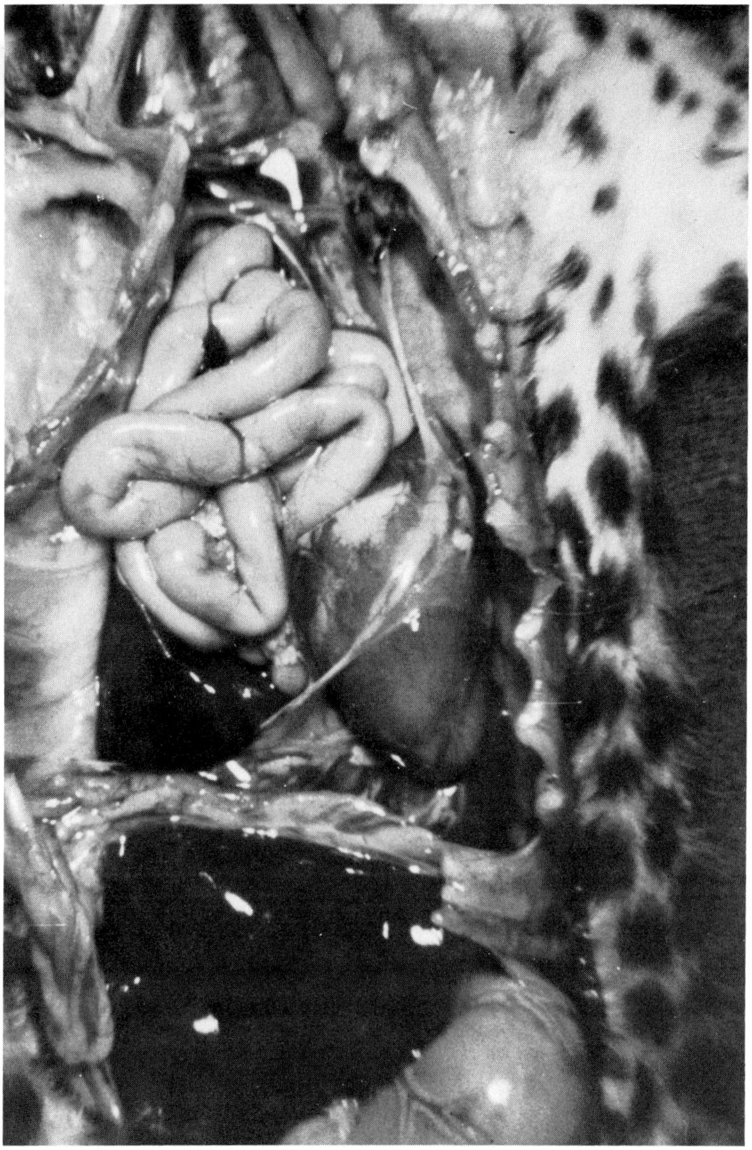

Fig. 14.5. Diaphragmatic hernia in a leopard cub, *Felis pardus.* This defect can be produced by avitaminosis A in the gravid female during early gestation.

of copious thick saliva, malodorous breath, and fever. As cats cannot synthesize niacin from tryptophan, they require between 2.6 and 4.0 mg/day in the diet.

Deficiency of pantothenic acid produces a disruption in fat metabolism with a resultant infiltration of fat into the liver. Dietary levels of 0.25 mg/day appear to be adequate in the small cats.

Folic acid, vitamin B_{12}, and biotin deficiencies have been incriminated with anemias in cats. Prolonged administration of oral sulfonamides also is thought to be a cause of anemia by suppressing the utilization of folic acid.

Deficiency of vitamin D is characterized by true rickets. Unsupplemented all-meat diets have repeatedly produced rickets in exotic cats. The daily vitamin D requirement of cats ranges from 50 to 100 IU.

Clinical signs of rickets include enlarged joints because of a widened epiphyseal plate that can be visualized radiographically. This should be differentiated from calcium deficiency which produces similar clinical signs and gross bone changes except that the epiphyseal plate is of normal width. Lameness, shortened long bones, curvature of long bones, and pathological fractures all may be observed with rickets.

Diagnosis of true rickets may be made from observing the clinical signs and dietary history and is confirmed by radiography. Microscopically, true rickets is characterized by an increase in the width of the zone of growing cartilage columns. There is a disruption and disorderly arrangement of the cartilage columns. Bony trabeculae are rare and are primarily composed of osteoid rather than calcifying bone.

Treatment of rickets should include an evaluation of the diet. The diet should be supplemented; preferably the animal should be placed on a commercially prepared diet. Parenteral administration of vitamin D_3 should be considered only if adequate calcium levels and the correct Ca:P ratio are present. Excessive vitamin D_3 in the presence of low dietary calcium or an imbalance of the Ca:P ratio will encourage fibrous osteodystrophy. Vitamin D_3 will also encourage the withdrawal of calcium from the bone in a deficient diet.

Hypervitaminosis D will produce calcification of soft tissue, including the media of elastic blood vessels, lungs, kidneys, and heart.

Deficiency of the vitamin E-selenium complex can result in muscular dystrophy, encephalomalacia, and steatitis as reported in lion, *Panthera leo;* jaguar, *Felis onca;* ocelots, *F. pardalis;* and snow leopards, *F. uncia* (Wallach et al., 1978). Vitamin E deficiency may be produced by feeding too much fish or oils with excesses of long-chained polyunsaturated oils. Clinical signs include anorexia, muscular weakness, depression, and torticollis. Hepatic disease typical of selenium deficiency in domestic species has been reported in the cheetah, *Acinonyx jubatus* (Dinnes, 1970).

Diagnosis of vitamin E deficiency may be made by finding the typical lesions in a muscle or fat biopsy or finding an elevated CPK level above 40 Sigma units/ml. Encephalomalacia is diagnosed by dietary history and finding the typical lesions at necropsy. Treatment of vitamin E deficiency should include parenteral administration at the rate of 25 IU vitamin E/day and a correction of the diet.

MINERALS. Free-ranging cats usually meet their mineral requirements by eating whole small carcasses. Captive cats are usually provided with supplemental vitamins, while mineral supplementation is usually omitted, thereby leading to overt deficiencies.

Calcium deficiency is the mineral problem most frequently encountered in free-ranging or captive felids. Clinical signs of the deficiency are characterized by lameness, pathological fractures, convulsions, and renal dysfunction. Bones from animals with calcium deficiency and uncomplicated by vitamin D deficiency demonstrate an epiphysis of normal width with a distinct peripheral "lipping." Fibrous osteodystrophy and pathological fractures and folding are commonly seen. Anemia resulting from chronic bone pathology is common. Excessive serum alkaline phosphatase activity develops in most cats as a result of a negative calcium balance before clinical or radiographic signs are definitive. If the diet is not corrected, the chronic demineralizing process may result in NSH in less than 30 days in growing animals. Diffuse renal fibrosis and renal cortical atrophy can appear in animals as young as 45 days old.

Renal cortical atrophy and fibrosing renal disease have been encountered for many years in the large carnivores fed only muscle meat. This renal disease is erroneously thought by some to be the result of "too much protein" in the diet. In fact, a simple adjustment of the mineral imbalance will lower the alkaline phosphatase activity to normal, often within two weeks, unless irreparable damage has occurred.

Muscle meat is notoriously low in calcium and phosphorus but especially low in calcium. This results in an imbalance of the Ca:P ratio to 1:5, as well as producing an absolute deficiency of calcium. Organ meat has an even worse Ca:P ratio, 1:44. The required Ca:P ratio is 2:1 or 1.5:1. Oily dietary supplements form insoluble calcium soaps in the alimentary canal rendering the calcium unusable by the cat.

Diagnosis of calcium deficiency and an imbalance of the Ca:P ratio or NSH may be made from observation of the animal at the time of its physical examination, history, dietary evaluation, blood chemistry, and radiography. Serum levels of calcium and phosphorus will remain approximately normal until severe collapse is imminent. Calcium deficiency is often misdiagnosed as rickets. Treatment of calcium deficiency may be made by adding sufficient levels of calcium carbonate to the diet, if the animal is being fed a commercially prepared diet. Excellent results may be expected within 30 days.

Iron deficiency anemia occurs in kittens on unsupplemented milk diets. The minimum iron requirement is 5 mg/day. Diagnosis of iron deficiency anemia is made by an evaluation of the blood picture, which will demonstrate a low PCV and hemoglobin level. Copper deficiency also occurs in kittens fed unsupplemented milk diets. The minimum copper requirement is 0.2 mg/day.

Iodine deficiency produces clinical signs of hypothyroidism within 30 weeks. The deficiency is characterized by stunted, sparse, short hair; thickened skin; broadening of the head; and slow deliberate movements. It may also produce open eyes at birth and cleft palate. Iodine should be supplemented in a range from 400 μg to 5 mg/day.

Excesses of dietary iodine will cause anorexia, severe weight loss, fever, rapid pulse, and hyperventilation.

The requirement for sodium is 20 to 30 mg/day and can be provided as salt supplemented to the diet at the rate of 0.5%. Potassium is required at 80 to 200 mg/day, while magnesium is required at 8 to 10 mg/day. Excesses of magnesium have produced urethral obstruction in laboratory cats (Scott, 1964).

Mustelids. Captive mustelids were early victims of nutritional abuse. The descriptions of these nutritional diseases reflected all-meat or all-fish diets being fed to the animals. Because of the economic importance of mustelid fur ranching, basic nutritional requirements have been established (Anon., 1953). The greatest volume of food is needed for the growth period, between 15 and 31 weeks of age, and during lactation.

PROTEIN. The protein requirement for mustelids is that the percentage of protein should be 10 percentage points above the fat level, with a minimum of 25% (Wallach, 1971a). Most commercial diets for mustelids contain 35 to 40% animal protein. Fat content of the diet should be 25% in the fall and drop to 20 to 22% during late winter-early spring. Excessive levels of dietary protein for extended periods produce overgrowth of claws.

VITAMINS. Vitamin A should be supplemented as vitamin A rather than carotene as the mustelids have a poor conversion rate of β-carotene to vitamin A. Clinical signs of vitamin A deficiencies include poor growth, dry dull hair coat, infertility, and birth defects in the kits. Chronic deficiency in adults produces anasarca. Treatment of vitamin A deficiency in mustelids includes parenteral administration of 500 IU of vitamin A and a correction of the diet.

Vitamin B_1 deficiency leads to the development of Chastek paralysis (Jubb and Kennedy, 1970). The deficiency is induced by a thiaminase present in certain types of fish. As the enzyme destroys dietary vitamin B_1, fish containing high levels of thiaminase should be avoided in the diet. If such fish must be fed, supplementation of vitamin B_1 at a rate of 25.3 to 26.4 mg/kg of fish should be administered.

Clinical signs may develop in two to four weeks after exposure to thiaminase or overt deficiency. The Chastek syndrome is characterized by anorexia, salivation, ataxia, incoordination, pupillary dilatation, and sluggish reflexes. Convulsions are easily induced and are characterized by a strong ventroflexion of the head. Even at this stage of the syndrome, animals will respond rapidly to parenteral vitamin B_1. After two to three days of the severe neurological signs, animals pass into an irreversible phase of semicoma, opisthotonus, continual crying, and spasticity.

Diagnosis of vitamin B_1 deficiency is made by utilizing the clinical signs, dietary history, and lesions. Postmortem lesions of the deficiency are characterized as emaciation, right ventricular dilatation, and terminal secondary infections. Microscopically, lesions of the central nervous system include edema, vascular dilatation, hemorrhage, and necrosis, especially in the periventricular gray matter. Treatment of vitamin B_1 deficiency should include correction of the diet and parenteral administration of vitamin B_1 at 5 mg/day until signs subside.

Biotin is an essential coenzyme that functions in the metabolic carbon cycles. Long-term deficiency of biotin results in a progressive paralysis. Raw eggs should not be fed regularly as the biotinase content of the albumin will result in biotin deficiency. Treatment includes parenteral biotin at the rate of 1 mg twice/week or 1 mg/kg of feed/day.

Vitamin E deficiency is produced by feeding a high percentage of long-chain polyunsaturated fatty acids as provided in fish oils and horse meat. The disease can be produced within two to nine months on diets low in vitamin E and containing polyunsaturated oils or rancid fish oil. Clinical signs are characterized by lethargy, lumpy subcutaneous fat, and death. Diagnosis of the deficiency is based on dietary history, physical examination, and fat biopsy. Postmortem lesions are generalized induration of adipose tissues with well-circumscribed lesions being heavily pigmented with a ceroid-lipofuscin. This yellow-brown pigment emits a yellowish orange fluorescence upon exposure to ultraviolet light. Microscopically, the lesion appears as an intracellular granuloma associated with the amorphous acid-fast ceroid. The reticuloendothelial cells and macrophages of the liver and spleen contain globules of ceroid pigment. Treatment is difficult and while parenteral administration of 10 IU of vitamin E and correction of the diet may arrest the disease, they will not reverse it.

MINERALS. The ash content of the mustelid diet should range between 7 and 8% on a dry matter basis. The calcium and phosphorus levels should be kept at about 0.4% of the diet on a dry weight basis. The Ca:P ratio should be 1:1. The NSH is a common syndrome in privately kept animals and in zoological specimens fed unsupplemented meat diets. Animals affected with NSH show posterior paresis, lameness, and pathological fractures. Metastatic calcification may occur with chronic renal disease, NSH, or hypervitaminosis D (Wallach et al., 1978).

Primates. Free-ranging primates are omnivorous, with many species actively seeking out small and medium-sized prey animals. In captivity, careful attention must be paid to the nutritional requirements of each species.

CARBOHYDRATES. The lack of calories is regarded as one of the greatest problems encountered by the newly acquired primate. Historically the initial captive diet began as a cafeteria style plate of fresh fruit and vegetables, with the caretaker noting the animal's preferences. This standard diet of fruit and vegetables is relatively low in calories and the caloric crisis would appear a few months later as the animal's fat deposits were exhausted.

Diagnosis of caloric exhaustion in the living animal is relatively easy and is based on a dietary history, low blood glucose, ketonuria, emaciated body condition, and depressed attitude. Treatment and prevention of caloric exhaustion include an increase of dietary calories in the form of mixed birdseed, hard-boiled eggs, whole wheat bread, and commercial primate diets. Animals that are anorexic should be given parenteral corticosteroids and lactated Ringer's solution intravenously. It is also prudent to administer parenteral vitamin B_1 and vitamin B complex to ensure the utilization of consumed calories.

PROTEIN. Primates require 15 to 25% protein of high biological value. Smaller forms of primates, including tree shrews, marmosets, and galago, *Galago* sp., derive a considerable amount of their daily energy requirements from the deamination of protein. Deficiencies of protein result in a chronic weight loss and lowered resistance to infectious disease.

FATS. Dietary fat levels of 3 to 5% appear to be adequate if sufficient amounts of carbohydrates are available as the major energy source. Excessive levels of fat will precipitate diarrhea and if continued over an extended period will interfere with the metabolism of calcium and vitamin E.

VITAMINS. Deficiencies of vitamin A produce stunted growth, xerophthalmia, keratitis, dermatitis, secondary infections, a dry dull hair coat, and stillbirths or birth defects in the primate. Recognition of a syndrome entirely related to a vitamin A deficiency is difficult clinically. Signs of avitaminosis A are normally related to a generalized malnutrition and should be treated as such. Treatment should include 5,000 IU vitamin A/day until signs subside.

The "cage paralysis" syndrome, including enteritis, dilatation of the right ventricle, emaciation, a marked plantigrade gait, and paraplegic state, may be produced by chronic deficiencies of vitamin B_1. This syndrome is produced in primates fed a high proportion of fruit and vegetables and may be particularly pronounced in the smaller primate species that have a limited stomach capacity. Parenteral administration of 25 mg of vitamin B_1 with a subsequent increase in dietary vitamin B_1 and energy levels usually produces a rapid clinical recovery.

Vitamin B_2 deficiency in primates produces retarded growth, dermatitis, alopecia, glossitis, cessation of the estrous cycle, and testicular atrophy. Dietary levels of 100 mg/day will reverse and prevent clinical signs.

Niacin deficiency in primates is characterized by hyperkeratosis, glossitis, enteritis, depression, and death. Large oral doses, such as 20 mg, will reverse the clinical disease.

Pyridoxine deficiency produces a hypochromic anemia, dermatitis, and convulsions. Dietary levels of 1.5 to 2.0 mg/day appear to be sufficient.

Pantothenic acid deficiency produces weight loss, tender feet, dermatitis, irritability, and convulsions. Ten to 15 mg/day appear to meet the primate requirements. Clinical signs of pantothenic acid deficiency in man are quickly reversed with parenteral doses of 20 to 40 mg of calcium pantothenate.

Biotin deficiency in primates includes alopecia, dermatitis, emaciation, hyperirritability, and death. Raw egg white and amphibian egg jelly have high levels of biotinase, which combines with biotin so it passes through the alimentary tract unchanged. Twenty mg/day will reverse the clinical course.

Folic acid deficiency produces neural tube defects, enteritis, macrocytic anemia, and megaloblastic anemia. Supplementation of the diet with 4.0 to 4.5 mg/day of folic acid will reverse the clinical signs.

Anemia is produced by a deficiency of vitamin B_{12}. Dry, brittle hair coats, depression, and ataxia may be associated with the syndrome. Prevention of vitamin B_{12} deficiencies can be accomplished by feeding commercial primate pellets or canned primate foods as the basic daily diet, using fruits and vegetables only as a supplement. If the owners insist on feeding table scraps as the basic diet, the diet should be supplemented with eggs or canned primate diet and an appropriate vitamin-mineral supplement.

Vitamin C deficiency produces scurvy and is observed in primates fed a "coffee and toast" diet. Clinical signs include diarrhea, capillary hemorrhaging of the gums and gingiva, failure to mineralize growing bones, and loss of teeth. The supplementation of 25 mg of vitamin C/day will reverse the clinical disease. The disease is not common in captive primates as most receive some form of green leafy vegetable or citrus fruit as a dietary supplement. Excessive intake of vitamin C will produce diarrhea.

Rickets caused by vitamin D deficiency is a common problem observed in the caged primate, especially immature individuals. Early clinical signs include lameness, enlarged painful articulations, anorexia, and stunted growth. Radiographic examination of the skeletal system at this time will reveal widened epiphyseal plates that may reach measurements of three to five times the normal width. Serum calcium and phosphorus levels are usually low while the alkaline phosphatase is within the nomal range. Rickets may appear in growing animals on a deficient diet in only 30 to 60 days. Deformities of the skeletal system, including the pelvis, pathological fractures, and paraplegia are associated with the chronic rickets syndrome. Complete demineralization with the production of "sickle shins" and "dropped wrist" and kyphosis syndromes will often occur with diets that are deficient in both vitamin D and calcium, in which case the alkaline phosphatase levels are very high.

Dietary levels of 10 IU vitamin D_2/gm of diet fail to arrest or reverse clinical cases of rickets, while 1.25 IU vitamin D_3/gm of diet prevented, arrested, and reversed clinical rickets in monkeys (Hunt et al., 1967). Marmosets require dietary levels of 8,800 IU vitamin D_3/kg of diet because of a limited gastric volume. Marmosets having free access to unaltered sunlight should be limited to 2,200 IU vitamin D_3/kg of food.

Excessive dietary levels of vitamin D_3 have produced interstitial nephritis in experimental baboons, *Papio* sp. Diets that are deficient in calcium and rich in phosphorus and have adequate or elevated vitamin D_3 content will produce a rapid demineralization of the skeletal system (Gerblich et al., 1977) and calcification of soft tissues, including elastic arteries and lungs (Wallach et al., 1978).

Clinical signs of the deficiencies associated with the vitamin E-selenium complex are only now being recognized in primates (Bartsch et al., 1977; Fitch and Dinning, 1963). Chronic cases demonstrate severe anemia and advanced fibrous muscular dystrophy of skeletal muscle. The creatinine levels and BUN values are usually within normal limits in the chronic stages; however, physical exertion will often produce the characteristic increase in these values. Treatment should include the parenteral administration of vitamin E-selenium preparation at the rate of 0.11 ml/kg of body weight. The dietary levels of vitamin E should be elevated to 50 to 60 IU/day. Animals that are being fed a diet rich in polyunsaturated fats should be given increased amounts of vitamin E.

MINERALS. Deficiencies of calcium or imbalance of the Ca:P ratio are among the more common of the nutritional disease syndromes of free-ranging and captive primates. The typical diet of fruits, vegetables, and bread offered to the captive primate is deficient in both phosphorus and calcium, but lower in calcium. This presents an absolute deficiency of calcium and an imbalance in the Ca:P ratio. This relatively uncomplicated calcium deficiency is characterized by skeletal demineralization, epiphyseal plates of a normal width, and pathological fractures. If the calcium deficiency is chronic, NSH results. This syndrome is characterized by elevated alkaline phosphatase levels, often reaching over 100 Bodansky units; normal to elevated calcium levels; and deforming fibrous osteodystrophy. Pregnancy and lactation place additional stress on calcium-depleted animals.

The "dropped wrist" and "sickle shin" syndromes, lordosis, scoliosis, and kyphosis are typical deformities associated with vitamin D_3 or calcium deficiency. A particularly common deformity in primates with chronic calcium deficiency is fibrous osteodystrophy of the maxilla and mandible with the associated separation and loss of teeth. The loss of teeth is often misdiagnosed as an infectious process or tumor (Wallach et al., 1978).

Treatment of calcium deficiencies and balances should be based on the administration of a calcium-enriched, phosphorus-inhibiting agent. Equal parts of calcium gluconogalactogluconate and basic aluminum carbonate gel may be administered orally at the rate of 2.2 ml/kg of body weight/day in two to three divided doses. As this suspension tends to settle, the agent should be shaken before being used. The diet should be corrected with proper levels of vitamin D_3 to efficiently utilize the supplemented calcium. Care should be taken to distinguish between rickets and calcium deficiency as the administration of parenteral vitamin D_3 preparations alone without the associated adjustments in calcium intake will only aggravate the syndrome and bring about a clinical crisis in the animal. Radiographs should be taken at 15- to 30-day intervals to monitor the mineralization process. The supplement should be discontinued when the bones become remineralized to normal densities. Deforming calcium deficiency may be at least be partially corrected in the young growing monkey, while deforming processes in the adult may be arrested but rarely completely reversed.

Deficiencies of iron produce a characteristic anemia syndrome in primates. The disease is seen in growing primates that are either being bottle-reared or remain with the parents. The clinical disease is characterized by depression, pale mucous membranes, and anorexia. Sudden death may occur in anemic primates that have become physically exhausted. A diagnosis is based on finding a low hematocrit and hemoglobin level. Treatment of iron deficiency anemia should include the oral or parenteral administration of iron products. The diet should be supplemented with iron and other hematinics, such as vitamin B_{12}, folic acid, and vitamin C.

Parakeratosis of the dorsum of the tongue characterizes zinc deficiency in the primate and there may or may not be an associated dorsal alopecia. Diets rich in calcium and vitamin D aggravate the syndrome by interfering with zinc absorption.

Hypochromotrichia is noticeable in guenons and marmosets on copper-deficient diets. Diets having only 9 mg/kg or less result in loss of orange and gold hair color. Excesses of dietary molybdenum and sulfates will increase the rate of copper loss from liver stores and interfere with utilization. Excesses of dietary copper produce liver dysfunction.

Suidae and Tayassuidae. The basic nutritional and dietary requirements of free-ranging swine and peccaries are identical to those of domestic swine (Whitehair, 1958). Free-ranging swine and peccaries are omnivorous and feed on both plant and animal material. The clinical manifestations of deficiencies are also identical. Commercial swine diets provide excellent complete diets for captive swine.

CARBOHYDRATES. High-energy rations are required because the simple stomachs of the swine and peccaries are incapable of efficiently utilizing cellulose. Excesses of carbohydrates in the diets of young animals precipitate diarrhea and, eventually, obesity and infertility in adults.

PROTEINS. Deficiencies of high-quality protein result in early fetal death and slow perinatal growth. Excesses of high-quality proteins cause excessive hoof growth in captive animals. The frequency of hoof growth problems is statistically higher in males due to the anabolic effects of testosterone.

FATS. Captive swine and peccaries require minimal levels of dietary fat if sufficient levels of carbohydrate are available. Excesses of dietary fats usually interfere with vitamin E absorption and utilization, which eventually produces muscular dystrophy, dietary liver necrosis, "mulberry heart disease," and steatitis.

VITAMINS. Vitamin A deficiency produces retarded growth, ataxia, torticollis, posterior paralysis, stiffness, lordosis, muscular spasms, corneal opacities, conjunctivitis, abortions, dead piglets at term, and congenital defects.

Vitamin B_1 is required for proper utilization and metabolism of carbohydrates. Deficiency produces anorexia, emesis, diarrhea, cyanosis, and sudden death. Classical lesions include cardiac dilatation and demyelination of nerve fibers.

The vitamin B complex deficiencies can lead to retarded growth, scaling and ulceration of the skin, alopecia, and anemia (vitamin B_2); anorexia, diarrhea, coughing, alopecia, ataxia of the hindlimbs, and edema of the colon (pantothenic acid); colitis, anemia, anorexia, and neurologic signs (niacin); alopecia, dermatitis, ulceration of the skin, and progressive paralysis (biotin); fatty infiltration of the liver with hepatic rupture and exsanguination (choline); anemia, neurologic disease, and emaciation (vitamin B_{12}); and stunted growth, anemia, convulsions, ataxia, and fatty degeneration of the liver (pyridoxine).

Exotic swine and peccaries are able to use both vitamin D_2 and D_3 equally well, provided that those receiving D_2 have access to sunlight for an hour or so each day. Deficiencies result in classic rickets with all of the characteristic clinical signs.

Deficiencies of the vitamin E-selenium complex result in muscular dystrophy, nutritional hepatic necrosis, "mulberry heart disease," and steatitis. The disease complex may also appear in exotic swine and peccaries fed rations adequate in vitamin E but heavily fortified with oily supplements, such as cod liver oil or fish meal.

True clinical deficiencies of vitamin K rarely occur. However, accidental ingestion of warfarin or other dicumarol-impregnated grain products will result in epistaxis and subcutaneous hematocysts of massive proportions.

MINERALS. Calcium and phosphorus deficiencies are usually associated with grain-based, home-mixed diets. The lameness-paralysis syndrome appears with some frequency in the growing animal and lactating female. The classical signs of osteodystrophy, osteoporosis, stiffness, lameness, unthrifty appearance, stunted growth, pathological fractures, and elevated alkaline phosphatase levels may be observed.

Iron and copper anemias are common in bottle-reared swine and peccaries. These dietary-induced anemias usually appear in animals between two weeks and six months of age. Clinical signs include dyspnea, pale mucous membranes, and drooping tails and ears. Swine and peccaries are prone to develop classical goiter on home-mixed rations unsupplemented with iodized salt. Iodine deficiencies result in slow growth and hypertrophic goiter in young animals. Females on iodine-deficient rations or rations contaminated with goitrogens produce dead, edematous newborn that are characteristically hairless. Low zinc diets produce stunted growth and hyperkeratosis. Increased dietary calcium levels produce an increased dietary requirement for zinc. Deficiencies of magnesium produce irritability and in the advanced stages produce tonic-clonic seizures that may be similar in clinical appearance to tetanus. Clinical deficiencies of potassium rarely occur in free-living or domestic swine. However, chronic gastroenteritis will deplete serum levels of potassium. Hyperirritability and paralysis are associated with depletion. Salt deficiencies produce polydipsia, urine drinking, and a propensity for licking walls and fences. Chronic deficiency results in unthriftiness and weight loss. Excesses of salt or water deprivation on normal rations containing 0.5% salt will produce poisoning.

Equines, Pachyderms, and Tapirs. The basic nutritional and dietary requirements for equines, pachyderms, and tapirs approximate those of the domestic horse, *Equus caballus* (Wallach, 1970). With the exception of the tapirs, all of the other animals are total herbivores.

WATER. Water is consumed in relatively large amounts by these animals and should be provided *ad libitum* for all captive species, except elephants kept indoors. The elephant will drink 132 to 151 liters of water/day, losing 40 liters daily in the urine and another 23 liters through vaporization from the lungs and skin.

CARBOHYDRATES. Carbohydrates and starches provide the major source of energy. The elephant requires 12 to 28 cal/kg of body weight/day for basic metabolic processes. This value is probably valid for the other species as well. Insufficient dietary calories in the growing animal will result in insufficient weight gains and stunted skeletal growth. Working animals, females in late pregnancy, lactating females, and weanlings require 50 to 100% more energy over and above the basal metabolic rate. Hay or good pasture alone are reported sufficient to provide enough calories for maintenance of a nonworking adult animal.

PROTEIN. Dietary protein requirements range from 8 to 10% in the mature animal for maintenance. Protein levels of 13 to 14% are required by growing animals and lactating females. The amino acid lysine is especially important to the animals presented in this section. A level of 0.6 to 0.7% of lysine in the diet is required for proper bone matrix development. Protein makes up 20% of fresh bone weight. Legume hays or pellets have adequate levels of protein and are high in their lysine content. Soybean meal contains more lysine than most of the vegetable proteins. Poor-quality protein in the diet will result in poor hair coats in equines and tapirs. Excess protein in the diet will produce accelerated rates of hoof growth and horn growth in rhinoceros.

FATS. The serum lipids of the elephant are found in concentrations similar to those of the rat and the rabbit, suggesting similar systems of fat metabolism. Insufficient levels of essential fatty acids will produce dry scaly skin. Most grain supplements contain sufficient levels of the essential fatty acids.

VITAMINS. Avitaminosis A produces skeletal fragility, fractures, and deformities. Vitamin A is required for the normal growth and development of the epiphyseal cartilage. Failure of resorption of endosteal bone results in relative reduction in caliber of the foramina. The failure of skeletal foramina to enlarge to accommodate the spinal cord and optic nerve may partially explain neuronal and cord pressure degeneration. Early clinical signs of avitaminosis A may include lacrimation, anorexia, progressive weakness, abscesses of the sublingual glands, ataxia, birth defects, and persistent reproductive problems. Vitamin A at 25 IU/kg/day is sufficient for maintenance, but requirements increase to 40 IU/kg/day for growth and 50 IU/kg/day for pregnancy and lactation.

A dietary level of vitamin B_1 at 0.14 mg/45 kg of body weight will maintain peak food consumption. Deficiency of this vitamin produces anorexia, weight loss, ataxia, hypertrophy, and dilatation of the heart. Parenteral administration of 50 to 100 mg/day of vitamin B_1 will reverse the clinical course in one to three days.

A dietary deficiency of vitamin B_2 produces periodic ophthalmia, catarrhal conjunctivitis, photophobia, and lacrimation. A level of 2.0 mg/45 kg/day will prevent and reverse clinical signs. Dietary deficiency of niacin rarely occurs in the equine; however, a dietary level of 0.10 mg/kg is recommended.

The vitamin C content of elephant milk is reported to be four times greater than in bovine milk. No supplementation is necessary in adult diets as normal intestinal flora are thought to produce adequate amounts.

Avitaminosis D produces rickets. Rickets has been reported several times in the hand-reared elephants and will undoubtedly occur in all animals of this group not offered sufficient dietary levels of vitamin D. The classical lesions of rickets have been reported in the Asian elephant, *Elephas maximus* (Fig. 14.6). Radiographic examination of the articulations of suckling animals will easily confirm the diagnosis of rickets. Prevention and treatment of rickets requires sufficient levels of dietary vitamin D at 200 IU/kg of feed/day.

Hypervitaminosis D can occur and should be considered. The syndrome is characterized by loss of weight, hypercalcemia, and lameness. There is extensive calcification of elastic tissues, including the elastic media of the aorta and suspensory ligament system.

Hypovitaminosis E-selenium complex has caused both nutritional muscular dystrophy and steatitis in Grevy, *E. grevyi,* and Burchell, *E. burchelli,* zebra (Harthoorn and Young, 1974; Higginson et al., 1973). There has been a great amount of discussion concerning the interrelationships of the hypovitaminosis E-selenium complex and capture myopathy in zebra. The reader is referred to Chapter 9 for a detailed account. Dietary levels of 44 IU of vitamin E and 0.2 ppm of selenium/kg of feed/day are required by the animals.

Clinical signs of vitamin E-selenium deficiency in the zebra, tapir, rhinoceros, hippopotamus, and elephant are characterized by weak or stillborn young, young unable to find the udder, weak pasterns in the front and hind limbs, ataxia, sudden collapse following exercise, dyspnea, icterus, anemia, and rapid weak pulse. The normal CPK level reported in equines is 20 Sigma units; increased levels of 400 Sigma units or more have been reported in zebra with muscular dystrophy following exercise.

Gross pathology of hypovitaminosis E-selenium includes the large skeletal muscle groups, especially the adductor muscles and cardiac muscle. Pale linear areas may be observed throughout the heart. There also are enlargement of the liver, hemorrhages of the adrenal cortex, subcutaneous edema, intramuscular edema, and cardiac ventricular septal defects.

Microscopic lesions are characterized by hyaline and granular degeneration of the skeletal muscle and cardiac fibers. There are coagulation and fragmentation of the sarcoplasma. Mineralization of dystrophic fibers, muscle fibers separated by edema, formation of "retraction caps," and interstitial fibroplasia have been reported in zebra and domestic horses.

MINERALS. Because of the large size of the animals presented in this section, the importance of dietary calcium and phosphorus throughout life cannot be overemphasized. Degenerative arthritis of low calcium has been described in elephant, zebra, black rhinoceros, *Diceros bicornis*, and even a fossilized rhinoceros discovered in a middle Miocene quarry (Wallach et al., 1978). The NSH syndrome occurs frequently in young elephants and zebra raised on high-phosphorus, low-calcium diets. Mineralized enteroliths have been described in mountain zebra, *E. zebra* (Decker et al., 1975).

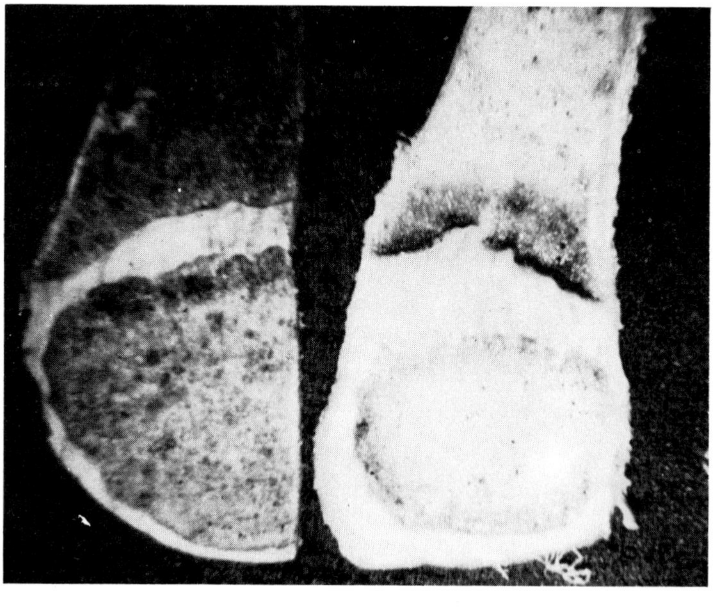

Fig. 14.6. Rickettic rib and humerus from a baby Asiatic elephant, *Elephas maximus.* Note the characteristic widening of the epiphyseal plates.

Clinical signs of calcium deficiency in young growing zebra, tapir, rhinoceros, and elephant are characterized by pica, lameness, pathological fractures, limb and facial deformities, and reluctance to move. The free-ranging elephant will eat limestone in road beds in calcium-deficient areas. Radiographic examination of calcium deficiency or NSH is characterized by "lipping" of an epiphysis of relatively normal width, folding fractures, and fibrous osteodystrophy. The normal alkaline phosphatase activity for an Asian elephant is 4 to 15 K-A units/ml; an elevation over 20 K-A units/ml is significant.

The dietary Ca:P ratio for all of the animals in this group should be considered as 1:1 as NSH occurs in horses on a diet with a Ca:P ratio of 0.8:1 for 6 to 12 months and will progress very rapidly when the dietary Ca:P ratio is 0.6:1.0. The NSH syndrome may be reversed by correction of the ratio to 1.4:1 until clinical recovery occurs, then it is returned to 1:1. As a rule of thumb 15 mg each of dietary calcium and phosphorus should be provided daily/45 kg of body weight.

Copper deficiency in the domestic equine and zebra and probably the other species presented in this section produces anemia, achromotrichia, spinal cord demyelination, myocardial fibrosis, and rickets-like bone disorders. Excessive dietary molybdenum causes a relative copper deficiency. The equine dietary requirement for copper is 5 to 10 ppm/day.

Iron is required in the diet of domestic equines at the rate of 40 ppm/kg of diet. Most high-forage diets contain sufficient iron.

Manganese is required for synthesis of chondroitin sulfate, an important constituent of cartilage and bone matrix. Deficiencies of manganese produce shortened, bowed limbs with enlarged joints and congenitally contracted tendons. Most high-forage diets contain sufficient manganese.

Zinc deficiency in equines produces poor growth, parakeratosis, and a lowered serum alkaline phosphatase level. Growing horses fed 0.54% zinc develop anemia, swelling of the epiphyses of the long bones, stiffness, and lameness; 40 ppm in the feed appears to meet the needs of the equine and probably the other animals in the group.

Selenium is an important trace mineral required for the health of skeletal muscle, cardiac muscle, liver, and fat; it was discussed with vitamin E. Excesses of selenium in the diet cause loss of the mane, tail hair, and a ring of disturbed growth on the hoof below the coronary band. In severe cases the hoof may slough off. Dietary levels of 0.2 ppm/kg of diet appear to be adequate.

Iodine deficiency results in abnormal growth rates, goiter, abortion, and brittle skeletal matrix. The iodine requirement may be considered around 0.1 mg/day. Weekly oral doses of 1 gm of potassium iodine may be useful in iodine-deficient areas.

Salt at 60 to 85 gm/day or 0.5% of the diet is required for the domestic horse and probably all animals in this section.

Cetaceans

WATER. Dolphins obtain most of their fresh water from the tissues of food animals; however, captive cetaceans will drink fresh water if it is made available. Because cetaceans obtain a relatively large amount of their daily water requirement from fish, dehydration and electrolyte imbalance are severe side effects of anorexia.

When cetaceans are in transit, or otherwise beached, hyperthermia must be anticipated. If the cetacean is not kept cool and moist, its core temperature may rise to 42° C. The dolphin's fins may have a surface temperature of up to 9° C higher than the flank. Since the cetacean skin is devoid of sweat glands it must be kept moist. Water conducts heat at a rate 27 times greater than does air; thus water provides an efficient cooling mechanism during evaporation. The heart rate will be increased in an effort to circulate greater amounts of blood through the surface capillaries in order to dissipate heat.

The blood picture of a cetacean subjected to travel stress is rather characteristic. A neutrophilia and an eosinopenia are marked. An increase in the hematocrit and elevation of the plasma are evident as a result of dehydration. Prevention of travel and heat stress is easy if the proper equipment is available and the animal is kept moist. During hot weather the cetacean should be packed with crushed ice or ice cubes. Treatment includes the administration of dexamethasone IM at the total dose of 5 to 10 mg, 10 ml of B complex with vitamin C IM, and 10 to 20 ml of penicillin-streptomycin. Fluids may be administered orally via stomach tube.

VITAMINS. Most cetaceans are fed frozen fish and are thereby subject to the possibility of vitamin B_1 deficiency as a result of the thiaminase levels found in certain fish. One of the more common fish fed to cetaceans is smelt, *Osmerus* sp. For each 1 gm of smelt fed to the animals, 44 μg of vitamin B_1 are destroyed (Geraci, 1968). Therefore, if 4.5 kg of smelt are fed, 118 mg of vitamin B_1 would have to be supplemented to the diet just to counteract the effects of the enzyme. The supplementation can be accomplished with

100 mg vitamin B_1 tablets. Five gm of vitamin B_1 should be added for each 1,000 calories in the diet to meet the basic metabolic requirements.

Vitamin B_1 deficiency in marine and fresh water cetaceans is characterized by anorexia, loss of body weight, secondary bacterial infections, cardiac dilatation, and demyelination of myelinated nerves (Fig. 14.7). The clinical signs and examination of the dietary program usually provide enough evidence to make a diagnosis. Treatment includes the parenteral administration of 2,000 mg of vitamin B_1, and a response may be expected within 45 minutes to 24 hours. Vitamin B_1 should be administered *per os* for one week at the rate of 1,000 mg/day and reduced to a maintenance dose of 500 mg/day.

In the early stages, vitamin C deficiency is characterized by gingivitis, glossitis, and pharyngitis. In advanced stages, the disease may appear as necrotic or ulcerative stomatitis. Fish stored at −18° C for more than six months will lose most of the vitamin C content. Symptomatic cetaceans respond to 1,000 mg of vitamin C/day. A prophylactic dose of 250 mg/day added to the diet is recommended.

Vitamin E-selenium complex deficiencies may be either acute or subacute and may be the cause of scoliosis and pale musculature in dolphins.

MINERALS. What appears to be a calcium deficiency is fairly common in cetaceans. The unsupplemented diet of cetaceans eating only fish has a Ca:P ratio of 1:2 or worse. The finding of numerous fractures of the ribs and vertebrae, in addition to phosphate or calcified microuroliths in tissue sections of the kidneys, tends to substantiate this theory. Calcium carbonate should be supplemented to a fish diet to bring the Ca:P ratio up to a 1.5:1 level. A series of postmortems on 60 pilot whales, *Globicephala melaena,* showed an age-related accumulation of calcified microliths and pathological fractures (Cowan, 1966). Whole fresh squid, the pilot whale's primary diet, has a Ca:P ratio of 1:10 with a low absolute amount of both minerals. If pathological lesions occur and analysis of the diet indicates that a negative calcium balance exists, then a calcium supplementation of the diet should be made for captive animals. For each kilogram of whole squid, 0.5 gm of calcium, such as 1.5 gm of oyster shell, should be added to bring the ratio up to 1:1.

Iron deficiency occurs in captive dolphins. The disease is characterized by hypochromic red blood cells. A rapid response is seen when the animal is treated with standard hematinics containing iron and vitamin B_{12}.

Pinnipeds

WATER. Dehydration and electrolyte imbalance are commonly associated metabolic problems of pinnipeds kept in fresh water. Although young pinnipeds do not lose water through sweating, they must feed regularly to ensure adequate intake. Adult animals may go for longer periods without feeding and partially maintain proper hydration by the production of metabolic water as

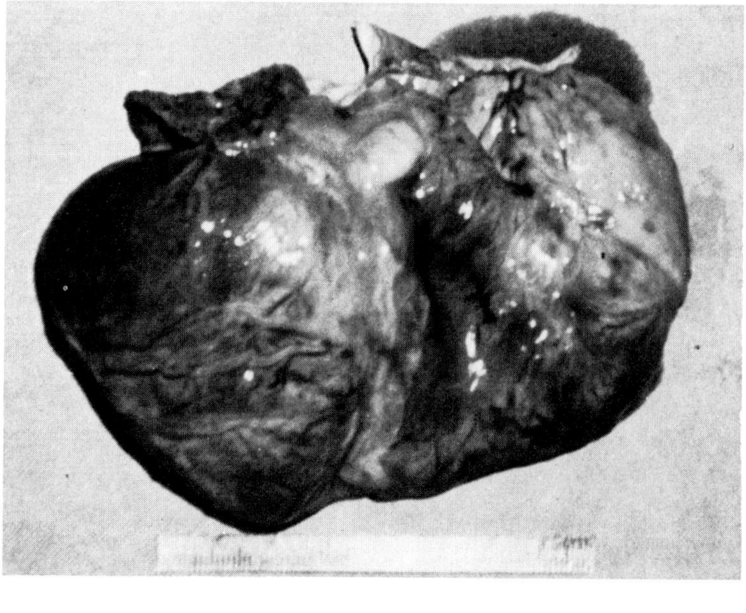

Fig. 14.7. Severe dilatation of the right ventricle of a fresh water dolphin, *Inia* sp., that died of a vitamin B_1 deficiency. This dolphin was fed a fish diet based on smelt.

a by-product of lipid oxidation. Blubber stores are often not adequate in the young orphan pinniped to provide proper hydration.

A second cause of dehydration in pinnipeds is the use of low-sodium diets with fresh water pools. Accidental ingestion of fresh water apparently results in sufficient "leaching" of electrolytes to cause clinical problems. The sodium level in marine fish ranges from 30 to 150 mg/100 gm of fish. Herring has sodium levels ranging from 100 to 110 mg/100 gm of fish. The practice of thawing fish in cold fresh water further reduces the sodium level in the feed fish at a rate of 25% in three hours.

Extreme muscular weakness, elevated hematocrit (up to 60%), and significantly lowered plasma sodium chloride levels are classic signs of dehydration. Replacement therapy with oral sodium chloride usually results in prompt recoveries. Most California sea lions, *Zalophus californianus,* and harbor seals, *Phoca vitulina,* tend to develop corneal opacities. However, these lesions have been observed in all species of pinnipeds and may be associated with chloramine levels in the water or hypervitaminosis A.

The addition of sufficient salt to the water to raise the sodium chloride level to 2.75 to 3.0% will normally reverse the corneal lesions. Where this is not possible, the diets should be supplemented with salt at the rate of 3 gm/kg of food/day. Plasma sodium chloride should be monitored and the salt level increased if indicated even to three times if necessary. If it is impossible to provide the pinniped with salt water swimming facilities, daily baths of the eyes with a 3% salt solution are recommended. Daily oral supplements of 500 mg of sodium chloride in the diet can be administered as an alternative. In general, acute electrolyte imbalances in pinnipeds should be treated with extracellular replacement solutions, but not saline. The administration of one-half to one-fourth strength saline is contraindicated and will produce electrolyte imbalances.

CARBOHYDRATES. Related to the clinical problem of pinniped neonatal exhaustion is hypoglycemia. Hypoglycemia occurs frequently in newly captive pups that have not yet begun to eat or have been offered an incorrectly prepared diet. Often the onset of signs will occur just prior to feeding and is precipitated by the sight of the keeper with the food.

Clinical signs of hypoglycemia include tonic-clonic seizures. Surprisingly, blood taken from pinnipeds showing acute signs may have a blood glucose level as low as 104 mg/100 ml (Keyes, 1968). The hypoglycemic animal may die following or during a seizure or recover spontaneously and immediately feed as though nothing had happened. Intraperitoneal administration of 25% glucose is the treatment of choice during an episode of hypoglycemic seizures. A 10-cm, 18-g needle should be used to ensure penetration of the blubber layer and the peritoneum. It may be necessary to add 1 gm of glucose to the diet to prevent a relapse.

VITAMINS. Hypovitaminosis A is characterized in pinnipeds by birth defects, arrested growth in the young, corneal opacities, copious lacrimation, and diffuse pustular dermatitis. The animals most often affected are those not offered a regular dietary supplement of vitamins or fed large quantities of long-chain polyunsaturated lipids. Administration of 25,000 IU of vitamin A/day in the diet, instillation of an ophthalmic ointment containing vitamin A into the conjunctival sac, and gentian violet applied topically for the pustular dermatitis will normally result in a reversal of signs.

Vitamin B_1 deficiency has been reported in several species (Wallach, 1972) and is undoubtedly a potential hazard for all pinnipeds. Dietary supplementation with vitamin B_1 should be the same as described above for cetaceans. Clinical signs of the deficiency in pinnipeds include anorexia, loss of body weight, and tremors. Blood levels of the thiamine-dependent enzyme, erythrocyte transketolase, is used to specifically diagnose vitamin B_1 deficiency. Transketolase activity is expressed as ThPP-E, a percentage. All values below 10% in pinnipeds are considered normal, whereas values of 12 to 31% are seen in vitamin B_1 deficiency.

Parenteral administration of vitamin B_1will arrest the signs in 45 minutes to 48 hours. If the correct dietary supplementation is not instituted, a relapse will occur within seven to ten days. The clinical disease should be treated with a minimum of 100 mg of vitamin B_1 given parenterally with a B complex-vitamin C product. The diet should then be properly supplemented to contain 100 to 500 mg of vitamin B_1/day over the level required to cancel the thiaminase activity.

Vitamin E deficiency has been reported in seals fed herring and is always a potential hazard in all pinnipeds because their fish diets are high in polyunsaturated lipids. The use of corn oil as the total calorie source for walrus calves, *Odobenus rosmarus,* has produced signs and lesions similar to those seen in domestic animals with vitamin E deficiency. There were cessation of blubber development, muscular dystrophy, arrested growth, desquamous dermatitis, and alopecia. Comparison of the lipid assay of livers from free-ranging walrus with livers of the clinically ill calves revealed considerable aberrations in the fatty acid ratios. This syndrome appeared despite the supplementation of 50 IU of vitamin E. The syndrome does not appear or is arrested and reversed in walrus calves fed whipping cream, which contains short saturated lipid chains, as the major source of calories. The recommended level of alpha-tocopherol is 50 to 100 IU/kg fish/day.

MINERALS. Calcium deficiency is commonly seen in young pinnipeds fed filleted fish or marine animals with minimal skeletal structure. The Ca:P ratio should be supplemented with 3,168 mg of calcium carbonate/kg of fish especially if vitamin D is supplemented in a multivitamin capsule or as cod liver oil.

The clinical disease appears as a reluctance to move, lameness, pathological fractures, fibrous osteodystrophy, and an elevated alkaline phosphatase. Laminated calcified microuroliths are a common finding in the renal tubules of sea lions at postmortem. These along with the dietary history, indicate chronic low-calcium diets with adequate sources of vitamin D. Triple phosphate calculi have been found in the renal pelvis of seals. The diagnosis of renal calculi may be made from a dietary history, radiographic examination, and clinical pathology. Treatment includes immediate correction of the diet, restricted activity, and surgery if warranted.

Marsupials. Captive and free-ranging marsupials are subject to the basic principles of nutrition as are all animals. The widespread use of commercially prepared diets for pet and laboratory marsupials has in large measure been responsible for the remarkable lack of reported nutritional disease in this group.

WATER. Water restriction in macropods does not influence nitrogen balance, but water-restricted animals will excrete less urea than controls and maintain higher plasma urea concentrations (Baker et al., 1970). Water-restricted animals excrete less water in the feces but the urine volume remains normal. Macropods recycle urea via saliva, which is swallowed and then used in the stomach.

PROTEIN. Kangaroos do not conserve energy or protein efficiently. When food is restricted to half of their voluntary intake, they enter a state of negative nitrogen balance and lose weight. When macropods are fed low-quality fiber diets, they will digest only 14 to 37% while sheep on this same diet will digest 52 to 58%.

VITAMINS. Deficiency of vitamin A results in infertility, causes a rough hair coat, and increases susceptibility to diseases of the skin and mucous membrane.

Deficiencies of vitamin D_3 have been reported in the young of several species, manifested by ataxia, paraplegia, fibrous osteodystrophy, and widened epiphyseal plates. Excesses of vitamin D_3 have produced medial calcifications of the elastic arterial tree.

Deficiencies of the vitamin E-selenium complex have been attributed to both low vitamin E diets and diets supplemented with cod liver oil (Munday, 1972). Clinical signs of hypovitaminosis E include hyperirritability, anorexia, muscular stiffness, progressive ataxia, elevated creatine phosphokinase, and symmetrical paleness of skeletal muscle masses, especially of the heavy muscle groups of the back and hindlimbs. Microscopically the lesions appear as hyaline degeneration, Zenker's necrosis, with scattered areas of calcification. Diagnosis of hypovitaminosis E may be made when the CPK level is above 40 Sigma units and may be confirmed with a positive biopsy. Treatment of vitamin E deficiency in marsupials should include a minimum of 25 mg alpha-tocopherol/day.

MINERALS. Deficiencies of calcium have been reported in free-ranging and captive animals fed all-meat diets. The bilateral bony changes of the maxilla and mandible are spectacular and may lead to the erroneous diagnosis of a tumor (Wallach, 1971b). Clinical signs include stiff gait, paraplegia, ataxia, and fibrous osteodystrophy of the facial and long bones, pathological fractures and an elevated alkaline phosphatase level of up to 100 K-A units or more. Correcting the calcium level of the diet to a 1.5:1 ratio with phosphorus and increasing the absolute amount will arrest the process in young animals.

CONTROL.

CONTROL. Individuals responsible for the nutrition of wild mammals have typically either followed tradition or extrapolated information from known species to unknown species (Sedgwick and Fowler, 1973). However to achieve proper nutritional guidelines for each species, normal parameters must be established in order to evaluate the health of the animals. The needs of individuals of a species at different stages of development can be more diversified than the needs at similar stages of different species. It is essential that proper nutritional standards be established for each species from 1) birth to weaning, 2) weaning to reproductive maturity, 3) calendar season for reproduction terminating in parturition, and 4) age of maturity until senility (Sedgwick and Fowler, 1973). In addition, environmental stresses must be considered.

REFERENCES

Abrams, J. T., 1968. Fundamental approach to the nutrition of the captive wild herbivore. Symp. Zool. Soc. Lond. 21:41–62.

Adams, C. E., F. C. Aitken, and A. N. Warden, 1967. The rabbit, *Oryctolagus cuniculus* L. In UFAW handbook on care and management of laboratory animals. 3rd ed. Williams & Wilkins, Baltimore.

Anon. 1953. Daily nutrient requirements per mink for growth. Natl. Acad. Sci. Natur. Res. Council, Washington.

______. 1965. Basic guide to canine nutrition. Gaines Dog Res. Center, White Plains.

Barker, S., S. M. Lintern, and C. R. Murphy. 1970. The effect of water restriction on urea retention and nitrogen excretion in the kangaroo island wallaby, *Protemnodon eugenii* (Desmarest). Comp. Biochem. Physiol. 34:883–893.

Bartsch, R. C., E. E. McConnell, G. D. Imes, and J. M. Schmidt. 1977. A review of exertional rhabdomyolysis in wild and domestic animals and man. Vet. Pathol. 14:314–324.

Basson, P. A., and J. M. Hofmeyr. 1973. Mortalities associated with wildlife capture operations. In E. Young. The capture and care of wild animals. Human and Rousseau, Cape Town.

______, R. M. McCully, S. P. Kruger, J. W. Van Niekerk, E. Young, V. De Vos, M. E. Keep, and H. Ebedes. 1971. Disease conditions of game in southern Africa: Recent miscellaneous findings. Vet. Med. Rev. 2:313–339.

Brady, P. S., and D. E. Ulrey. 1975. Protein requirements of weaned aoudads, *Ammotragus lervia*. J. Zoo Anim. Med. 6:24–28.

Church, D. C. 1971. Digestive physiology and nutrition of ruminants. Vol. 1–3. Oregon State Univ. Press, Corvallis.

Cowan, D. F. 1966. Pathology of the pilot whale, *Globicephala melaena.* Arch. Pathol. 82:178–189.

Crawford, M. A., J. M. Patterson, and L. Yardley. 1968. Nitrogen utilization by the cape buffalo, *Syncerus caffer*, and other large mammals. Symp. Zool. Soc. Lond. 21:367–379.

Decker, R. A., and A. M. McDermid. 1977. Nutritional myopathy in a young camel, *Camelus dromedarius*. J. Zoo Anim. Med. 8:20–21.

______, T. L. Randall, and J. W. Prideaux. 1975. Enteroliths in a confined Hartman's mountain zebra. J. Wildl. Dis. 11:357–359.

Dieterich, R. A. 1969. Medial arterial sclerosis in captive beavers, *Castor canadensis,* Kuhl. Bull. Wildl. Dis. Assoc. 5:115–116.

______, and R. W. Van Felt. 1972. Juvenile osteomalacia in a coyote. J. Wildl. Dis. 8:146–148.

Dinnes, M. R. 1970. Liver disease in cheetahs: A preliminary report. Proc. Annu. Meet. Am. Assoc. Zoo Vet., East Lansing.

Farrell, R. K. 1974. Canine rickets. In R. F. Kirk. Current veterinary therapy. Vol. V. W. B. Saunders, Philadelphia.

Fisher, H. 1976. Protein and amino acid requirements of the laboratory rabbit. Lab. Anim. Sci. 26:659–663.

Fitch, C. D., and J. S. Dinning. 1963. Vitamin E deficiency in the monkey. J. Nutr. 81:69.

Fleming, W. J., W. M. Haschek, W. H. Gutenmann, J. W. Caslick, and D. J. Lisk. 1977. Selenium and white muscle disease in woodchucks. J. Wildl. Dis. 13:265–268.

Flynn, A., A. W. Franzmann, P. D. Arnesan, and J. L. Oldemeyer. 1977. Indications of copper deficiency in a subpopulation of Alaskan moose. J. Nutr. 107:1182–1189.

Geraci, J. R. 1968. Diet induced thiamine deficiency in captive marine mammals. Proc. 2nd symp. on diseases and husbandry of aquatic mammals. St. Augustine.

Gerblich, A. A., S. M. Genuth, and J. G. Haddad, Jr. 1977. A case of idiopathic hypoparathyroidism and dietary vitamin D deficiency: The requirement for calcium and vitamin D for bone but not renal responsiveness to PTH. J. Clin. Endocrinol. Metab. 44:507–513.

Giroud, A. 1968. Nutrition of the embryo. Fed. Proc. 27:163–184.

Harthoorn, A. M., and E. Young. 1974. A relationship between acid-base balance and capture myopathy in zebra, *Equus burchelli*, and an apparent therapy. Vet. Rec. 95:337–341.

Higginson, J. A., R. J. Julian, and A. A. Van Drumel. 1973. Muscular dystrophy in zebra foals. J. Zoo Anim. Med. 4:24–27.

Howard, D. A. 1964. The copper content of the liver of some game animals in Kenya. East Afr. Wildl. J. 2:47–50.

Hunt, R. D., F. G. Garcia, and G. M. Hegsted. 1967. A comparison of vitamin D_2 and D_3 in New World primates. I. Production and regression of osteodystrophia fibrosa. Lab. Anim. Care 17:222–234.

Jubb, K.V.F., and P. C. Kennedy. 1970. Pathology of domestic animals. Vol. 2. 2nd ed. Academic Press, New York.

Keyes, M. C. 1968. The behavior and physiology of pinnipeds. Appleton-Century-Crofts, New York.

Kurtz, H. J., and P. D. Karns. 1969. Polioencephalomalacia in white-tailed deer. Pathol. Vet. 6:475–480.

Mitchell, G. E. 1967. Vitamin A nutrition of ruminants. J. Am. Vet. Med. Assoc. 151:430–436.

Munday, B. L. 1972. Myonecrosis in free-living and recently captured macropods. J. Wildl. Dis. 8: 191–192.

Nordan, H. C., I. Mc. T. Cowan, and A. J. Wood. 1968. Nutritional requirements and growth of black-tailed deer, *Odocoileus hemionus columbianus,* in captivity. Symp. Zool. Soc. Lond. 21:89–96.

Porter, G. 1967. The Norway rat, *Rattus norvegicus*. In UFAW handbook on care and management of laboratory animals. 3rd ed. Williams & Wilkins, Baltimore.

Reed, D. E., H. Shave, M. E. Bergeland, and C. E. Gates. 1976. Necropsy and laboratory findings in free-living deer in South Dakota. J. Am. Vet. Med. Assoc. 169:975–979.

Rogerson, A. 1968. Energy utilization by the eland and wildebeest. Symp. Zool. Soc. Lond. 21:153–161.

Sargent, A. P, 1974. Spontaneous arteriosclerosis in a brown hare. J. Wildl. Dis. 10:130–134.

Scott, P. P. 1964. Nutritional requirements and deficiencies. In E. J. Catcott. Feline medicine and surgery. Am. Vet. Publ., Inc., Santa Barbara.

———. 1968. The special features of cats with observations on wild Felidae nutrition in the London Zoo. Symp. Zool. Soc. Lond. 21:21–36.

Sedgwick, C. J., and M. E. Fowler, 1973. Methods of feeding mammals. Proc. Annu. Meet. Am. Assoc. Zoo Vet., Columbus.

Sheldon, W. G. 1971. Alopecia of captive flying squirrels. J. Wildl. Dis. 7:111–114.

Smith, J. C., E. D. Brown, and W. A. Cassidy. 1977. Zinc and vitamin A: Interrelationships of zinc metabolism: Current aspects in health and disease. Alan R. Liss, Inc., New York.

Steen, E. 1968. Some aspects of the nutrition of semidomestic reindeer. Symp. Zool. Soc. Lond. 21:117–128.

Treus, V. D., and N. V. Lobanov. 1971. Acclimatization and domestication of the eland, *Taurotragus oryx,* at Askanya-Nova Zoo. Int. Zoo Yearbook 11:147–156.

Ulrey, D. E. 1974. Nutrition of herbivores in the zoo. Proc. Annu. Meet. Am. Assoc. Zoo Vet., Atlanta.

Van Fleet, J. F. 1975. Experimentally induced vitamin E-selenium deficiency in the growing dog. J. Am. Vet. Med. Assoc. 166:769–774.

Wackernagel, H. 1966. Feeding wild animals in zoological gardens. Int. Zoo Yearbook 6:23–37.

Wallach, J. D. 1970. Nutritional diseases of exotic animals. J. Am. Vet. Med. Assoc. 157:583–599.

———. 1971a. The nutrition and feeding of captive ruminants in zoos. In D. C. Church. Digestive physiology and nutrition of ruminants. Oregon State Univ. Press, Corvallis.

———. 1971b. Lumpy jaw in captive kangaroos. Int. Zoo Yearbook 11:13.

———, L. Marcus, and R. Altman. 1978. The diseases of exotic animals: Medical and surgical management. W. B. Saunders, Philadelphia.

Whitehair, C. K. 1958. Diseases of swine. Iowa State Univ. Press, Ames.

Wobeser, G., and W. Runge. 1975. Arthropathy in white-tailed deer and a moose. J. Wildl. Dis. 11: 116–121.

Woodward, D. L., and P. M. Newberne. 1966. Relation of vitamin B_{12} and one-carbon metabolism to hydrocephalus in the rat. J. Nutr. 88:375–381.

———, and D. J. Reed. 1969. Effect of magnesium deficiency on electrolyte distribution in the rabbit. Am. J. Physiol. 217:1477–1482.

Woolf, A., D. Krodel, and H. Rothenbacher. 1976. Prevalence of renal urolithiasis in a large captive white-tailed deer herd. J. Wildl. Dis. 12:306–309.

Yerganian, G. 1967. The Chinese hamster, *Cricetulus griseus.* In UFAW handbook on care and management of laboratory animals. 3rd ed. Williams & Wilkins, Baltimore.

Yoshimura, K., Y. Nishibe, Y. Indue, S. Hirono, K. Toyoshima, and T. Minnesita. 1976. Animal experiments on thiamine avitaminosis and cerebral function. J. Nutr. Vitaminol. 22:429–437.

15 *Metabolic and Nutritional Diseases of Reptiles*

JOEL D. WALLACH
GERALD L. HOFF

THE BASIC DIFFERENCE between the poikilothermic vertebrate and the homothermic vertebrate is the inability of the poikilotherm to maintain an optimal core body temperature by means of involuntary controls. This unique feature of poikilotherm physiology requires the individual animal to use an environmental source of energy in order to reach optimal core temperatures during periods of activity to ensure the proper function of subcellular metabolic and digestive enzyme systems. The basic metabolic processes and subcellular pathways found in homotherms are present in the poikilotherm; therefore, the requirements for the basic macronutrients and micronutrients are the same. The nutritional state of free-ranging reptiles is directly affected by the nutritional health of the prey animals that make up the bulk of their food intake. Radical departures from environmental norms, for example, drought, flooding, heat waves, and hard winters, have both direct and indirect effects on the nutritional health of reptiles.

TEMPERATURE. Free-ranging reptiles withstand unfavorable seasonal changes by reducing metabolic rates and becoming torpid (Bellairs, 1970). The dramatic effects of temperature on the basal metabolic rate of poikilotherms is illustrated by experiments utilizing the American alligator, *Alligator mississipiensis* (Coulson and Hernandez, 1964). Oxygen consumption was measured in resting alligators subjected to environmental temperatures ranging from 5 to 30° C. The results produced a curve that approached the horizontal below 20° C and became almost vertical between 20 and 30° C. The total oxygen consumption at the alligator's optimal temperature was one-tenth that expected for a similar-sized mammal. A similar experiment conducted with chuckwallas, *Sauromalus obesus*, indicated that their metabolic rate was only one-seventh that of similar-sized mammals (Bellairs, 1970).

Reptiles have a relatively high ratio of surface area to body volume, and as a result they gain or lose core temperature rapidly. Basking is raise the core temperature to the preferred optimum. Lizards and chelonians commonly employ a prominent structure of the environment within their home territory as a basking site. The structure permits the animal to align itself perpendicularly to the rays of the sun. Many species of lizards and snakes climb high onto the tops of shrubs and low trees, especially in the shaded areas found in woods and forests. In the absence of a vertical surface many reptiles press themselves against a warm substrate. They are able to increase their surface area by drawing their ribs forward and outward, thus flattening their bodies dorsoventrally. On cool days small reptiles can gain heat very rapidly while larger species and individuals may require a considerable amount of basking time to significantly raise their core temperature. A 1.5 meter long alligator requires 7.5 minutes of basking time to increase its core temperature 2° C (Bellairs, 1970).

Preferred optimal (PO) temperature reflects temperatures for which a poikilotherm is physiologically adapted. The PO temperature for most reptiles falls between 20 and 39° C (Bellairs, 1970; Brattstrom, 1965; Peaker, 1969; Stebbins and Barwick, 1968; Wallach, 1971a). The known exception to this generalization is the tuatara, *Sphenodon punctatus*, of New Zealand that has a PO temperature of 12.8 to 21.0° C (Hoessle, 1969).

There is evidence to indicate that a constant exposure to the PO temperature produces pathological changes. A group of sceloporus lizards, *Sceloporus occidentalis*, exposed to their PO temperature for 13 weeks showed thyroid hypertrophy and death (Bellairs, 1970). Those exposed to temperatures above the PO temperature range developed anorexia, muscle atrophy, and failure of spermatogenesis (Licht, 1965). Similar results have been observed in iguanids constantly exposed to their PO temperature (Bellairs, 1970).

Certain lizards are capable of maintaining a core temperature of 38.5° C with only minor fluctuations, despite radical changes in the environmental temperature (Bellairs, 1970). This efficiency is the direct result of behavioral response. The reptilian skin is devoid of sweat glands and is an inefficient cooling mechanism. Reptiles cool themselves by altering body posture, panting, or entering a cool microenvironment or water. Panting occurs in the desert iguana, *Dipsosaurus dorsalis*, and collared lizard, *Crotaphytus collaris*, when their core temperatures reach 43° C.

Captive reptiles have been maintained for one or two years without ever reaching their PO temperature; however, they failed to eat or otherwise function normally (Kauffeld, 1968, 1969a; Pawley, 1969; Wallach, 1971a, b). It is generally agreed that captive poikilotherms should have the opportunity to reach their PO temperature for a portion of each day so the basic functions of life can be carried out.

LIGHT QUALITY. Light quality and temperature requirements for reptiles are interrelated (Bellairs, 1970; Kauffeld, 1969b; Licht, 1965; Murphy, 1969). Although many species are nocturnal feeders, seasonal changes in light quality and length of day are required to initiate endocrine systems that directly or indirectly control feeding behavior. Feeding may never occur in captive reptiles, despite the availability of the PO temperature, if proper light quality is not available. Experience has shown that animals which have refused to feed for many months with incandescent lights as the only light source will feed almost immediately when a simulated source of sunlight is provided (Laszlo, 1969).

PHYSICAL ADAPTIONS. All modern reptiles are carnivorous or partially so for at least a portion of their development (Bellairs, 1967, 1970; Kauffeld, 1968, 1969b; Wallach, 1971a, b). Adaptions of the mouth, teeth, and head are related to the types of prey animals generally eaten. Some of the more specialized adaptions include an elastic mandibular symphysis in snakes so they can consume prey animals that are larger than the diameter of their own heads. Another useful adaption is the conversion of salivary glands into poison glands for the immobilization of potentially dangerous prey.

The stomachs of reptiles are in general simple structures. In snakes the stomach is a long tubular organ that fits into a long tubular body. Chelonians and most lizards have simple stomachs that are saclike dilatations at the junction of the anterior and middle one-third of the alimentary canal. The stomachs of crocodilians have two distinct chambers. The anterior chamber (gizzard) is thick walled and lacks digestive glands and may contain a considerable number of rocks and other foreign bodies. The posterior chamber is thin walled and is lined by gastric glands. It is thought that both hydrochloric acid and pepsin or its precursor are produced by the same cells in reptiles (Bellairs, 1970).

The small intestine of reptiles is comparatively longer in species that consume a significant amount of plant material, for example, tortoises. The small intestine produces enzymes of diges-

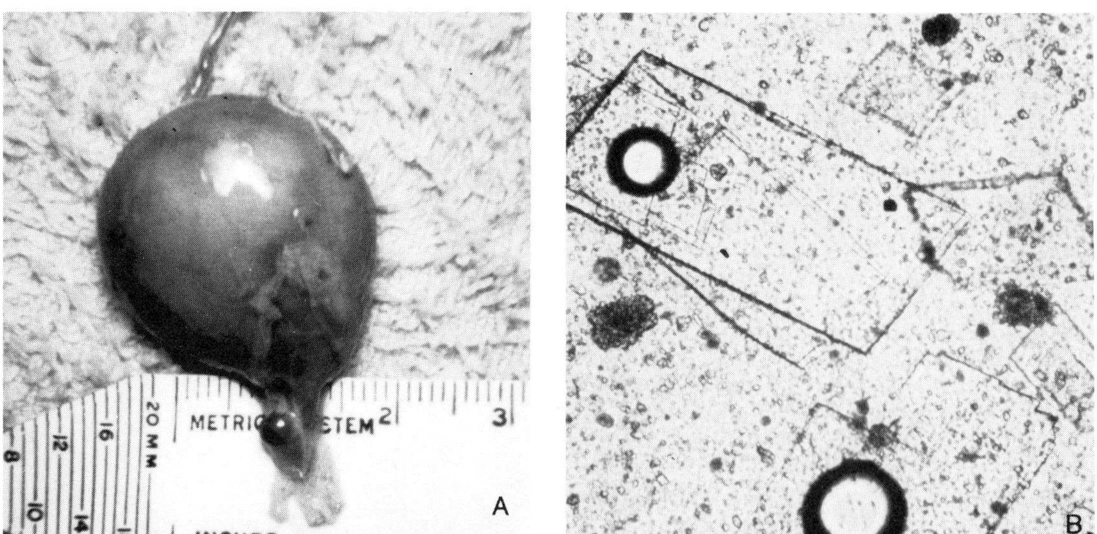

Fig. 15.1. (**A**) Gallbladder of a black-tailed rattlesnake, *Crotalus molossus,* showing a gallstone obstructing the common bile duct. (**B**) Photomicrograph of cholesterol crystals in a crush preparation of the gallstone illustrated above (×940).

tion similar to those found in avian and mammalian species and is very efficient in absorbing amino acids.

The livers of snakes are of a single-lobed, fusiform shape, while those of the remainder of the reptiles are bilobed. The gallbladder of snakes is located at the caudal pole of the liver and possesses a long common bile duct that courses caudally to the duodenum. Captive reptiles with high-fat, high-cholesterol diets are subject to the production of cholesterol gallstones (Fig. 15.1).

The pancreas produces both enzymes for digestive processes and insulin for control of blood and cellular glucose levels. The pancreas of snakes is intimately associated with the spleen. The colon is primarily for absorbing water and water-soluble vitamins from the fecal mass. The cecum is prominent in chelonians and some species of lizards. The function of the cecum in large herbivorous tortoises is thought to parallel that of the equine cecum.

Reptiles are intermittent feeders in nature because of the availability of food. Captive reptiles tend to become obese when kept under optimal conditions and fed regularly. Obese reptiles have a lowered tolerance to elevated environmental temperatures, a greater rate of infection, and the males tend to become infertile. Failure to feed eventually leads to death from caloric exhaustion (Fig. 15.2) when body reserves are depleted. A 2.4 meter long Indian python, *Python molurus*, reportedly lost 10% of its body weight following a 140-day fast (Bellairs, 1970). A 2.7 meter long boa constrictor, *Constrictor constrictor,* lost 50% of its body weight during a fast of 506 days. Gila monsters, *Heloderma suspectum,* and chelonians have reportedly survived fasts of 365 days.

Environmental temperatures directly affect the digestive process of poikilotherms (Bellairs, 1970; Wallach, 1971a). A 2.4 meter long python was able to digest a rabbit completely after five days at a temperature of 28° C and in seven days at a temperature of 22° C. At 18° C an ingested rabbit was not digested after 15 days. Lizards kept in PO temperatures digest insects in 12 hours. Normal feces from snakes will often contain undigested material, such as feathers, horns, and scales. Teeth of the host snake or ingested prey may also be found in the feces.

ETIOLOGY, PATHOLOGY, DIAGNOSIS, AND TREATMENT

Carbohydrates. Reptiles are capable of digesting and metabolizing simple carbohydrates. Excesses of carbohydrates above the immediate requirements are converted to glycogen and body fat and stored.

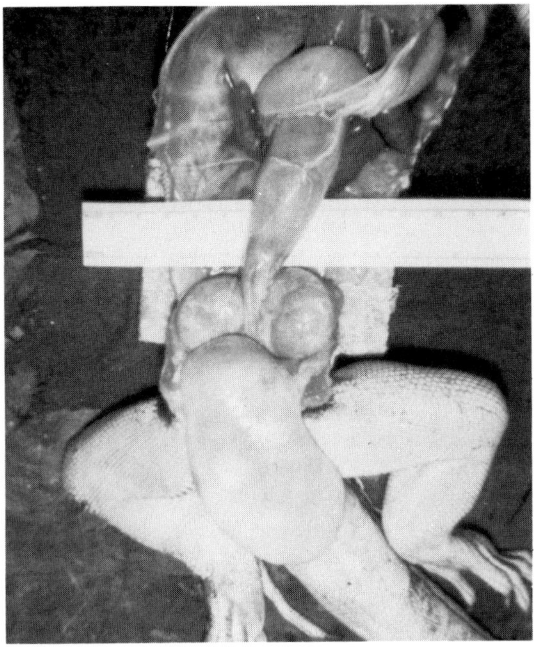

Fig. 15.2. An emaciated green iguana, *Iguana iguana,* that has died as a result of caloric exhaustion. Note the complete absence of abdominal and subcutaneous fat.

The alligator has a seasonal physiological periodicity of blood glucose levels ranging from 50 to 100 mg/100 ml. This variation appears in both the free-ranging and captive alligator (Black et al., 1963; Coulson and Hernandez, 1964). The normal endogenous sources of energy for the alligator are glucose (blood glucose levels of the alligator are directly related to the metabolic rate), lactate, and acetate. Summer levels of blood glucose in alligators invariably exceed those of the winter. The lowest levels of 50 mg/100 ml appear in the fall, followed by a gradual return to the summer levels of 100 mg/100 ml. This is followed by another, but less dramatic, decline in spring. Prolonged fasting in the alligator does not alter the expected seasonal levels of blood glucose (Black et al., 1963; Coulson and Hernandez, 1964).

In mammals, the resultant hypoglycemia of a fast elicits a hunger sensation, while the alligator is hungry only when it has high blood glucose levels (Coulson and Hernandez, 1964). The oxygen consumption rates (QO_2) of normal alligators are nine times greater than those of alligators with naturally occurring and artificially produced hypoglycemic shock. Hypoglycemic shock in alligators is characterized by mydriasis, star gazing,

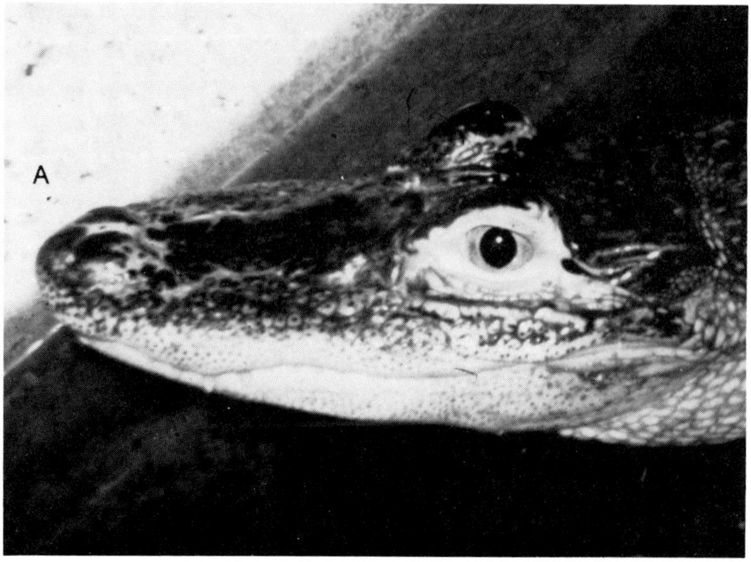

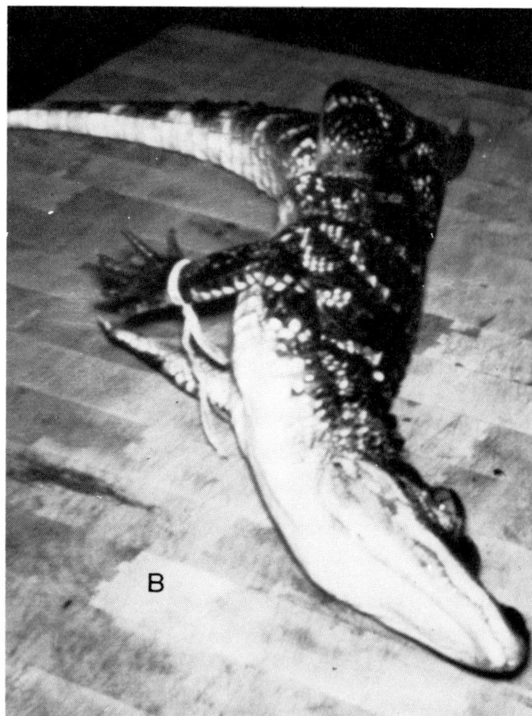

Fig. 15.3. (**A**) An American alligator, *Alligator mississipiensis,* showing mydriasis in the early stages of hypoglycemic shock. (**B**) An American alligator in extreme opisthotonos produced by advanced hypoglycemic shock.

and circular swimming patterns in the early stages and torticollis, opisthotonus (Fig. 15.3), catatonic seizures, and death in advanced stages (Coulson and Hernandez, 1964; Wallach, 1971a, b; Wallach et al., 1967). This condition has been recorded in alligators; caiman, *Caiman crocodylus;* and gavial, *Tomistoma* sp., and may occur in other reptiles with seasonal fluctuations in blood glucose levels.

The onset of the disease is usually preceded by a population density stress or relocation of an individual. Agitation of a mildly affected animal will result in the progression of the signs to a more severe level. The resulting epinephrine release appears to deplete the low levels of liver glycogen, precipitating a hypoglycemic shock. The same stresses during spring and summer do not have any clinical effect.

Clinical signs identical to those of naturally occurring hypoglycemic shock can be reproduced in alligators by the administration of regular insulin at the rate of 1,000 IU/kg of body weight. After an initial rise to 150 mg/100 ml, the blood levels drop slowly almost to zero so as "to raise doubts as to whether any was present" (Coulson and Hernandez, 1964; Wallach et al., 1967). Despite the alligators' severe hypoglycemic state there are no signs of shock for almost 24 hours. Clinical cases of hypoglycemic shock are treated by administering glucose parenterally at the rate of 3 gm/kg of body weight (Wallach et al., 1967).

Protein. In general, terrestrial reptiles are uricotelic (having uric acid as the principal compound of the nitrogenous waste), whereas alligators may be uricotelic or ammonotelic (having ammonia as the principal compound of the nitrogenous waste), depending on their state of hydration (Coulson and Hernandez, 1964). Ingested protein is hydrolyzed in the small intestine to amino acids. The essential amino acids are absorbed unchanged while glutamic acid is converted into alanine in the intestinal wall and the residual α-ketoglutaric acid is further degraded in the intestine. Aspartic acid is partially deaminated in the intestinal wall with oxaloacetic acid and alanine the primary metabolic products. Most of the nonessential amino acids are converted in the tissues to glycine, alanine, and glutamine, which are transported to the liver, muscle, and kidneys where they are deaminated, deamidated, or transaminated. The α-ketoglutaric derivatives formed in the deamination process are used rapidly and the fragments converted to fat, glucose, or glycogen. The essential amino acids, with the exception of arginine and lysine in the alligator, are deaminated slowly and are used primarily for protein synthesis.

Uric acid is the metabolic end product of both protein and purine metabolism in reptiles. Investigators have demonstrated that the rates of uric acid excretion in the alligator were just as great with purine-free diets as they were with high-purine diets. The normal excretion rates of nitrogenous wastes in alligators are 20% urea, 10% uric acid, and 70% ammonium salts; these rates are subject to change, depending on the animal's state of hydration. In alligator embryos these values are 46.2, 7.3, and 46.5% respectively (Clark et al., 1967). Other studies have shown the percentage of uric acid wastes in normal reptiles to be 93 to 98% in lizards, 89% in a python, and 63% in an unidentified snake (Neiland et al., 1956). The excretion rates for black snake embryos, *Coluber constrictor,* are 60% urea, 20% uric acid, and 10% ammonium salts (Bellairs, 1967).

Overt protein deficiency occurs in reptile populations during extended droughts and in the aftermath of a hard winter. Captive reptiles frequently suffer from protein deficiency when they are fed high-cellulose, low-protein diets, for example, lettuce and fruits. Chronic protein deficiency in reptiles is characterized by a wasting disease and death after body stores of fat and muscle mass are exhausted. Secondary infections are common in the terminal stages of this process and should be identified as such; however, they are often blamed as the primary cause of death. Borderline deficiencies of protein produce disrupted growth patterns in shells and beaks, and disrupted reproduction. Commercial diets containing 13% crude protein proved adequate for growth and maintenance in snakes and snapping turtles (Goellner, 1976).

Gout occurs in captive and free-ranging reptiles. Both the arthritic and visceral forms are common (Appleby and Siller, 1960; Bellairs, 1967; Coulson and Hernandez, 1964; Kauffeld, 1968; Wallach, 1969, 1970, 1971a,b; Wallach and Hoessle, 1967). The arthritic form is most often recognized in the living reptile while the visceral form is most often discovered at autopsy after a sudden death. Naturally occurring cases of gout have been observed in all forms of reptiles without the presence of primary renal disease. The high-protein diets of reptiles and concurrent dehydration are thought to contribute to the etiology of gout.

Investigators have artificially reproduced gout in alligators by means of intraperitoneal injections of the amino acid, *d*-serine (Coulson and Hernandez, 1964). An increase in uric acid excretion could be obtained when *dl*-alanine, *b*-alanine, and *l*-arginine were administered at the rate of 15 mg/kg of body weight. Glycine and *dl*-arginine were ineffective in altering uric acid excretion in the alligator because of rapid renal deaminization to ammonia.

Gout is characterized by the deposition of uric acid crystals in the joint or periarticular tissue (tophi) in the articular form and on the serosa and in the parenchyma of organs in the visceral form (Fig. 15.4). Microscopic appearance of the lesions is characterized by deposits of uric acid which are arranged in a radial pattern and often surrounded by inflammatory cells, including plasma cells and multinucleated giant cells. The normal concentration of uric acid in the blood of alligators ranges from 1.0 to 4.1 mg/100 ml. In alligators with gout, the plasma uric acid levels are increased to 70 mg/100 ml or more.

Water. Water makes up 70 to 73% of the body in terrestrial and freshwater reptiles and 65% in marine forms (Thornson, 1968). Reptiles conserve considerable amounts of water by utilizing relatively humid microenvironments for protection against severe desiccating heat. The efficient use of metabolic water by reptiles is questionable. Increased oxygen requirements incurred during β-oxidation cause panting, but the respiratory tract gives up more water than cells produce.

Terrestrial chelonians and all lizards and snakes excrete the greater part of their nitrogenous wastes as uric acid. Uric acid is relatively insoluble and requires large amounts of water to stay in solution. Uric acid is carried by the blood from the liver to the renal glomeruli and the renal tubules for excretion (90% by the latter route in iguanids). The concentrated uric acid in the collecting ducts precipitates out of solution as a chalky white or peach-colored sludge for excretion.

Renal constipation occurs in reptiles as a result of fatal desiccation (Wallach, 1969). Superficially the postmortem appearance of the affected reptile looks like gout in that urates precipitate and plug the renal tubules producing an acute renal shutdown. The disease is characterized by a series of peach-colored radiations that correspond to the collecting duct anatomy of the kidney. However, unlike the uric acid crystals of

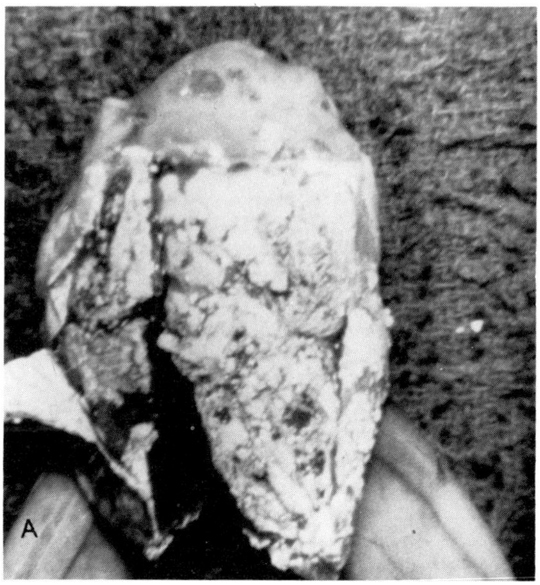

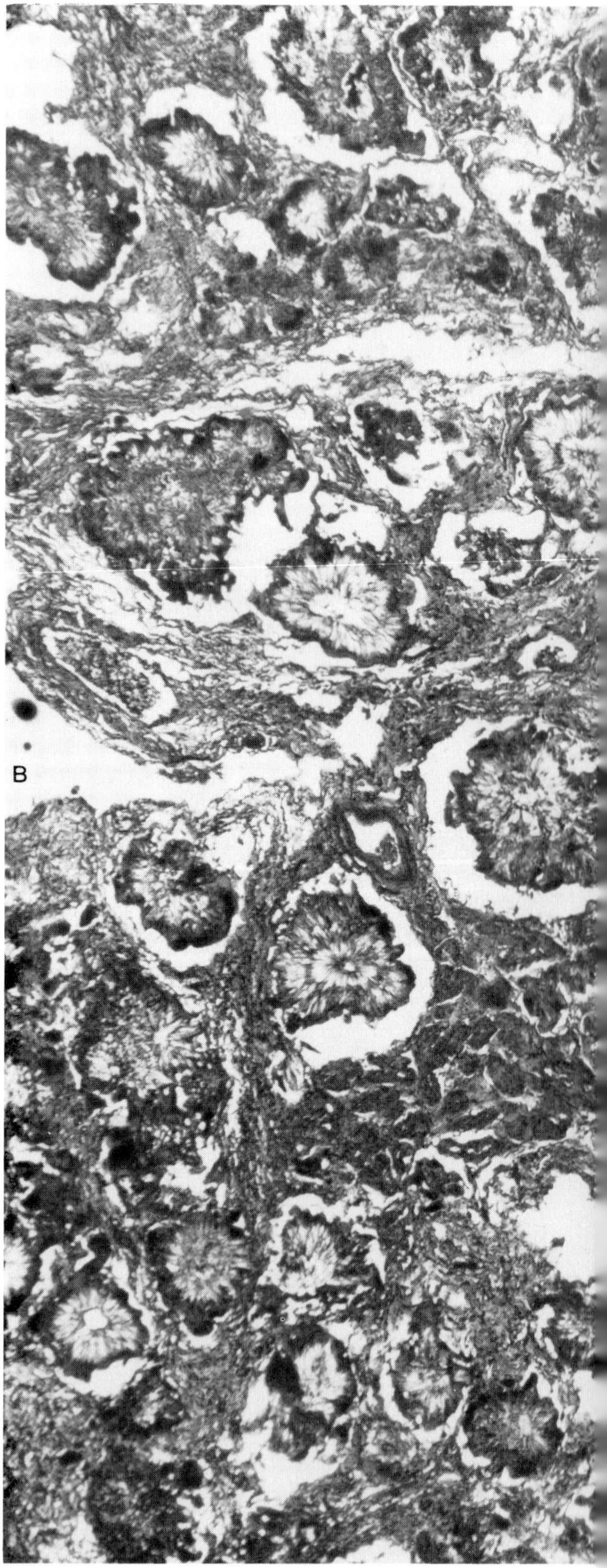

Fig. 15.4. (**A**) Pericardial sac and heart from a tegu lizard, *Tupinambis teguixin,* with visceral gout. Note the heavy accumulation of uric acid crystals in the pericardial sac and epicardium. (**B**) Numerous tophi in the kidney of a black-tailed rattlesnake, *C. molossus.* Note the multinucleated giant cells associated with the radiating deposits of uric acid crystals.

gout, the urates do not evoke an inflammatory response and are not trapped in the tissue. The urate crystals are dissolved into solution when the tissues are being prepared for miscroscopic examination, leaving behind a microscopically normal kidney.

Vitamins. Deficiencies occur in both the free-ranging populations of reptiles and captive individuals. The sometimes subtle evidence of vitamin deficiencies is often overshadowed by the more obvious secondary bacterial and parasitic infections that often end the life of the deficient animal. A definite clue to the rate of vitamin deficiencies in the field is the relatively high rate of hatching defects in reptile embryos, for example, cleft palates, two-headed individuals, alterations of scale patterns, and so on. These anomalies indicate the strong possibility of nutritional deficiency in the gravid female.

Vitamin A deficiency occurs in all types of reptiles but has been most frequently recognized and reported in chelonians (Reichenbach-Klinke and Elkan, 1965; Wallach, 1971a, b). Avitaminosis A is characterized by stunted growth, palpebral edema, anasarca (generalized edema), hyperkeratosis, and metaplasia of epithelial surfaces.

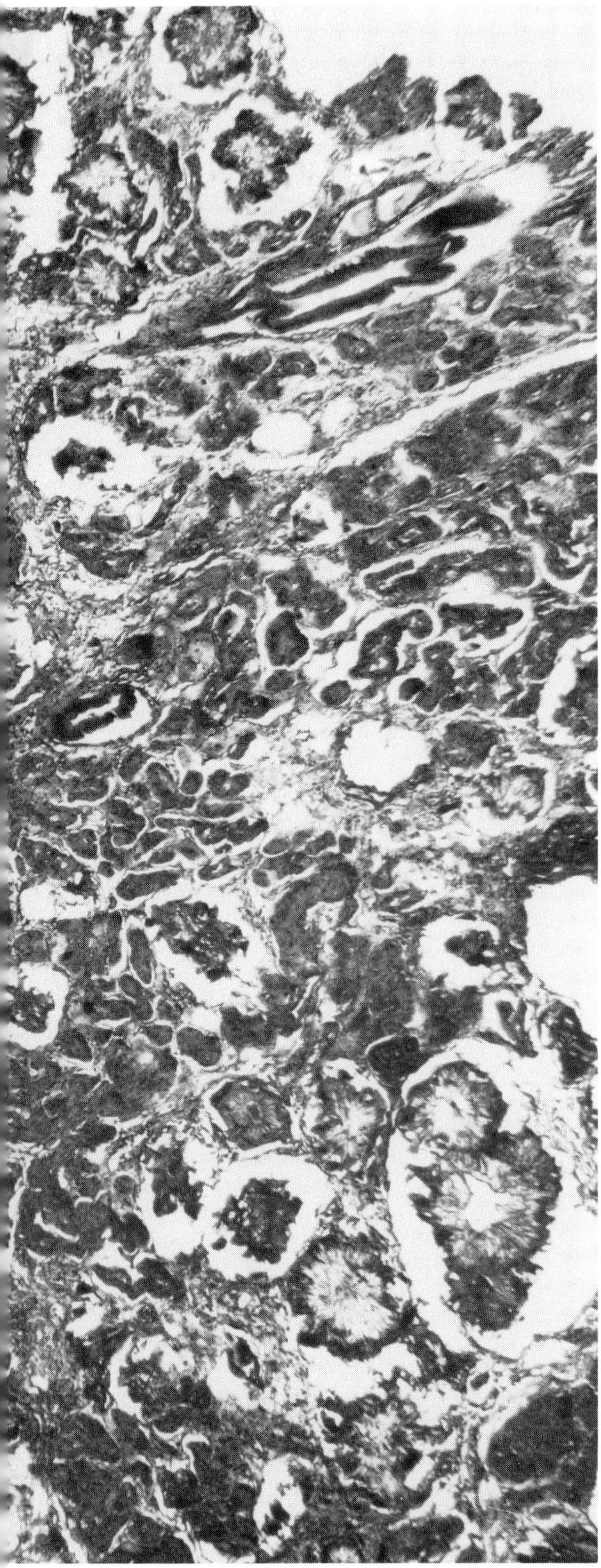

Table 15.1. Common Food Fishes Containing Thiaminase

Common Name	Scientific Name	Thiaminase Activity*
Fresh water smelt	*Osmerus mordax*	4,400
Milkfish	*Chanos chanos*	690
Green snapper	*Aprion virescens*	370
Black cod	*Moridae* sp.	354
Jack	*Caranx ignoblis*	185
Gray mullet	*Mugil cephalus*	184
Goldfish	*Carassius auratus*	+
Herring	*Clupea harengus*	+
Whitefish	*Coregonus clupeaformis*	+

* Micrograms of Vitamin B_1 destroyed/100 gm fish/hour

Commercial reptile diets having 4,850 IU vitamin A/kg of diet have proved adequate for growth and maintenance of snakes and snapping turtles (Goellner, 1976).

Vitamin B_1 deficiency can occur in all reptiles but is most common in species that feed on prey animals containing the enzyme thiaminase (Wallach, 1970). Thiaminase is found in a variety of fishes (Table 15.1); therefore, water snakes, *Nerodia* sp., aquatic chelonians, and crocodiles are most frequently affected. Vitamin B_1 deficiency in reptiles is characterized by chronic weight loss despite adequate food consumption. A flaccid dilated heart and enteritis may be associated findings. Commercial diets providing 4.4 to 11 mg of vitamin B_1/kg of diet have proved adequate for growth and maintenance in snakes and snapping turtles (Goellner, 1976). Thiaminase levels of a kg of smelt will deactivate 25.4 mg of dietary vitamin B_1; it is recommended that 33 mg of vitamin B_1 be supplemented for each kg of smelt fed. The parenteral injection of 50 to 500 mg of vitamin B_1 will produce a rapid and dramatic clinical recovery from the clinical signs; however, the diet must be corrected for continued improvement and prevention of relapse.

Many reptile forms may have bacterial production of vitamin C in the colon and cecum; however, stress or disruption of the intestinal flora can produce vitamin C deficiency (Nelson, 1971; Wallach, 1971a, b). The disease is characterized by subcutaneous and submucosal hemorrhages that often become secondarily infected with resident microorganisms that produce a necrotic stomatitis (Fig. 15.5). Dietary levels of vitamin C at 5 to 30 mg/day appear adequate under normal conditions. Parenteral injections of 50 to 100 mg/day have increased the recovery rate of reptiles with necrotic stomatitis when compared with reptiles treated only with topical or parenteral antibodies.

Vitamin D deficiency in reptiles produces classical rickets (Reichenbach-Klinke and Elkan,

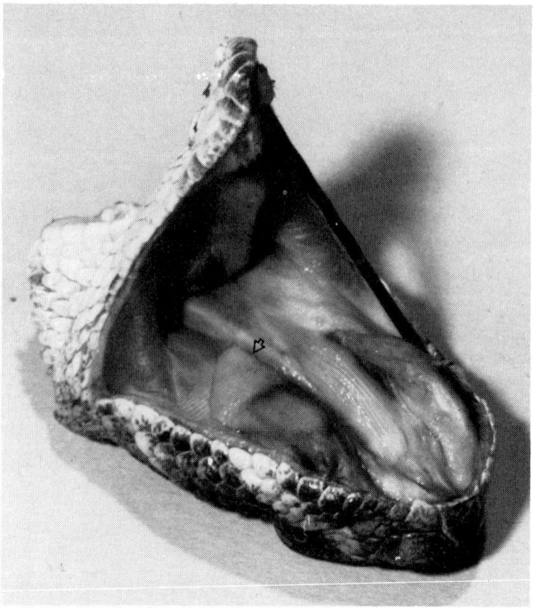

Fig. 15.5. Early edema and hemorrhage in the fang sheath of a rattlesnake, *Crotalus* sp., with uncomplicated vitamin C deficiency (above). Severe necrotic stomatitis secondary to vitamin C deficiency in a boa constrictor, *Constrictor constrictor* (below).

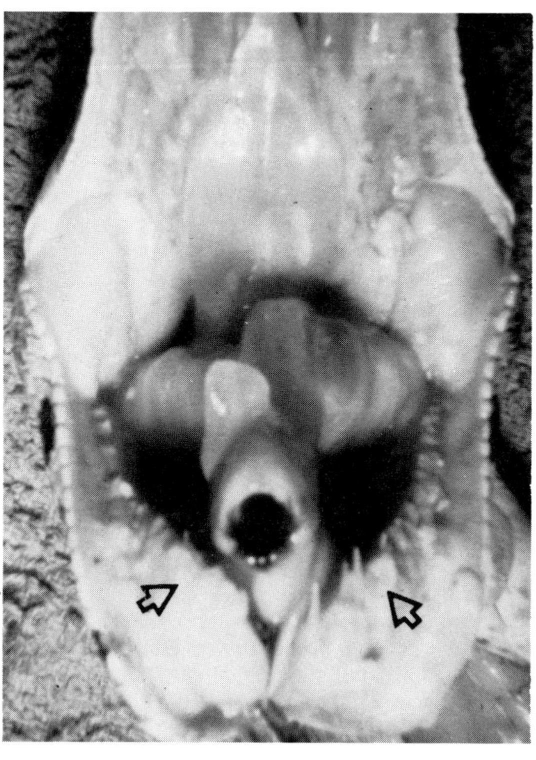

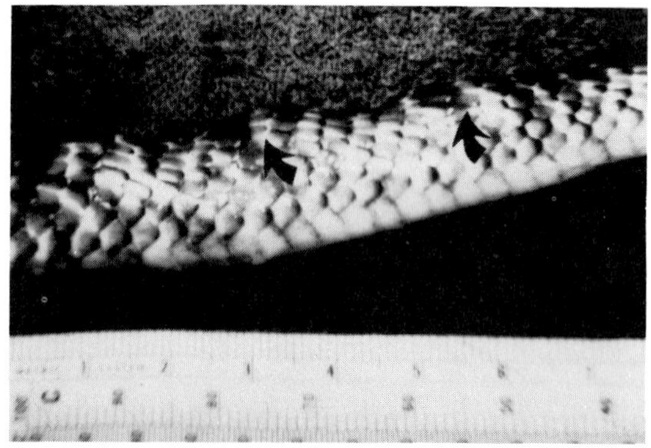

Fig. 15.6. Cobra, *Naja* sp., with enlarged costovertebral articulations (arrows) produced by rickets.

1965; Wallach, 1971a, b). The disease is characterized by depression, ataxia, anorexia, enlarged articulations (Fig. 15.6), malformed limbs, and soft and malformed shells. Dietary levels of 608 IU/kg of diet have proved adequate for growing snakes and snapping turtles (Goellner, 1976).

Excess of dietary vitamin D can produce classical disease in all reptiles, but it has been reported most often in the green iguana, *Iguana iguana* (Pallaske, 1962; Schuchman and Taylor, 1970; Wallach, 1969, 1970, 1971a, b; Wallach and Hoessle, 1966). Hypervitaminosis D is characterized by a medial calcification of the elastic arteries, including the aorta (Fig. 15.7) and renal arteries. Advanced cases are easily visualized radiographically. Hypervitaminosis D is characterized clinically by anorexia, lameness, and an increase in the serum and urine levels of calcium and phosphorus. Vitamin D taken orally enhances both the absorption of calcium and phosphorus from the intestine and the resorption of calcium by the proximal convoluted tubules of the kidneys. When excessive vitamin D is present, the degree of intoxication is affected by the amounts of calcium and phosphorus in the intestine. Vitamin D administered parenterally mobilizes calcium stores from the skeletal system and does not appear to affect intestinal absorption. Hypervitaminosis D is characterized microscopically by a deposition of calcium salts in soft tissue, especially in the fibroelastic components, renal tubular necrosis with renal calcium deposition, and an osteomalacia if there is a concurrent calcium deficiency.

Vitamin E deficiency can occur in all reptiles (Wallach, 1969, 1970, 1971a, b; Wallach and Hoessle, 1966, 1968). Vitamin E deficiency is potentiated or precipitated by diets high in polyunsaturated fats, including diets containing significant amounts of mackerel, *Scomber scom-*

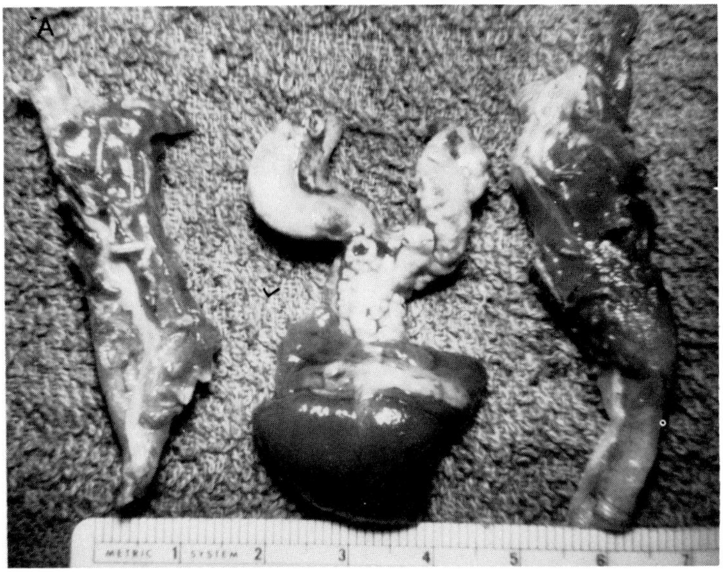

A

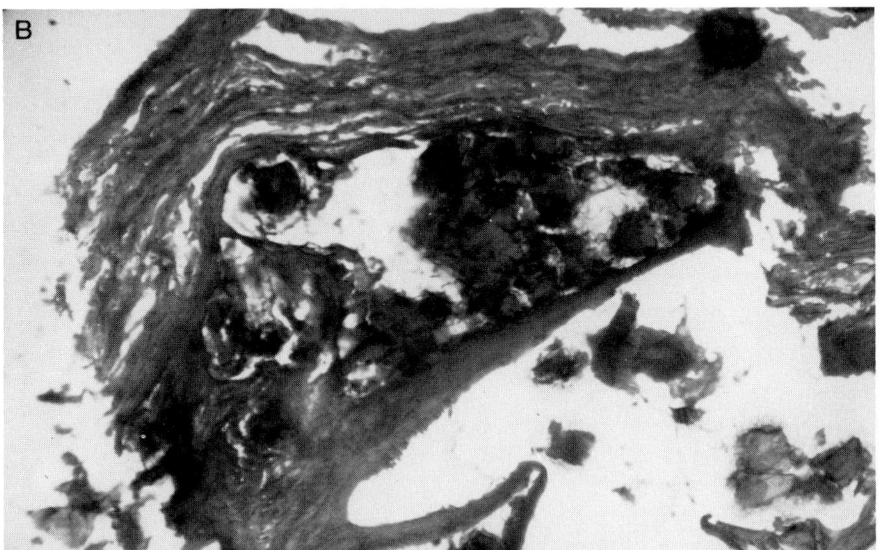

Fig. 15.7. (**A**) Heart and lungs of a green iguana, *I. iguana,* that show severe calcification of the aorta and pulmonary artery produced by hypervitaminosis D. (**B**) Cross-section of same aorta as above showing medial calcification characteristic of hypervitaminosis D (H & E, ×105).

brus; red tuna; or laboratory rodents that have been fed experimental diets rich in polyunsaturated fats. The disease is characterized by skeletal muscle dystrophy and steatitis. Steatitis in reptiles is manifested by a well-circumscribed induration of fat. The lesions are heavily pigmented with ceroid lipofuscin and may be found in any fat depot (Fig. 15.8). The pigment emits a yellowish orange fluorescence when exposed to ultraviolet light. The microscopic examination of such lesions reveals an acid-fast positive, basophilic amorphous material surrounded by fibroblasts and macrophages. The reticuloendothelial system of the liver and spleen are often laden with pigment. Anorexia may be the only clinical sign of vitamin E deficiency presented; therefore, the disease is only diagnosed by muscle biopsy, laparotomy, or at autopsy.

Minerals. Mineral deficiencies rarely occur in free-ranging reptiles living in their normal environment. Conversely, mineral deficiencies are among the most commonly recognized and reported of the nutritional problems of captive reptiles (Ippen, 1965; Reichenbach-Klinke and Elkan, 1965; Wallach, 1969, 1970, 1971a, b; Wallach and Hoessle, 1968; Zwart and Van de Watering, 1969). The basic requirements for

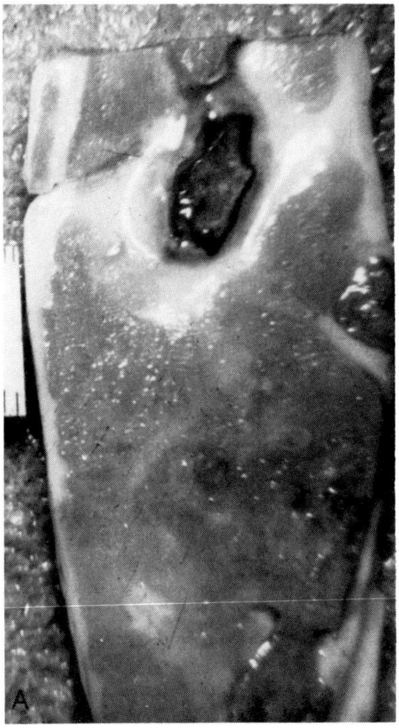

Fig. 15.8. (**A**) Renal fat depot of an American alligator, *A. mississipiensis,* that died from steatitis. Note the heavily pigmented accumulation of ceroid characteristic of chronic vitamin E deficiency. (**B**) Longitudinal section of tail muscle from the same alligator. Note well-circumscribed steatitis lesions. (**C**) Photomicrograph of the liver from the same alligator. Note ceroid pigment in the reticuloendothelial cells and histiocytes (H & E, ×750).

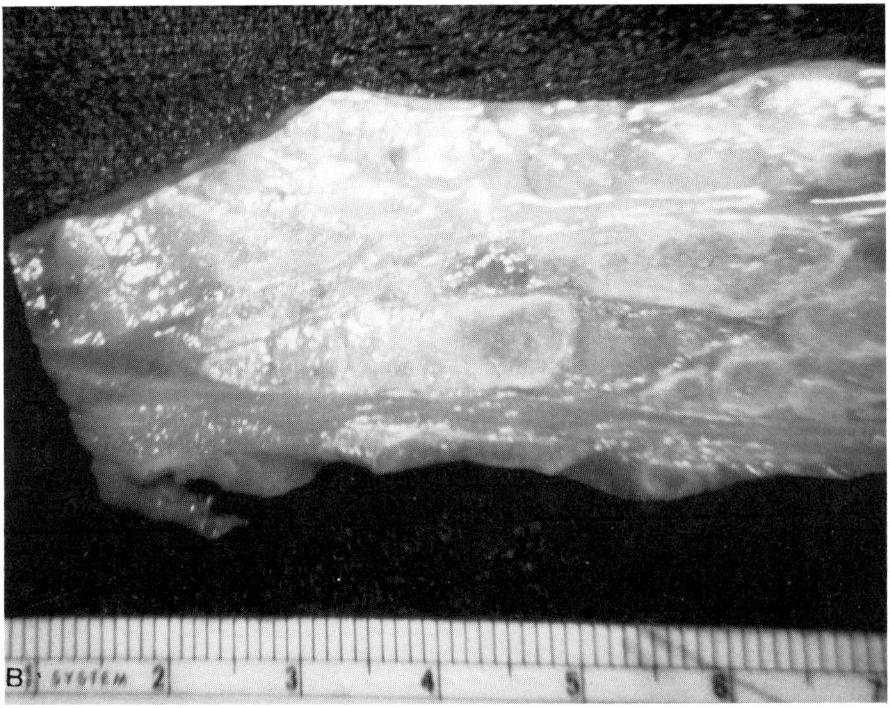

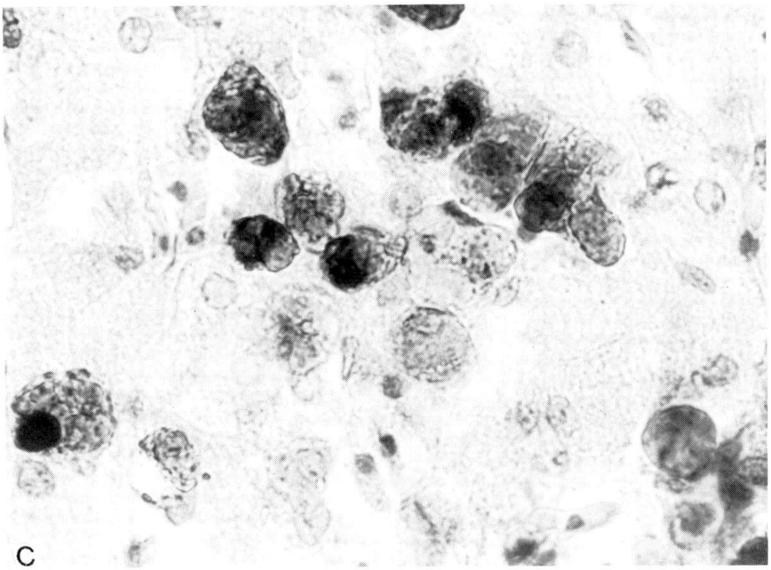

C

calcium and phosphorus are twofold: 1) absolute quantities and 2) calcium to phosphorus ratio (Ca:P). Commercial reptile diets containing 0.3% calcium and 0.2% phosphorus have proved adequate for the growth and maintenance of snakes and snapping turtles.

Fibrous osteodystrophy, long recognized as a sequela to chronic renal disease, also results from a diet chronically deficient in calcium or rich in phosphorus. This syndrome, also known as nutritional secondary hyperparathyroidism (NSH) is characterized by extensive osteoclastic resorption of cortical bone and its subsequent replacement with connective tissue. Lesions of NSH may affect one bone more severely than others (monostotic) because that bone is growing most rapidly during the peak of the imbalance or deficiency. In a very young animal NSH is more generalized (polystotic). The presence of adequate levels of vitamin D potentiates the disease because of accelerated withdrawals of calcium from skeletal stores to maintain serum calcium levels. Many whole prey animals and meats fed to captive reptiles are deficient in absolute calcium and phosphorus levels and also have a Ca:P ratio that is severely out of balance (Table 15.2). Large muscular fishes, insects, and muscle meats are the foods most often incriminated. If horsemeat must be fed out of necessity, the diet should be supplemented with calcium carbonate at the rate of 400 mg/100 gm of meat. Fish and liver diets require up to 900 mg/100 gm of meat to correct the Ca:P ratio (Collins, 1971). Nutritional secondary hyperparathyroidism is characterized by the loss of teeth, fibrous osteodystrophy of long bones, grossly misshapen vertebral bodies and enlarged parathyroid glands, and cystic calculi. Cystic and urinary calculi occur in all reptiles subjected to chronic calcium deficiencies or phosphorus excess, especially in those obtaining adequate levels of vitamin D. Cystic calculi are only found in reptiles that have urinary bladders. Overt dietary deficiency of calcium or excess dietary phosphorus in a formerly well-nourished reptile causes a negative calcium balance in the animal, requiring withdrawal from body stores and increased urinary excretion of phosphorus. Parenteral injections of vitamin D at this time aggravate the process as the skeletal stores are further drawn upon. It is this endogenous calcium and phosphorus that is the bulk of the mineral calculi. The onset of other nutritional problems and dehydration further favors the formation of urinary calculi.

Iodine deficiency can occur in all reptiles but is most often observed in chelonians and lizards fed a large quantity of plant material (Reichenbach-Klinke and Elkan, 1965; Wallach, 1969, 1970, 1971a, b).

Table 15.2. Calcium and Phosphorus Content of Common Reptile Feeds

Food	Calcium (%)	Phosphorus (%)	Ca:P Ratio
Meal worms	0.0008	0.0024	1:3
Sardines	0.150	0.975	1:6
Horsemeat	0.010	0.0024	1:15
Beef muscle	0.011	0.188	1:16
Chicken muscle	0.012	0.201	1:17
Mackerel	0.008	0.274	1:34
Beef liver	0.008	0.352	1:44

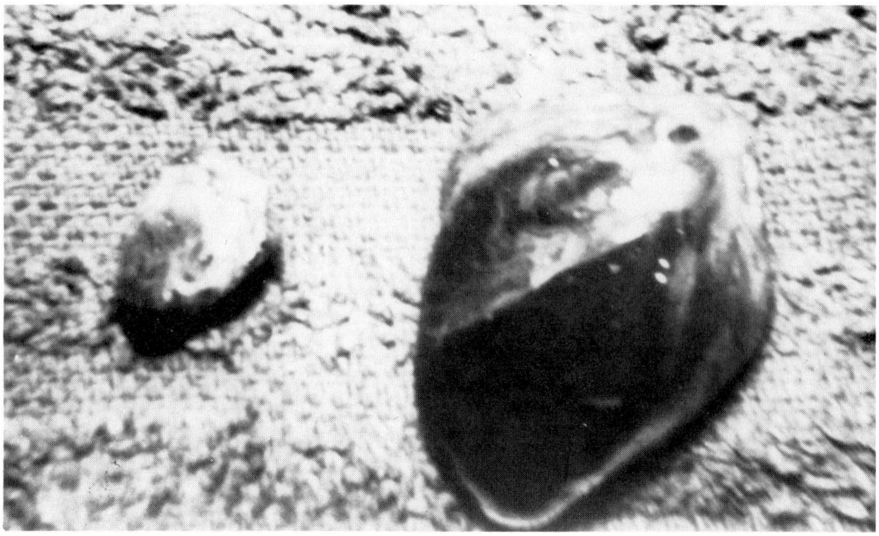

A

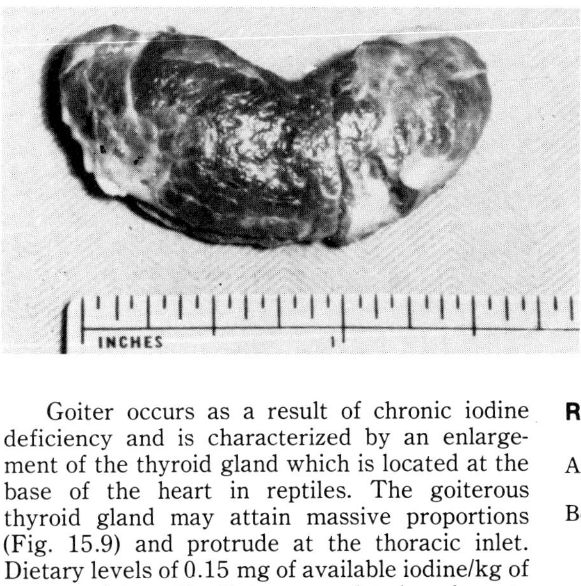

B

Fig. 15.9. (**A**) Thyroid glands from young green sea turtles, *Chelonia mydas.* Thyroid from iodine-deficient turtles (R) compared with the thyroid from a normal turtle (L) of the same age. (**B**) Thyroid gland from an iodine-deficient iguana, *Cyclura cornuta.* The gland is enlarged more than 20 times normal (note the scale is in inches).

Goiter occurs as a result of chronic iodine deficiency and is characterized by an enlargement of the thyroid gland which is located at the base of the heart in reptiles. The goiterous thyroid gland may attain massive proportions (Fig. 15.9) and protrude at the thoracic inlet. Dietary levels of 0.15 mg of available iodine/kg of commercial reptile diet appeared to be adequate for growth and maintenance of snakes and snapping turtles.

PREVENTION. Mismanagement of captive reptiles is a common prelude to nutritional disease, especially with the amateur herpetologist, but unfortunately also occurs in zoological collections. Realizing that many nutritional disease problems are at least partially a result of errors in management, it is necessary to evaluate the habitat and management of an ailing reptile as well as the clinical signs in order to formulate a diagnosis, institute therapy, and initiate appropriate changes in management practices.

REFERENCES

Appleby, E. C., and W. G. Siller. 1960. Some cases of gout in reptiles. J. Pathol. Bacteriol. 30:427–430.

Bellairs, A. 1967. Reptiles. In UFAW handbook on the care and management of laboratory animals. 2nd ed. Williams & Wilkins, Baltimore.

______. 1970. The life of reptiles. Vol. 1. Universe Books, New York.

Black, A. L., M. G. Simesen, and J. C. Bortley. 1963. Glucose and acetate metabolism in *Alligator mississipiensis.* Comp. Biochem. Physiol. 8:299–310.

Brattstrom, B. H. 1965. Body temperature of reptiles. Am. Midland Natur. 73:376–422.

Clark, H., B. Sishen, and J. E. Shannon. 1967. Excretion of nitrogen by the alligator embryo. J. Cell Comp. Physiol. 50:129–134.

Collins, D. 1971. Quantities of calcium carbonate needed to balance calcium:phosphorus ratios of various meats. J. Zoo Anim. Med. 2:25.

Coulson, R. A., and T. Hernandez. 1964. Biochemistry of the alligator. Louisiana State Univ. Press, Baton Rouge.

Goellner, R. 1976. Experiences in reptilian and amphibian nutrition. Annu. Proc. Am. Assoc. Zoo Vet., St. Louis.

Hoessle, C. 1969. Display of tuatara, *Sphenodon punctatus*, at St. Louis Zoological Park. Int. Zoo Yearbook 9:32–33.

Ippen, R. 1965. Considerations on the comparative pathology of the bone diseases in reptiles. Zentralbl. Allg. Pathol. 108:424–434.

Kauffeld, C. 1968. Nutrition of reptiles. Proc. Zoo Vet. Short Course. Michigan State Univ., East Lansing, Dec. 10–11, 1968.

______. 1969a. The keeper and the kept. Doubleday, Garden City.

______. 1969b. The effect of altitude, ultraviolet light and humidity on captive reptiles. Int. Zoo Yearbook 9:8–9.

Laszlo, L. 1969. Observations on two artificial lights for reptile displays. Int. Zoo Yearbook 9:12–13.

Licht, P. 1965. Decreases in spermatogenesis in lizards exposed to elevated temperatures. Copeia 1965 (4): 428–436.

Murphy, J. B. 1969. Notes on iguanids and varanids in a mixed exhibit at Dallas Zoo. Int. Zoo Yearbook 9:39–41.

Neiland, K. A., B. T. Sheer, and H. M. Sinclair. 1956. Excreted nitrogen partition: Animals. In Handbook of biological data. W. B. Saunders, Philadelphia.

Nelson, L. 1971. Subepidermal hemorrhages in a tegu. J. Zoo Anim. Med. 2:19.

Pallaske, G. 1962. Hypervitaminosis D in a lizard. Berl. Muench. Tieraerztl. Wochenschr. 74:132.

Pawley, R. 1969. Observations on a prolonged food refusal period of an adult fer-de-lance, *Bothrops atrox asper.* Int. Zoo Yearbook 9:58–59.

Peaker, M. 1969. Some aspects of the thermal requirements of reptiles in captivity. Int. Zoo Yearbook 9:3–8.

Reichenbach-Klinke, H., and E. Elkan. 1965. The principal diseases of lower vertebrates. Academic Press, New York.

Schuchman, S. M., and D. O. N. Taylor. 1970. Arteriosclerosis in an iguana, *Iguana iguana.* J. Am. Vet. Med. Assoc. 157:614–616.

Stebbins, R. C., and R. E. Barwick. 1968. Radiotelemetric study of thermoregulation in a lace monitor. Copeia 1968(4):541–547.

Thornson, T. B. 1968. Body fluid partitioning in Reptilia. Copeia 1968(4):592–601.

Wallach, J.D. 1969. Medical care of reptiles. J. Am. Vet Med. Assoc. 155:1017–1031.

______. 1970. Nutritional diseases of exotic animals. J. Am. Vet. Med. Assoc. 157:583–599.

______. 1971a. Diseases of reptiles and their clinical management. In R. F. Kirk. Current veterinary therapy. Vol. IV. W. B. Saunders, Philadelphia.

______. 1971b. Environmental and nutritional diseases of captive reptiles. J. Am. Vet. Med. Assoc. 159: 1632–1643.

______, and C. Hoessle. 1966. Hypervitaminosis D in green iguanas. J. Am Vet. Med. Assoc. 149:912–914.

______, and ______. 1967. Visceral gout in captive reptiles. J. Am. Vet. Med. Assoc. 151:897–899.

______, and ______. 1968. Steatitis in captive crocodilians. J. Am. Vet. Med. Assoc. 153:845–847.

______, ______, and J. Bennett. 1967. Hypoglycemic shock in captive alligators. J. Am. Vet. Med. Assoc. 151:893–896.

Zwart, P., and C. C. Van de Watering. 1969. Disturbance of bone formation in the common iguana, *Iguana iguana:* Pathology and etiology. Acta Zool. et Pathol. Anat. 48:333–356.

Index